3D Printing in Radiation Oncology

3D Printing in Radiation Oncology: Personalization of Patient Treatment Through Digital Fabrication presents a comprehensive and practical view of the many forms in which 3D printing is being integrated into radiation oncology practice. Radiation oncology employs among the most sophisticated digital technologies in medicine. Until recently, however, the "last mile" of treatment has required manually produced or generic devices for patient set up, positioning, control of surface dose, and delivery of brachytherapy treatment. 3D printing is already offering enhancements in both precision and efficiency through the digital design and fabrication of patient photon and electron bolus, customized surface and gynecological brachytherapy applicators, proton beam compensators and range shifters, patient immobilization, novel radiation detectors, and phantoms. Various innovations are disrupting decades-old practices in radiation therapy (RT) facilities, resulting in vital improvements in personalization of treatment and patient experience.

An essential read for radiation oncologists, medical physicists, radiation therapists, oncology nurses, hospital administrators, engineers, and medical educators, this book is an indispensable resource for those bringing 3D printing to the RT clinic, looking to expand the role of 3D printing in their practice, or embarking upon related research and development.

James L. Robar, PhD, FCCPM is a globally recognized medical physicist, the Chief of Medical Physics at Nova Scotia Health, a professor of radiation oncology at Dalhousie University and a specialist in the high technology of radiotherapy—a treatment technique used for roughly half of all patients with cancer. He is also co-founder and CSO at Adaptiiv Medical Technologies, a medical-tech firm in Halifax, with the mission of improving the accuracy of cancer treatment. As a scientist, inventor, and entrepreneur, Dr. Robar has pioneered multiple advancements improving imaging and treatment delivery for radiotherapy. These technologies include enhanced imaging to improve the accuracy of targeting tumors with radiation, hardware and software detecting submillimeter motion of patients to improve the precision of treatment, planning algorithms to provide improved sparing of healthy tissues and organs, and turnkey solutions allowing intelligent design of 3D printed, patient-specific accessories used during radiotherapy. For his contributions in this field, he became a Canadian Governor General's Innovation Laureate in 2021.

3D Printing in Radiation Oncology

Personalization of Patient Treatment Through Digital Fabrication

Edited by
James L. Robar

CRC Press
Taylor & Francis Group
Boca Raton London New York

CRC Press is an imprint of the
Taylor & Francis Group, an **informa** business

Designed cover image: James Robar

First edition published 2024
by CRC Press
2385 NW Executive Center Drive, Suite 320, Boca Raton FL 33431

and by CRC Press
4 Park Square, Milton Park, Abingdon, Oxon, OX14 4RN

CRC Press is an imprint of Taylor & Francis Group, LLC

© 2024 James Robar

ISBN: 9781032261959 (hbk)
ISBN: 9781032264578 (pbk)
ISBN: 9781003288404 (ebk)

DOI: 10.1201/9781003288404

Typeset in Minion
by Newgen Publishing UK

Contents

Acknowledgments

I wish to thank my lovely family, my wife Fiona, and kids Finlay and Keira, for your patience and support while I worked on this project. You always add levity, laughter and perspective.

Of course, this book would not have been possible without the pioneers and champions of 3D printing and radiation oncology. Your ingenuity and creativity shine in the pages that follow. I am grateful to those from this community who produced chapters herein. Thank you for enduring my editorial persistence.

I am extremely grateful to Ms. Angela Henry for her assistance in producing this book. Thank you, Ange.

Finally, a big shout-out to everyone on the publishing team, including Carolina and Hailey, for entertaining a novel topic for a book and for guiding me along the way.

James L. Robar, PhD, FCCPM

Contributors

Stéphane Bedwani
University of Montreal Hospital
　　Research Centre
Montreal, Canada

Daniel Cail
Brigham and Women's Hospital
Boston, Massachusetts, U.S.A

Amanda Cherpak
Dalhousie University
Halifax, Nova Scotia, Canada

Fallon Chipidza
Dana-Farber Cancer Institute
Boston, Massachusetts, U.S.A

Tsuicheng David Chiu
UT Southwestern Medical Center
Dallas, Texas, U.S.A

Krista Chytyk-Praznik
Dalhousie University
Halifax, Nova Scotia, Canada

Daniel Craft
MN Oncology
St Paul, Minnesota

Joshua Hempstead
Dana-Farber Cancer Institute
Boston, Massachusetts, U.S.A

Cornelia Hoehr
TRIUMF
Vancouver, Canada

Yuji Kamio
University of Montreal Hospital
　　Research Centre
Montreal, Canada

Astrid Langoe
Boston College
Boston, Massachusetts, U.S.A

Clay Lindsay
BC Cancer
Victoria, B.C., Canada

Thalat Monajemi
Dalhousie University
Halifax, Nova Scotia, Canada

Peter Orio
Dana-Farber Cancer Institute
Boston, Massachusetts, U.S.A

Brian Overshiner
RICOH
Exton, Pennsylvania, U.S.A

David Parsons
UT Southwestern Medical Center
Dallas, Texas, U.S.A

Tiffany Phillips
Cedars Sinai
Los Angeles, California, U.S.A

Jennifer Pretz
Dana-Farber Cancer Institute
Boston, Massachusetts, U.S.A

Robert Reynolds
Atrium Health
Charlotte, North Carolina, U.S.A

James L. Robar
Nova Scotia Health
Halifax, Nova Scotia, Canada

Mutlay Sayan
Dana-Farber Cancer Institute
Boston, Massachusetts, U.S.A

James W. Stasiak
Digital Materials Engineering LLC
Portland, Oregon

Laura Warren
Dana-Farber Cancer Institute
Boston, Massachusetts, U.S.A

Zhenyu Xiong
Rutgers Cancer Institute of New Jersey
New Brunswick, New Jersey, U.S.A

You Zhang
UT Southwestern Medical Center
Dallas, Texas, U.S.A

CHAPTER 1

Introduction and Clinical Perspective

Mutlay Sayan, Astrid Langoe, Laura Warren, Joshua Hempstead, Daniel Cail, Fallon Chipidza, Jennifer Pretz, and Peter Orio

INTRODUCTION

The past decade has seen significant integration of additive manufacturing, commonly known as 3D printing, into both the research and practice of radiation oncology. An early catalyst for this development was proliferation of 3D printing technology following the expiry of foundational patents. This suddenly allowed integration of 3D printing within various fields and industries, while stimulating awareness of 3D printing methods and materials for advanced manufacturing based on digital designs. For decades radiation oncology has been among the most technology-intensive fields of medicine, employing multi-modality anatomical and functional imaging, advanced software for treatment planning, and versatile hardware devices for delivery of external beam therapy and brachytherapy. However, a number of steps in the radiation therapy (RT) process have remained decidedly low-tech. One of these has been the use of patient bolus, which is required in the treatment of a range of superficial tumors by photon or electron beam therapy. Although 3D printing presents a diverse range of applications in radiation oncology, in this chapter we begin by using patient bolus as an exemplar of the utility of 3D printing in enabling the transition from manual to automated, from analog to digital, and from generic to personalized, in creating a customized device that improves both the accuracy and efficiency of treatment. The bolus use case highlights the strengths of the current state of 3D printing technology and also points to areas for further development. Finally, we introduce various other exciting and creative innovations in radiation oncology that promise to enhance patient care, many of which are detailed in subsequent chapters of this book.

DOI: 10.1201/9781003288404-1

RATIONALE FOR BOLUS IN CLINICAL PRACTICE

RT is a critical tool in the treatment of a variety of malignancies. The main intention of RT is to cause damage to the DNA of cancerous cells, which restricts their ability to divide. RT can be used as focal local treatment to a visible gross tumor, or as adjuvant treatment after a surgery for the eradication of potential residual occult disease. It serves roles in both treatment with curative intent and in palliation of symptoms. Additionally, it can be used in combination with other cancer therapies such as chemotherapy and immunotherapy in order to increase treatment efficacy.

External beam radiation can be directed anywhere in the body, and there are many indications for radiation to be directed at or near the skin surface. In the definitive setting, for tumors involving the skin or subcutaneous tissue such as primary skin cancers, cancers of the head and neck, or soft tissue sarcomas, high radiation doses are required to eliminate the disease. In the adjuvant setting, post-mastectomy RT is frequently recommended to eradicate potential microscopic tumor cells in the residual breast glandular tissue, skin, and subcutaneous lymphatics. Because RT is not selective to cancer cells, it is vital that the correct dose is delivered to achieve optimal efficiency. Careful precautions need to be taken to limit unwanted radiation exposure. For example, organ spacers can be used to push away sensitive organs, which can significantly reduce the risk of radiation exposure to unwanted areas.

In situations where the intended radiation target is superficial, i.e., close to the body surface, special attention must be paid to ensure that the prescribed radiation dose covers the target region appropriately. This is because radiation is commonly delivered using megavoltage photon beams that exhibit a low surface dose, e.g., below 30%, and a depth of maximum dose ranging between 0.5 and 3 cm, for example, depending on energy. While this dose buildup effect spares the skin surface and is advantageous when targeting a deep internal tumor, it is problematic when the target area is at or near the surface itself. The skin-sparing effect of megavoltage photon treatment will reduce the dose to a superficial target, thus potentially reducing the efficacy of treatment. For this reason, when delivering RT for treatment of a superficial target, it is necessary to apply a tissue-equivalent material called a *bolus* to the patient surface. In doing this, the dose buildup can occur within the thickness of the bolus, allowing for a near maximal dose to be delivered to the skin surface of the patient. This is illustrated schematically in Figure 1.1.

In addition to increasing the surface dose, application of bolus to a patient surface shifts the entire dose distribution toward the skin. Through careful choice of the bolus thickness, the prescription radiation dose region can be adjusted to suit an individual tumor and patient anatomy and may advantageously move radiation dose away from non-target tissue that is deep to the area of interest. When designing a radiation treatment plan, the primary goal is to maximize the dose coverage of the target volume by the prescribed dose, while simultaneously sparing non-target nearby tissue. This serves to optimize the therapeutic window, i.e., to maximize tumor control while minimizing normal tissue complication. Bolus is an important tool when treating superficial targets to modulate and optimize radiation dose at or near the surface.

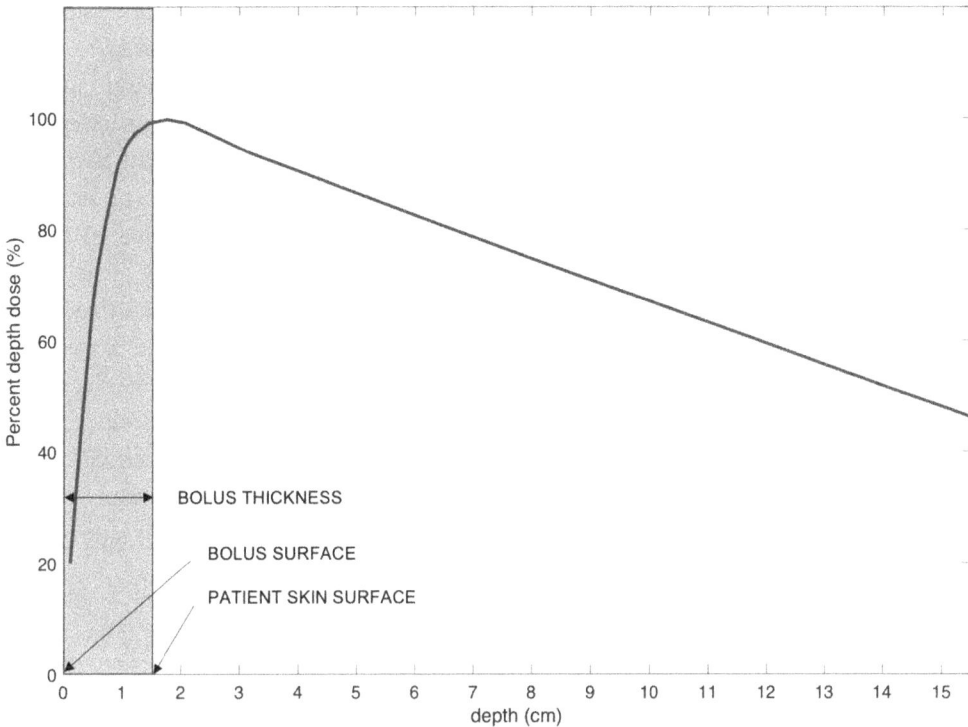

FIGURE 1.1 Percent depth dose for a megavoltage photon beam with application of bolus to the surface of the patient. This allows the buildup region of the percent depth dose curve to occur in the bolus material and the maximum dose to occur near the skin surface.

CLINICAL NEED TO REDUCE AIR GAPS

The dose delivered to the patient's skin will depend on several factors, including photon beam energy, field size, the presence of beam modifiers such as wedges or collimation, angle of beam incidence, and source to skin distance, as well as the thickness of bolus used. As described above, the accurate delivery of radiation doses, particularly at or near the skin surface, has important implications for both tumor coverage and potential radiation-related toxicities.

One important factor to consider when calculating radiation dose is the presence of air–tissue interfaces within the radiation field. An air cavity (or gap) can occur naturally in the body, e.g., at the interface of a sinus and surrounding tissue, or may be introduced to the anatomy, e.g., on the external surface of the patient, through the use of a bolus that does not fit the patient surface accurately. Many investigators have studied the perturbation of the radiation dose at air–tissue interfaces and report a significant underdosing effect due to loss of electronic equilibrium for megavoltage photon beams. The magnitude of the impact of the air cavity on the dose depends on several factors and will be greater with smaller field size, increased photon energy, and increased size and depth of the air cavity [1–3]. Many studies have focused on air cavities that result from normal human anatomy, such as air within the nasal cavity or the larynx [1, 4, 5]. However, the introduction of treatment devices, such as inflatable catheters or bolus, can create inadvertent air cavities with resultant implications on the radiation dose delivered.

Attention to potential air gaps created with the application of bolus during radiation delivery is required for safe and effective treatment. Minimizing air gaps between the bolus and skin surface increases the likelihood of achieving the intended goal by minimizing unintended underdosing and variability in dose distribution [6, 7]. As an example, for patients receiving post-mastectomy RT, bolus is frequently prescribed to ensure adequate surface dose given that the target volume includes any remaining breast tissue in the mastectomy flap. Boman and colleagues demonstrated that for patients receiving post-mastectomy RT with volumetric modulated arc therapy (VMAT), the presence of air gaps 5 or 10 mm in thickness under the bolus reduces the surface dose by nearly 14% compared to a case with no air gaps [8]. To address this unwanted effect, some investigations report that custom 3D printed bolus, in comparison to commercially available (non-customized) bolus, reduces air gaps and therefore may achieve more accurate dose delivery [9, 10]. This development will be discussed in greater detail later in this chapter.

BOLUS SOLUTIONS USED COMMONLY IN CLINIC

Several different types of bolus are available in today's RT departments, and each offers strengths and weaknesses, depending the treatment site. All fall short of providing a universal solution but certain types perform well in specific scenarios. Some available options, as shown below in Figure 1.2, are brass mesh, vinyl sheet (Superflab), bolus material that is mixed from powder (Super Stuff), thermoplastic sheets, thermoplastic pellets, and wax sheets. These various materials function similarly in that, following application to the patient skin and during treatment with a megavoltage radiation beam, they cause the maximum dose to be shifted toward the patient surface. However, as described above, any non-conformality of the bolus to the patient's surface may cause air cavities and thus loss of accuracy and uniformity of the delivered dose. While all bolus types may work well if they are sufficiently conformal to the patient, all involve individual shortcomings.

Brass mesh bolus, shown in Figure 1.2a, is effective in molding to surface anatomy but the higher density material introduces the risk of neutron contamination, thus introducing a radiation safety risk for both the patient and the handling therapist when beams of high energy (10 MV or above) are used. An advantage afforded by the density of brass is that a smaller thickness is required in order to achieve a given tissue equivalent thickness (TET) over which dose buildup will occur. This is in part due to low energy electrons created from interactions with the brass contributing to the surface dose. For a bolus of 5 mm of added tissue, two layers of 1.5-mm thick brass mesh are used, with each layer having a TET of about 2 to 3 mm. Another advantage of brass mesh bolus is that while the surface dose is increased due to electron interactions, the dose distribution at greater depths is not altered significantly. This allows for a single treatment plan to be used as opposed to creating separate plans with and without bolus.

One of the most common bolus types used is vinyl sheet bolus (trade name Superflab), seen in Figure 1.2b. This material is a pliable, allowing for it to be placed on an uneven surface for treatment. For this reason, it is a common bolus for a post-mastectomy chest wall therapy, which requires delivery of the prescription dose to superficial depths. This bolus is available in two forms, with or without a so-called 'skin'. A skin on the surface of the bolus allows for it to be reused between patients after proper cleaning protocols are followed. A vinyl sheet bolus without the skin has a sticky finish that will adhere to the surface to which it is applied. This bolus is meant for single use and therefore is sometimes shaped by cutting to customize to a specific area of treatment. One limitation of this type of bolus is that it is available only in several standard thickness increments. Therefore, as illustrated in Figure 1.1, this means that for a given beam energy, control of the dose produced at the skin surface will be limited by this selection. It also exhibits limited shaping to complex patient surfaces [9], which often prompts radiation therapists to use, e.g., adhesive tape or rolled linens to force conformation to concavities, thus limiting efficiency of set up and reproducibility among fractions of treatment.

Another pliable bolus option is a material mixed from a powder (trade name Super Stuff), seen in Figure 1.2c. Addition of water to the powder produces a bolus ranging in viscosity from 'slime' to putty. Composed mostly of water, this bolus will exhibit near-tissue equivalence after mixing but even with proper storage will dehydrate over time. This makes it more dense and less tissue equivalent, so it is best for shorter therapies and should be replaced for use over longer durations. It is suited to irregular patient surfaces, where a slab of bolus may not deform properly leaving unwanted air gaps. One common application is in treatment of skin cancers on the face, such as the nose or the ear, where the bolus can be placed into a crevice with a slab of vinyl sheet bolus on top of that to build a more regular treatment surface. It is advisable to build this bolus prior to the patient's computed tomography (CT) simulation, so that the scan can accurately take into account the variable thickness of the formed bolus.

A thermoplastic sheet, as shown in Figure 1.2d., is a viable option to conform to an irregular surface such as the ear or nose, while maintaining density and rigidity for the entirety of the treatment. Thermoplastic sheets begin as hard materials but soften in a heated water bath and are then formed to a surface. Once dried and hardened, this material will not deform over time and will consistently align to a rigid target on a daily basis for easy alignment. A popular area of use is the placement onto a face mask to then be included in the scan. The mask is then placed daily with the bolus in the same location. In addition, rigid areas such as the nose are suited to this type of bolus. In contrast, an expanded post-mastectomy chest wall may not be an appropriate application for rigid thermoplastic because of anatomical changes with motion or variations in patient posture.

Another option is thermoplastic in pellet form, seen in Figure 1.2e, that is similarly softened in a hot water bath and melted together. The pellets may be formed into any shape before hardening into a final permanent shape. This is suited to irregular surfaces that require bolus. One notable downside to hard thermoplastic bolus is that the final

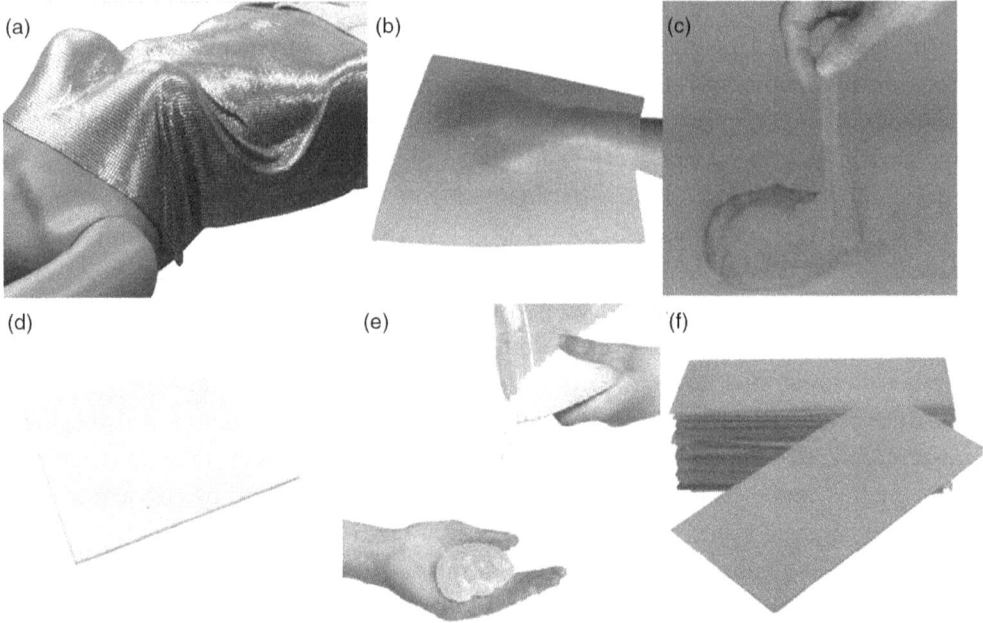

FIGURE 1.2   Commonly used boluses include (a) brass mesh, (b) vinyl sheet bolus (Superflab), (c) mixed bolus (Super Stuff), (d) thermoplastic sheets, (e) thermoplastic pellets, and (f) wax sheets.

product can be uncomfortable for the patient when placed into certain areas, such as within the concha of an ear.

Another material used frequently is paraffin wax, as shown in its common sheet form in Figure 1.2f. This is malleable following application of heat to allow forming, however the process introduces variability in thickness after softening and forming. Often used on the scalp, wax hardens and maintains its shape and thickness throughout a treatment. It can be fragile, however, and may bend or break without too much force even after hardening. Paraffin wax has an electron density similar to that of water, thus offering similar TET.

Finally, a historic method of adding bolus, e.g., in treatment of the post-mastectomy chest wall, is the use of layers of wet towel. The desired TET needs to be roughly approximated for the type of towel used. For example, one may use four and eight layers of wet towel, approximately equivalent to 5 mm and 10 mm respectively of tissue. Tap water may be used to soak the towels but not to the point of dripping. An obvious downside of this approach is that the degree of saturation with water, and in turn, the TET of the bolus is not easily controlled or monitored [11].

These examples demonstrate several options used in RT. Common to all of these bolus types is the need for human intervention (and skill) either in hand-crafting the bolus or in attempting to apply a non-customized bolus to the patient in a relocatable fashion. A common drawback is that handmade bolus cannot be fashioned according to regular, planned geometries, and thus cannot be specified in a radiotherapy treatment planning system without CT imaging the device on the patient. Different bolus types can be used in combination, in an attempt to make a more suitable product, but each type involves its own limitations. Thus, there remains is a need of a singular bolus technology that offers appropriate conformality, radiological properties, mechanical properties, and ease of use, providing consistent and accurate dosimetry throughout a course of radiotherapy.

NEED FOR BETTER CLINICAL SOLUTIONS

While numerous products and materials with different densities are commercially available as described above, finding an optimal bolus for all clinical applications remains challenging in practice. Examples of barriers include (i) a sparsity of materials that are tissue-equivalent, (ii) a lack of biocompatible, antibacterial, and antiphlogistic materials [12, 13], (iii) bolus materials with mechanical properties or geometries causing incomplete contact with tissue surfaces such as ears, nose, eyes, gluteal folds, or surgical defects, thus resulting in air gaps, and iv) the time and labor associated with manual fabrication of custom boluses. Depending on the scenario, these challenges may introduce heterogeneity and inconsistency in dose delivery as well as inefficiencies in the clinic due to manual fabrication and uncertainties by the radiation therapist in applying the bolus at each treatment fraction.

3D PRINTING: DIGITIZING AND AUTOMATING METHODS FOR BOLUS IN THE CLINIC

Given that each patient presents a unique anatomy, personalized RT accessories must be created with sufficient conformity to the patient surface such that air gaps are not created [14]. Fortunately, the standard RT treatment planning process already involves the acquisition of 3D imaging data, e.g., with CT or magnetic resonance imaging, as a step in the workflow. In addition to providing the essential data for treatment planning, this information can be used as input to allow design of bespoke patient devices. Thus, the input data may be sourced 'for free' and additional imaging steps may not be needed to obtain the source information for the design of the device. Once a patient device is fabricated, 3D printing provides a digital approach with improved accuracy [15, 16]. Moreover, if the design process is digitized, the 3D model of the device can be made available in the treatment planning system without the need to image it on the patient.

Personalized 3D printed bolus, for example, offers not only more efficacious treatment, but a more comfortable and tolerable patient experience. Patient-specific 3D printed bolus is applicable to multiple treatment sites such as skin cancer involving nose, ear, or cheek [17]. In these cases, application of bolus is necessary to deliver prescribed dose to the skin surface. Given the wide range of anatomies and the limitations of traditional bolus, 3D printed custom bolus can be designed to achieve optimal dose distribution to the target while sparing healthy distal tissue [15, 18]. In the setting of post-mastectomy RT, custom boluses improve the fit of the bolus to the chest wall relative to traditional bolus [9]. In addition, 3D printed bolus has been shown to reduce the patient setup time compared to standard bolus, making the process more efficient for both therapists and patients.

BENEFITS AND LIMITATIONS OF 3D PRINTING IN RADIATION ONCOLOGY

The application of 3D printing to clinical radiation oncology has already proven advantageous in the delivery of radiation dose to superficial targets, and many new applications will be forthcoming. As the bolus example demonstrates, 3D printing is capable of advancing the mission of personalization of treatment. Through precise modeling of personalized devices, 3D printing removes the operator dependency that has been pervasive in the fabrication of common patient devices such as bolus. As already demonstrated by multiple institutions, this allows daily treatment setup to become impressively consistent and the discrepancy between the planned radiation dose and the delivered dose may be reduced significantly. Finally, 3D printing alleviates workload and inefficiency upstream of treatment delivery. Once imaging data are acquired for a patient, 3D printing is an automated process that does not require the patient or operator to be present throughout the manufacture of the device. In typical clinical workflows, this automation introduces the potential to shorten the interval between CT planning and the start of radiation treatment. Finally, the additive manufacturing approach of 3D printing (as opposed to subtractive milling from a volume of material) has been shown to be cost-effective as there is little to no waste, potentially reducing environmental footprint.

As a relatively recent technology at least in the medical domain, at present the use of 3D printing does involve a few limitations. First, there is a finite selection of materials that can be used in device fabrication, and not all material options will satisfy the mechanical, radiological, and patient-related requirements. However, the field of material science focused on 3D printing has been prolific over recent years, with new printable media appearing continuously for almost all 3D printing technologies, including fused deposition modeling, stereolithography, jet fusion, and others. Second, the 3D printing approach will be new to many radiation oncology departments, and a learning curve must be expected as clinical teams transition from historical manual methods. Finally, establishment of 3D printing resources within existing radiotherapy departments can be resource intensive, with associated upfront cost. This can, however, be circumvented by outsourcing printing to existing 3D printing companies with an 'on-demand' model, to achieve the same outcome at a lower setup and maintenance cost.

EMERGING APPLICATIONS OF 3D PRINTING IN EXTERNAL BEAM THERAPY AND BRACHYTHERAPY

Use of 3D printing in the creation of photon bolus improves both accuracy and efficiency of treatment preparation and delivery by creating a personalized device. However, for other forms of RT, such as electron therapy, the 3D printed device itself can function to tailor and optimize the dose distribution in order to improve dose coverage of targets and sparing of normal tissues. For example, the treatment of mycosis fungoides involving forehead, eyelid, and nose with standard bolus may result in a high dose to underlying healthy tissue. In this scenario, the topology of a patient-specific bolus can be designed to be thicker over the ocular structures, allowing adequate dose delivery to the eyelids and sparing of the eyes and optic structures (Figure 1.3) [17]. By optimizing the variation of bolus thickness, the device modulates the mean electron energy reaching the surface of the patient, and thus the range of electrons below the skin. Similarly, in the case of treating the scalp, VMAT and electron therapy with a uniform thickness bolus may result in significant volume of normal brain receiving an intermediate dose. A custom-fit, modulated thickness electron bolus can provide a better isodose conformity and sparing of healthy tissues, and reduce hotspots compared to VMAT and electron treatment plans using conventional bolus [19, 20]. In the case of treating a finger with squamous cell carcinoma, customized modulated electron bolus allows delivering a uniform dose to the tumor volume while sparing a large amount of the underlying bone [21]. In addition, the custom electron bolus offers reproducible setup of the patient in unconventional position.

3D printing also promises significant new developments for brachytherapy. Patient-specific high dose rate (HDR) brachytherapy applicators provide an excellent fit to the patient anatomy and allow for simple daily setup. For example, treatment of multiple skin lesions with external beam radiation can be challenging due to possible overlapping of isodose lines and the patient's sloping contours when treating extremities. Customized HDR surface brachytherapy applicators can be created using the patient's external body contour; these devices have been shown to offer excellent fit to the patient's contour as well as simplification of daily treatment delivery. Furthermore, development of patient-specific surface or interstitial/intracavitary brachytherapy applicators provides opportunity to customize shape, size, and direction of source trajectory paths with respect to specific patient anatomy [22, 23]. This represents another application where the 3D printed innovation not only personalizes the geometry of the device, but also introduces the capacity for improved dosimetry by controlling the spatial distribution of the radiation source.

Proton therapy is a specialized but expanding approach in the field of radiation oncology. The main dosimetric benefit of the proton beam is the steep dose falloff distal to the target beyond the spread-out Bragg peak, allowing significant normal tissue sparing. Additional dosimetric benefits of proton radiotherapy include a low to medium entrance

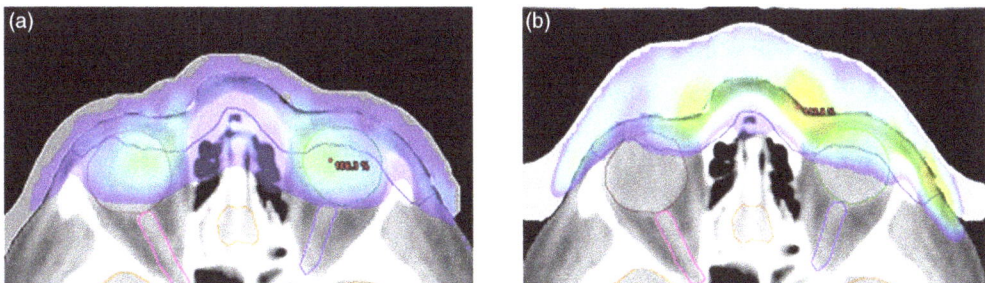

FIGURE 1.3   Axial planning CT slice shows dosimetry comparison between (a) standard bolus and (b) patient-specific modulated bolus plan for electron therapy of a mycosis fungoides of the face. Figure sourced with permission from [17].

dose and homogeneous dose distribution within the target [24, 25]. When proton therapy is delivered with a double scattering treatment technique, patient-specific compensators are needed to modify proton beams to shape the dose distribution to the distal end of the target. Emerging 3D printing technologies provide an alternative method to producing these compensators with an accessible fabrication technology and materials that offer appropriate radiological characteristics [26–28].

With more advanced 3D printing technologies, multiple materials may be combined in a single device, for example, including both tissue-equivalent and high-density shielding materials. This will find clinical application, for example, in treating superficial cancers in the head region, where the use of shielding limits unnecessary radiation to underlying tissue. Internal shields need to be coated with tissue equivalent material to absorb unwanted electron backscatter from the surface of the shielding, and 3D printing will allow this. This same concept of in-printed shielding can be applied to brachytherapy applicators to offer improved sparing of organs-at-risk. Here, automated algorithms will be able to determine the spatial distribution of the shielding with knowledge of the 3D geometry of surrounding anatomy [29].

Another promising application is the digitization of the previously manual process of fabricating patient immobilization. For decades, patient immobilization has been employed to ensure relocatable accuracy and stability of the cranium, head-and-neck, breast, and various other anatomical sites such as extremities. A status quo immobilizer device consists of a solid or mesh plastic shell that is manually formed around the patient's anatomy after heating in a hot water bath or oven. Despite the presence of image guidance on modern radiotherapy treatment units, immobilization remains essential in reducing intra-fractional error and to ensure accuracy of treatment delivery. Manual methods of fabricating immobilization, such as forming thermoplastic mesh are subject to the skill of the operator in determining the quality of the product, and thus the performance of the device in immobilizing the patient will be variable. The fabrication process is time consuming, claustrophobia-inducing for many patients, and consumes significant human and capital resources (e.g., in the CT scanner suite) during the fabrication. Recent developments [30, 31] have used 3D printing to produce patient immobilization, offering automation and excellent spatial accuracy relative to the 3D imaging input data. This approach also introduces the new capability of reducing unwanted surface dose causing skin toxicity through the development of low-density printable materials [31]. Importantly, fabrication of immobilizers using 3D printing may be achieved without the presence of the patient or the therapist, potentially lowering operational costs and increasing efficiency.

Finally, 3D printed patient devices can integrate functional capabilities such as *in vivo* dosimetry. For example, by in-printing pockets in bolus, one may include thermoluminescent dosimeters (TLDs) or optically stimulated luminescent dosimeters (OSLDs) to allow measurement of delivered dose during radiotherapy [9]. This incorporates an important quality assurance tool into the device itself. Although the technology is still in development, the printed medium itself may act as a dosimeter [32], for example, when scintillating materials are used to print regions within a device [33]. This creates a personalized patient device that emits visible light in proportion to the radiation dose absorbed. Collection of this light by cameras may allow continuous and spatial dosimetric measurement.

CONCLUSION

Considering that 3D printing has entered radiation oncology relatively recently, the progress in this area to date has been significant. The conversion of manual or analog processes to automated and digital methods has been in keeping with the general technological evolution of RT. The majority of innovations using 3D printing share a common goal of increasing personalization of treatment of patients. Several developments, such as customized photon bolus, modulated electron bolus, and surface brachytherapy applicators are in widespread use in RT already. This adoption has motivated the establishment of quality assurance methods to ensure the accuracy of treatment delivery with these new innovations. This need has been recognized by American Association of Physicists in Medicine (AAPM) who has formed Task Group No. 336 – Quality Assurance for 3D Printing in Medical Imaging and Radiation Therapy Applications (TG336). Continued advancement of 3D printing technologies and printable materials will introduce new options in the radiation oncology field and practice. Future developments may include digital design and 3D printing of gynecological brachytherapy applicators, patient immobilization, and other personalized devices. To ensure widespread adoption, these innovations must be accompanied by development of software design technologies and 3D printing methods that become readily accessible by clinicians, including radiation oncologists, medical physicists, dosimetrists, and radiation therapists.

REFERENCES

[1]   Epp ER, Boyer AL, Doppke KP. Underdosing of lesions resulting from lack of electronic equilibrium in upper respiratory air cavities irradiated by 10MV x-ray beams. *Int J Radiat Oncol Biol Phys*. 1977;2:613–619.

[2]   Klein EE, Chin LM, Rice RK, et al. The influence of air cavities on interface doses for photon beams. *Int J Radiat Oncol Biol Phys*. 1993;27:419–427.

[3]   Li XA, Yu C, Holmes T. A systematic evaluation of air cavity dose perturbation in megavoltage x-ray beams. *Med Phys*. 2000;27:1011–1017.

[4]   Niroomand-Rad A, Harter KW, Thobejane S, et al. Air cavity effects on the radiation dose to the larynx using Co-60, 6 MV, and 10 MV photon beams. *Int J Radiat Oncol Biol Phys*. 1994;29:1139–1146.

[5]   Kan WK, Wu PM, Leung HT, et al. The effect of the nasopharyngeal air cavity on x-ray interface doses. *Phys Med Biol*. 1998;43:529–537.

[6]   Butson MJ, Cheung T, Yu P, et al. Effects on skin dose from unwanted air gaps under bolus in photon beam radiotherapy. *Radiat Meas*. 2000;32:201–204.

[7]   Bahhous K, Zerfaoui M, Rahmouni A, et al. Enhancing benefits of bolus use through minimising the effect of air-gaps on dose distribution in photon beam radiotherapy. *J Radiotherapy Pract*. 2021;20:210–216.

 [8] Boman E, Ojala J, Rossi M, et al. Monte Carlo investigation on the effect of air gap under bolus in post-mastectomy radiotherapy. *Phys Medica*. 2018;55:82–87.

 [9] Robar JL, Moran K, Allan J, et al. Intrapatient study comparing 3D printed bolus versus standard vinyl gel sheet bolus for postmastectomy chest wall radiation therapy. *Pract Radiat Oncol*. 2018;8:221–229.

[10] Ha J-S, Jung JH, Kim M-J, et al. Customized 3D printed bolus for breast reconstruction for modified radical mastectomy (MRM). *Prog Med Phys*. 2016;27:196–202.

[11] Benoit J, Pruitt AF, Thrall DE. Effect of wetness level on the suitability of wet gauze as a substitute for Superflab as a bolus material for use with 6 mv photons. *Vet Radiol Ultrasound*. 2009;50:555–559.

[12] Herpel C, Schwindling FS, Held T, et al. Individualized 3D-printed tissue retraction devices for head and neck radiotherapy. *Frontiers Oncol*. 2021;11:628743.

[13] Lu Y, Song J, Yao X, et al. 3D printing polymer-based bolus used for radiotherapy. *Int J Bioprinting*. 2021;7:414.

[14] Sharma SC, Johnson MW. Surface dose perturbation due to air gap between patient and bolus for electron beams. *Med Phys*. 1993;20:377–378.

[15] Kim S-W, Shin H-J, Kay CS, et al. A customized bolus produced using a 3-dimensional printer for radiotherapy. *PLos One*. 2014;9:e110746.

[16] Park K, Park S, Jeon M-J, et al. Clinical application of 3D-printed-step-bolus in post-total-mastectomy electron conformal therapy. *Oncotarget*. 2016;8:25660–25668.

[17] Zhao Y, Moran K, Yewondwossen M, et al. Clinical applications of 3-dimensional printing in radiation therapy. *Med Dosim*. 2017;42:150–155.

[18] Dyer BA, Campos DD, Hernandez DD, et al. Characterization and clinical validation of patient-specific three-dimensional printed tissue-equivalent bolus for radiotherapy of head and neck malignancies involving skin. *Phys Medica*. 2020;77:138–145.

[19] Low JM, Lee NJH, Sprow G, et al. Scalp and Cranium Radiation Therapy Using Modulation (SCRUM) and bolus. *Adv Radiat Oncol*. 2020;5:936–942.

[20] Kudchadker RJ, Antolak JA, Morrison WH, et al. Utilization of custom electron bolus in head and neck radiotherapy. *J Appl Clin Med Phys*. 2003;4:321–333.

[21] Dipasquale G, Poirier A, Sprunger Y, et al. Improving 3D-printing of megavoltage X-rays radiotherapy bolus with surface-scanner. *Radiat Oncol Lond Engl*. 2018;13:203.

[22] Biele‚da G, Marach A, Boehlke M, et al. 3D-printed surface applicators for brachy-therapy: a phantom study. *J Contemp Brachyther*. 2021;13:549–562.

[23] Cunha JAM, Mellis K, Sethi R, et al. Evaluation of PC-ISO for customized, 3D printed, gynecologic 192-Ir HDR brachytherapy applicators. *J Appl Clin Med Phys*. 2014;16:5168.

[24] Pearlstein KA, Chen RC. Comparing dosimetric, morbidity, quality of life, and cancer control outcomes after 3D conformal, intensity-modulated, and proton radiation therapy for prostate cancer. *Semin Radiat Oncol*. 2013;23:182–190.

[25] Prasanna PG, Rawojc K, Guha C, et al. Normal tissue injury induced by photon and proton therapies: Gaps and opportunities. *Int J Radiat Oncol Biol Phys*. 2021;110:1325–1340.

[26] Polf JC, Mille MM, Mossahebi S, et al. Determination of proton stopping power ratio with dual-energy CT in 3D-printed tissue/air cavity surrogates. *Med Phys*. 2019;46:3245–3253.

[27] Zou W, Fisher T, Zhang M, et al. Potential of 3D printing technologies for fabrication of electron bolus and proton compensators. *J Appl Clin Med Phys*. 2014;16:4959.

[28] Michiels S, D'Hollander A, Lammens N, et al. Towards 3D printed multifunctional immobilization for proton therapy: Initial materials characterization: 3D printed immobilization for proton therapy: Materials characterization. *Med Phys.* 2016;43:5392–5402.

[29] Semeniuk O, Cherpak A, Robar J. Design and evaluation of 3D printable patient-specific applicators for gynecologic HDR brachytherapy. *Med Phys.* 2021;48:4053–4063.

[30] Haefner MF, Giesel FL, Mattke M, et al. 3D-Printed masks as a new approach for immobilization in radiotherapy – a study of positioning accuracy. *Oncotarget.* 2018;9:6490–6498.

[31] Robar JL, Kammerzell B, Hulick K, et al. Novel multi jet fusion 3D-printed patient immobilization for radiation therapy. *J Appl Clin Med Phys.* 2022;23:e13773.

[32] Lynch N, Monajemi T, Robar JL. Characterization of novel 3D printed plastic scintillation dosimeters. *Biomed Phys Eng Express.* 2020;6:055014.

[33] Lynch N, Robar JL, Monajemi T. Camera-based radiotherapy dosimetry using dual-material 3D printed scintillator arrays. *Med Phys.* 2023;50:1824–1842.

A Brief Introduction to 3D Printing

James W. Stasiak

INTRODUCTION

Since its introduction in the 1980s, three-dimensional printing (3DP) technologies have revolutionized how products are conceptualized, designed, prototyped, and manufactured. As a result, many different industries that once relied on analog fabrication methods that were slow, wasteful, and expensive are adopting new digital and additive methods that are redefining product development and manufacturing. These new digital fabrication approaches have substantially impacted manufacturing efficiencies and scale. In parallel with new digital fabrication methods, new computer-aided design (CAD) data management methods have rapidly developed, such as 3D Systems' invention of the Standard Tessellation Language (STL) [1]. In addition, STL and newer file formats have made CAD design files more portable and compatible across 3DP platforms.

Consequently, the digitization of design, fabrication, and manufacturing has made it easier to modify, customize, and personalize products without impacting manufacturing costs or throughput. While the ability to modify product features and mix unique designs in every production run has influenced many industries, it has had a significant and critical impact on medicine and healthcare. As a result, 3DP and digital fabrication techniques are being adopted in many different medical specialties, including cardiovascular medicine, orthopedics, and joint reconstruction, and the development of patient-specific surgical guides. Over the next few decades, digital fabrication will become an increasingly important tool in 3D biofabrication and regenerative medicine.

This chapter aims to provide medical physicists, physicians, radiation therapists, and medical imaging professionals with an introduction to the history of 3D printing, a review of conventional 3DP technologies, and printing materials. While it is impossible to provide a comprehensive overview of 3DP technology and additive manufacturing (AM) in a single chapter, the references and links at the end can provide further and more detailed information.

DOI: 10.1201/9781003288404-2

A SHORT HISTORY OF 3D PRINTING TECHNOLOGIES

This section provides a brief history of the evolution and commercialization of 3DP and AM technologies. It is not a comprehensive retrospective. Detailed historical perspectives and reviews can be found online and in the reference section at the end of the chapter. For example, the 'History of Additive Manufacturing,' published by Wohlers Associates, provides an excellent historical review, beginning with the commercialization of stereolithography (SLA) in 1987 through April 2014 [2]. In 2022, Wohlers published an updated report on the current state of the technology in 'Wohlers Report 2022' [3].

Before discussing specific printers and processes, it is helpful to establish a working definition. In the context of this chapter, 3DP and AM are defined as automated procedures that involve the systematic addition of material (or materials) resulting in the fabrication of a freestanding 3D object. The first technologies satisfying this definition involved the photochemical processing of liquid resins. Although there had been experimental research investigating the use of photochemistry to harden or polymerize photosensitive resins in the 1960s, the first patents describing the development of a 'photochemical machining' process were filed by Wyn Swainson in 1977 in US 4,041,476, 'Method, medium, and apparatus for producing three-dimensional figure product' [4]. The patent described a process for polymerizing a system of reactive monomers using two lasers operating at different wavelengths. Photochemical hardening occurred when the laser beams intersected in the liquid resin. Following the 1977 patent, Swainson filed three additional patents (US 4,288,861, US 4,333,165, and US 4,466,080) with co-inventor Stephen Kramer describing improvements on the initial invention. All patents were later assigned to Formigraphic Engine Corporation. However, the technology was never commercialized. In the late 1970s, Hideo Kodama, a researcher at the Nagoya Municipal Industrial Research Institute in Japan, was also investigating laser-induced photochemical hardening. He simplified the dual-wavelength requirement and developed a new resin system that could be hardened using a single laser. Later, in 1981, Kodama published a paper entitled 'Automatic method for fabricating a three-dimensional plastic model with photo-hardening polymer' in the *Review of Instruments* but failed to patent the invention [5]. Although the early embodiments of SLA by Swainson and Kramer, and Kodama were foundational, they were largely focused on exploiting photochemical processes using tailored resins and used for rapid prototyping applications.

In 1986, Charles (Chuck) Hull filed US 4575330 A, 'Apparatus for production of three-dimensional objects by stereolithography,' in which he describes a process for patterning and hardening selected areas of layers of liquid polymers using ultraviolet (UV) light [6, 7].

In the patent, he describes computer-controlled automation to repeatedly cure successive layers of photosensitive resins using a UV light source, as illustrated in Figure 2.1. Computer-controlled UV exposure and resin processing automation established this invention as a benchmark for future industrial 3D printers. Hull's invention of SLA is often considered the beginning of commercial 3DP technology, earning him a place in the National Inventors Hall of Fame in 2014. Hull commercialized the first SLA 3D printer in 1987 and later became one of the founders of the company 3D Systems.

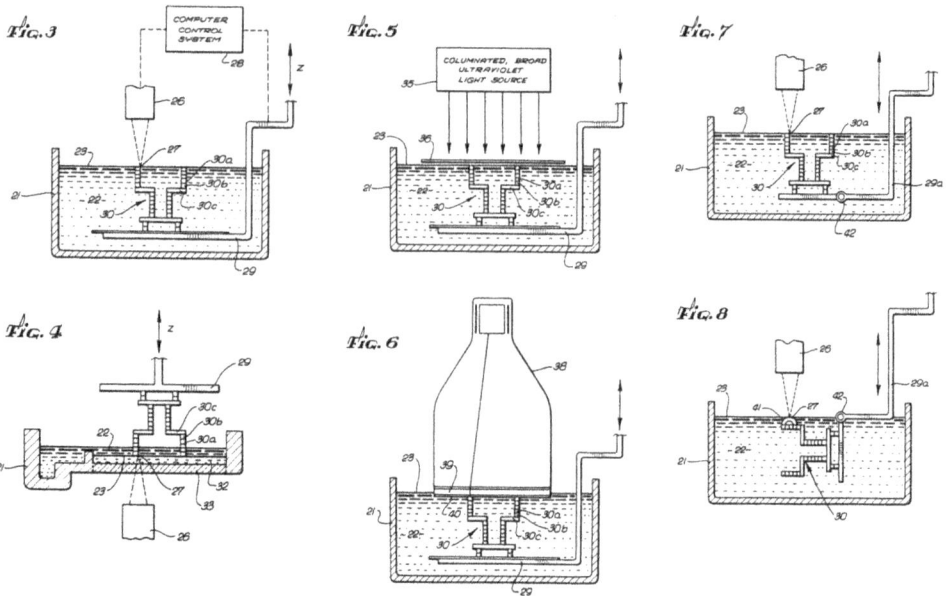

FIGURE 2.1   Figure from Hull's 1984 stereolithography (SLA) patent.

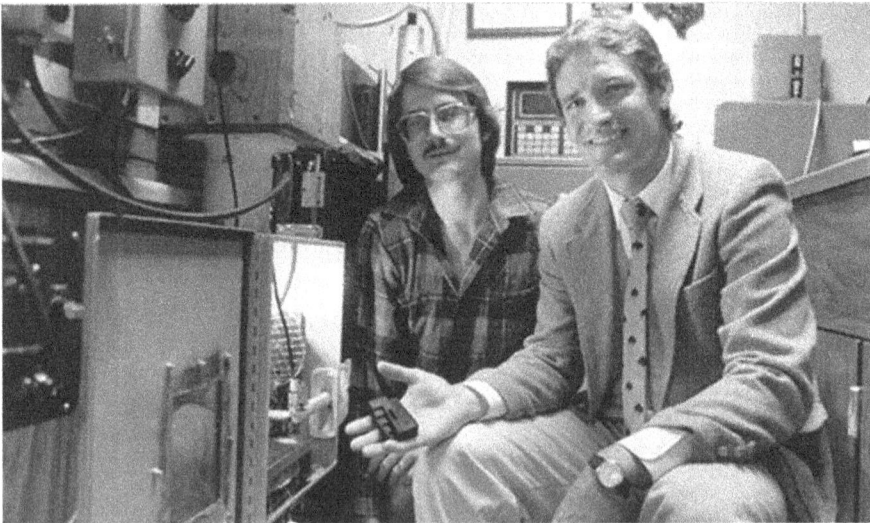

FIGURE 2.2   Photograph of Carl Deckard and Dr. Joe Beaman with one of the first Selective Laser Sintering (SLS) 3D printers circa 1988. Photo credit: Ralph Barrera.

Selective laser sintering (SLS) was developed in the mid-1980s by Carl Deckard, an undergraduate engineering student, and his academic advisor Joe Beaman at the University of Texas at Austin (Figure 2.2).

Unlike earlier methods that utilized photochemical hardening, the SLS process leveraged new developments of high-powered industrial lasers to melt or sinter thin powder media selectively. Physical features were created in the polymer powder layer by modulating or pulsing the on-and-off state of the laser as the beam was precisely and systematically scanned across the powder bed. In 1997, Deckard filed US 5,597,589 'Apparatus for producing parts by selective sintering' [8]. Deckard co-founded Desk Top Metal (DTM) which 3D Systems would later acquire.

In the early 1990s, several important alternatives to SLA technology emerged. Notably, S. Scott Crump filed the patent US 5,121,329, 'Apparatus and method for creating three-dimensional objects,' in 1989 [9]. The patent described a method for fabricating 3D objects using a layer-by-layer approach using a continuous thermoplastic material filament as feedstock. The method is called fused filament fabrication (FFF) and would later be trademarked by Crump *et al.* using the acronym fused deposition modeling (FDM). In 1988, Crump became a co-founder of the company Stratasys. Although FDM is used for industrial-scale fabrication, the simplicity of the process (compared to stereolithography) and the availability of different thermoplastic feedstock materials and desktop-sized printers have made the method popular with hobbyists and small businesses.

Powder bed, binder jetting, and drop-on-demand 3DP represent other foundational AM technologies. The original technology was developed at the Massachusetts Institute of Technology, patented by Emanuel Sachs in 1993, and commercialized by the start-up Z Corporation. In 1996, ExOne was granted an exclusive field-of-use patent for the technology. Most recently, the technology was acquired by 3D Systems. Although the technology has many variations and can accommodate a wide range of powder materials, the basic operating principle is the same. For example, a drop-on-demand process such as inkjet printing dispenses a binder fluid into a thin powder layer spread across a surface. The fluids dispensed into the powder layer are determined by the type of powder material and designed to bind or consolidate the powder particles in selected areas. Only the areas or features that have been patterned become part of the final object, and powder that has not been patterned is removed during post-processing. The powder spreading and patterning process is repeated until the completed 3D object is finished. Although the original technology was designed to use polymer powders, the basic process of powder spreading, drop-on-demand patterning, and binding (or fusing) is the basis for many different materials, such as metal powders, ceramic powders, and sand.

Similarly, the fluids (inks) that bind the powder particles are formulated based on deposition technology, powder material, and consolidation or fusing methods. As discussed above, this section provides a cursory review of the evolution and history of 3DP and AM. Additional material providing detailed discussions of the technologies and the adoption and commercialization of 3DP and AM can be found in the References section. For example, the Wikipedia '3D Printing' page is maintained, up to date, and an excellent source for references and external links [10].

3DP METHODS

This section provides a review of commercial 3DP technologies. In the three decades following Hull's introduction and subsequent commercialization of his SLA technology, the growth and adoption of 3DP technologies have been widespread. As a result, they continue to influence the future of manufacturing and how products are designed, fabricated,

Taxonomy of Conventional 3D Printing Technologies

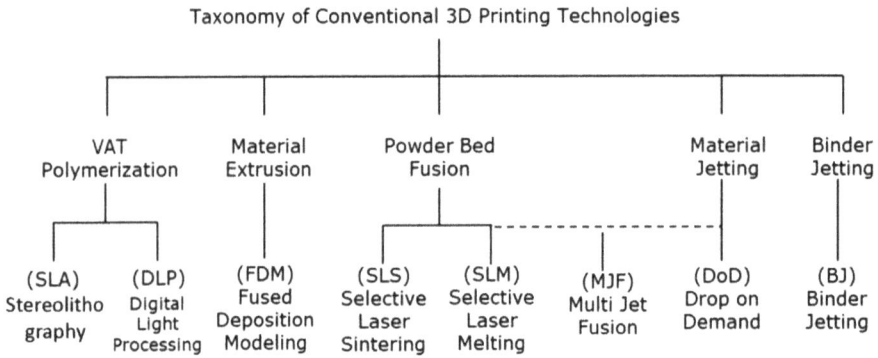

FIGURE 2.3   Taxonomy of conventional 3D printing technologies. Figure sourced with permission from: HUBS.

and distributed. Moreover, the technology domains and applications that exploit and benefit from their use are too numerous to discuss in this overview spanning desktop prototyping to new uses in healthcare and medicine. Consequently, this discussion will be limited to the most common methods and processes currently used in commercial applications and focused on those influencing the domains of healthcare and medicine. For detailed discussions of 3DP technologies and how they are utilized, references are given at the end of this chapter that provide comprehensive reviews and in-depth analyses of the different implementations and adaptations.

For this introduction, dividing 3DP technologies into five categories is convenient. Each category fabricates 3D objects using fundamental and functionally different physical mechanisms and processes. Specifically, each section below describes the different energy methods used to form solid layers and feedstock materials compatible with each approach. In Figure 2.3, a simple taxonomy is constructed based on these five methods.

Stereolithography

As discussed in the previous section, most histories of 3DP technology regard the vat polymerization method as the first modern 3DP technology. Although several approaches using photopolymerization were being developed concurrently by Kodama and others, Hull's SLA process represents the first 3DP technology to evolve from laboratory investigations to commercialization. In general, photopolymerization uses a wavelength-specific light source to initiate photochemical-induced modifications to the polymers' chemistry and physical properties. Typically, the starting material for the SLA process is a volume of the liquid resin contained in a shallow tank (or vat).

The photopolymer resin, exposure wavelength, and processing are engineered to selectively polymerize the liquid resin in the areas addressed by the light source, such as a laser, leaving the unexposed resin unaffected in the reservoir. The generic SLA process is schematically illustrated in Figure 2.4.

Fabricating a solid object involves incrementally raising the build platform using a computer-automated elevator and repeating the selective exposure of the next layer. A variation of the SLA process involves using a digital light projector to expose a digital

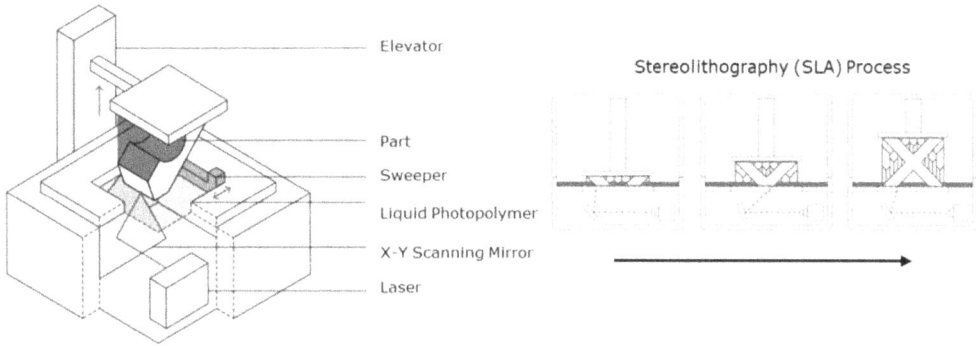

FIGURE 2.4   Schematic of a stereolithography (SLA) printer and fabrication process. Figure sourced with permission from: HUBS.

image of each layer using an exposure wavelength that polymerizes the layer. The subsequent steps of the Digital Light Processing (DLP) process are functionally similar to the SLA process. Exposing a complete image rather than rastering the laser results produces faster print times and throughput. Modern DLP printers use Digital Micromirror Device (DMD) technology to rapidly direct the focused light beam onto the build surface using Micro Electronic Mechanical Systems (MEMS) actuated micromirrors. An additional advantage of DMD-based SLA is the freedom to replace expensive wavelength-specific lasers with high-intensity UV lamps.

Compared to other 3DP technologies, SLA provides versatility, smooth surface properties, high throughput, and resolution. These advantages have made the technology especially useful for anatomical and dental modeling [11]. However, the cost of specialized photosensitive resins can be high, and post-processing the tacky surface of freshly finished components is often required. In summary, SLA-based printers have many configurations, including systems that can print from the top and bottom of the build platform and systems that use mask-based direct laser writing methods. Detailed information describing the variations and applications can be found in the reference section [12].

Material Extrusion

Compared to the SLA process, material extrusion technologies are less complicated and do not involve sophisticated photochemical chemistry to transform liquid resins into solid objects. The material extrusion process is schematically illustrated in Figure 2.5, which shows the components of a FFF printer. The fabrication process involves continuously feeding a polymer filament through a heated nozzle onto a temperature-controlled build platform. In most printer configurations, the filament is stored on a spool. Although FFF is significantly more precise and versatile, the basic process is analogous to depositing a bead of glue onto a surface using a hot-glue gun. First, an object is fabricated by scanning the heated nozzle across the build surface and depositing a pattern of parallel lines using an automated rastering procedure. After depositing a single layer of filament, the build platform is incrementally lowered, and the process is repeated until the fabrication of

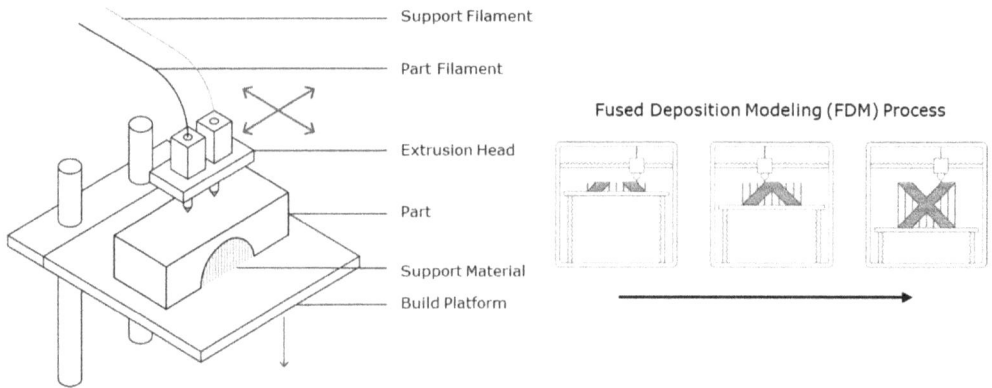

FIGURE 2.5 Schematic of a Fused Filament Fabrication (FFF) printer and fabrication process. Figure sourced with permission from: HUBS.

the object is completed. Deceptively simple, the FFF process is remarkably versatile and produces components with fine features and dimensional accuracy.

Note that the abbreviation FDM was trademarked by the company Stratasys, but the terms FFF and FDM have become ubiquitous and are often used interchangeably. The apparent simplicity of the FDM process provides a significant advantage to the designer or engineer. In addition, unlike the costly resins used in the SLA process, polymer filament materials are relatively inexpensive. Moreover, printers configured with multiple extrusion heads can use different filaments with different material properties or diameters. Discussed in more detail in subsequent sections, the ability to mix materials enables engineers to fabricate components with complex physical properties. The filaments used in the material extrusion process are typically thermoplastics such as acrylonitrile butadiene styrene (ABS) and polylactic acid (PLA). As mentioned above, these materials are relatively inexpensive, and spools can be purchased from many suppliers for US $20–$40. It is important to note that, unlike other 3DP technologies such as powder bed fusion (PBF), material extrusion printers can accommodate semi-crystalline (e.g., PLA) and amorphous thermoplastics (e.g., ABS), adding more versatility, functionality, and design freedom to the process. However, higher-performance thermoplastic materials such as polyetheretherketone (PEEK) and polyaryletherketone (PAEK) spools can exceed US $500/kg. It is also possible to produce filaments composed of composite materials such as polymers with embedded nanoparticles. These polymer nanocomposite materials can possess unconventional electromagnetic properties and are the subject of academic and industrial research organizations. This topic will be addressed more completely in the next section. Unsurprisingly, the simplicity of the extrusion process and the lower supply costs make FDM an economical entry point for hobbyists and other users who require prototypes or low-volume part production. However, industrial-scale FDM printers with large build volumes are used commercially for various applications.

Powder Bed Fusion

PBF 3DP is a broad category usually subdivided into two different processing approaches. Although both technologies are fundamentally similar, they were developed to process different feedstock materials. The SLS process was designed to process polymer powder feedstock, while selective laser melting (SLM) is almost exclusively used to process metal powders feedstock. Both processes involve using a high-power laser to selectively sinter or selectively melt powder particles that have been smoothly and uniformly spread across the surface of a temperature-controlled powder bed. Each process will be discussed in the next sections.

Selective Laser Sintering

The SLS process begins with the deposition of polymer powder onto the surface of the powder bed that has been heated to a temperature slightly below the polymer powder's melting point. Layer uniformity and smoothness are critical parameters achieved by drawing the recoating blade across the powder layer. Typically, the thickness of the powder layer is 100 microns or roughly the thickness of two stacked 50-micron diameter powder particles. A high-power laser beam is scanned across the layer surface, selectively sintering areas intended to become part of the finished object. Once the selected area is sintered, the powder bed is incrementally lowered, and fresh powder is spread using the recoater blade. The SLS process is schematically illustrated in Figure 2.6.

The scanning and sintering steps are repeated until the object is fabricated and the unfused powder is removed in a post-processing step. To achieve dimensional accuracy, each processing step is tightly controlled. For example, the laser spot size and energy must remain constant. In addition, as mentioned above, the thickness of the powder layer and the surface properties and smoothness of the layer must be carefully controlled. The surface properties largely depend on the quality and uniformity of the raw powder purchased from the supplier.

Direct Metal Laser Sintering and Selective Laser Melting

Direct metal laser sintering (DMLS) and SLM technologies follow the same processing steps as the SLS process discussed above. Both DMLS and SLM are used to fabricate

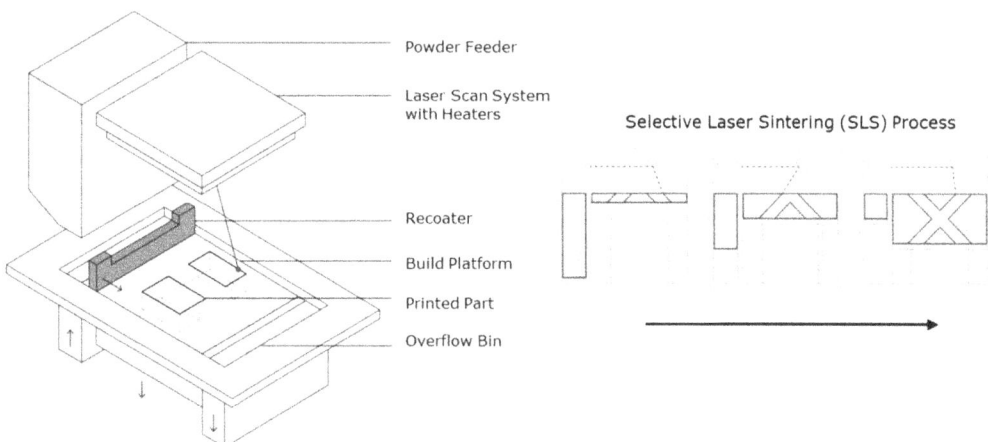

FIGURE 2.6   Schematic of a selective laser sintering (SLS) printer and fabrication process. Figure sourced with permission from: HUBS.

metal parts. However, they differ in how the metal powder particles are joined. DMLS uses a high-energy beam to heat the metal–alloy powder particles to temperatures high enough to cause the particles to fuse. SLM also uses a high-energy laser beam to produce temperatures high enough to cause the metal particles to melt fully.

Like SLS, metal components are fabricated using a layer-by-layer process. However, because large thermal gradients can develop in the molten regions of the piece, distortion and warpage can occur. Therefore, metal support structures are often required during the build process to minimize the effects of thermally induced forces. Support structures help to dissipate heat in critical areas and fix the component securely to the build platform. Like SLS, the final product's quality depends critically on the metal powder properties, such as uniformity and average particle diameter. The high quality required increases the cost of the powder feedstock. For example, a kilogram of stainless steel 316L powder can cost US $400 or more. Other metals and alloys compatible with both processes include aluminum, copper, nickel, and titanium. In addition to DMLS and SLM, electron beam melting (EBM) is also classified as a PBF technology. EBM printers incorporate directed electron beams to fuse the metal powder particles. Although accommodating an electron beam subsystem into the printer architecture adds considerable complexity, there are important benefits and advantages. Since the electron beam creates a higher energy beam and spot, the quality of the printed components is significantly higher. Moreover, the improved surface properties reduce the time required for post-process machining and finishing reducing overall process times. More information about DMLS, SLM, and EBM can be found in the reference section.

Binder Jetting

The binder jetting process is like SLS and involves the fabrication using powder feedstock and various methods for consolidating layers of powder materials to form 3D objects. The process has been developed to accommodate different powder materials, including polymers, metals, and different types of sand (sandstone or gypsum). The binder jetting process is schematically illustrated in Figure 2.7. Other applications include fabricating

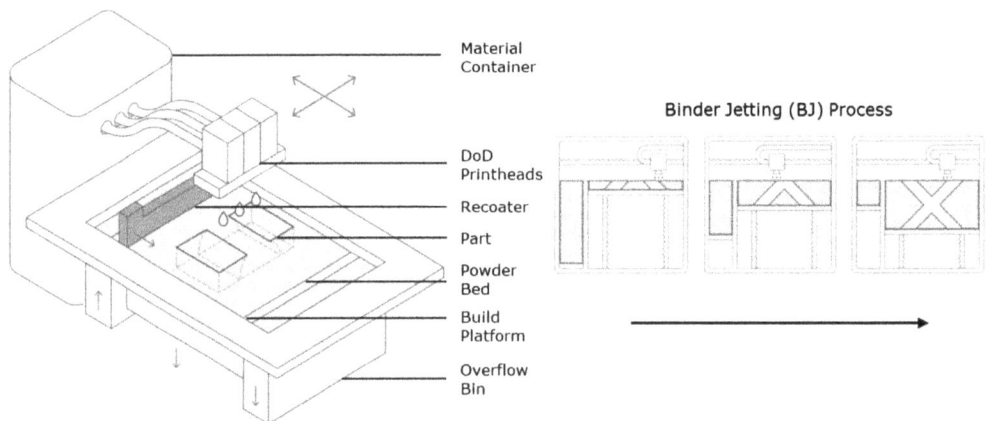

FIGURE 2.7   Schematic of a binder jet printer and fabrication process. Figure sourced with permission from: HUBS.

sand-casting forms and molds. However, unlike SLS processing which relies on lasers or electron beams to melt or fuse particles, binder jetting typically uses a liquid agent to bind particles together. After each layer is defined, fresh powder is spread over the previous layer and repeated. Once completed, the unbound powder is removed in a post-processing step.

Metal Jet 3D Printer Technology

In 2022, HP announced the commercialization of its Metal Jet 3D S100 printing technology [13, 14]. The Metal Jet 3DP process uses a water-based binding agent formulated with a polymer that binds metal particles together wherever the agent is deposited. The agent's fluid properties were engineered for delivery using HP thermal inkjet printheads. The process flow for the Metal Jet process is illustrated in Figure 2.8.

Once dispensed onto a layer of metal powder, capillary forces draw the agent into the pores and voids between the particles. Next, a thermal curing step causes the fluid to evaporate, leaving the polymer component behind, which acts like an adhesive holding the metal particles together. Once the layer is cured, a fresh layer of metal particles is spread and leveled, and the process is repeated until the fabrication of the object is finished. Finally, the unbound metal particles are removed in a post-processing step. After de-powdering, the 'green' object is moved into a sintering oven.

The sintering oven operates at temperatures high enough to cause atomic diffusion between the metal particles and drive off the remaining polymer. HP developed the Metal Jet 3DP technology to compete with metal injection molding (MIM). The Metal Jet process can achieve 96% solid density, equivalent to MIM solid densities. When the HP S100

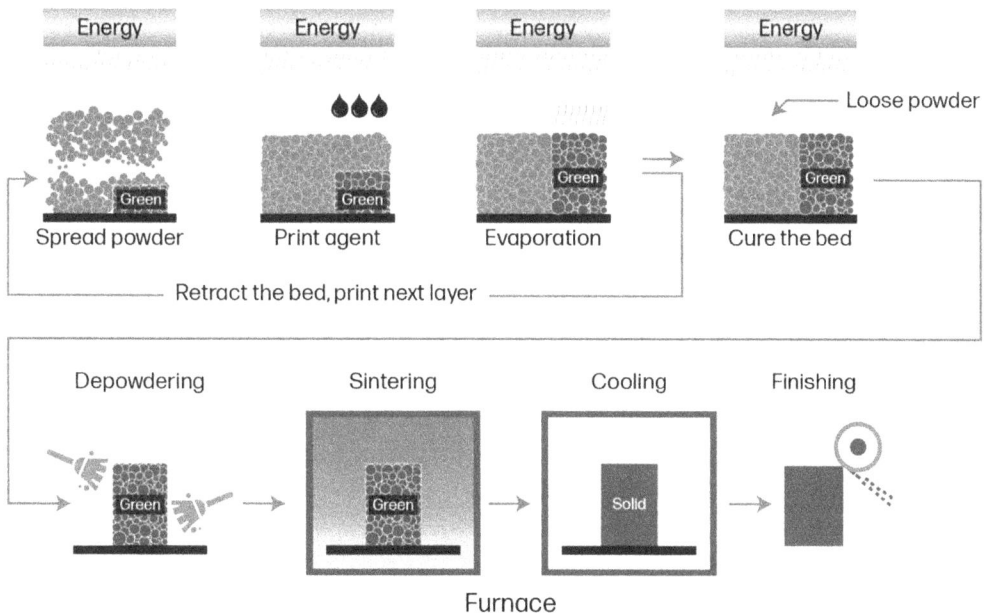

FIGURE 2.8 HP's Metal Jet 3D printing technology and fabrication process. Figure sourced with permission from: HP.

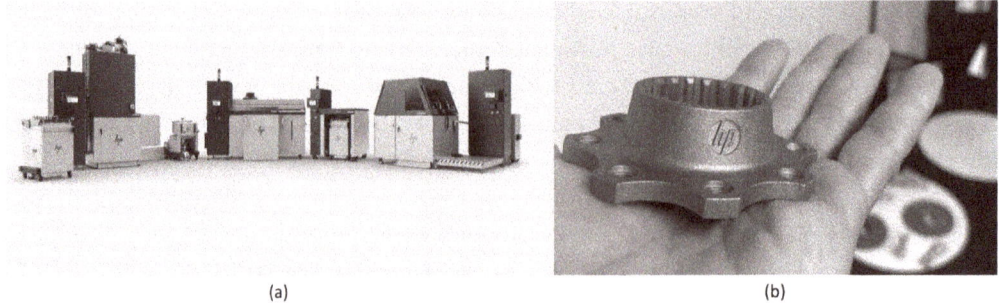

FIGURE 2.9   (a) HP's Metal Jet S100 3D additive manufacturing system. (b) Flange printed with HP's S100 printed using 316L stainless steel powder. Figure sourced with permission from HP.

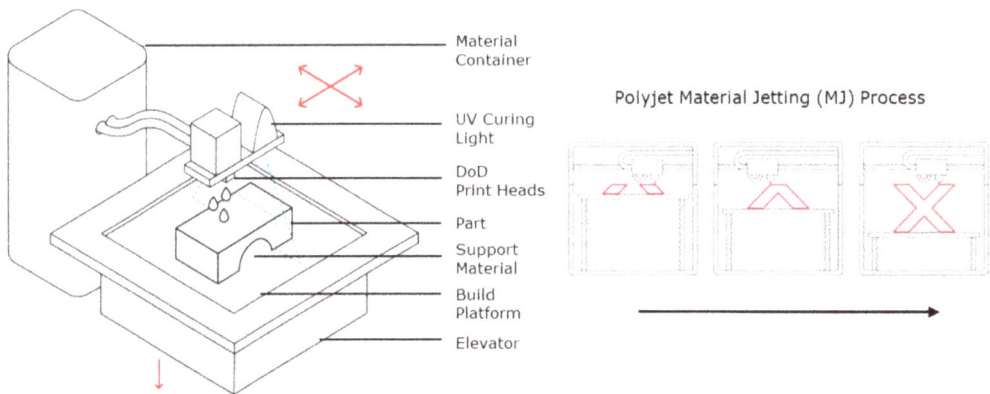

FIGURE 2.10   Schematic of the PolyJet Material Jetting (MJ) printer and fabrication process.

was announced in 2022, it could process 316L and 17-4PH stainless steel powders. A complete HP S100 Metal Jet 3DP system is shown in Figure 2.9a, and an example of a component printed using the S100 with 316L stainless steel powder is shown in Figure 2.9b. Other companies have commercialized metal binder jet technologies, including Xometry, ExOne, Markforged, and Desktop Metal.

Material Jetting

Material jetting 3DP uses inkjet deposition methods to dispense small droplets of thermoset photopolymer resin that are cured using UV light. The material jetting process is illustrated in Figure 2.10.

The process requires two different types of resin. One resin is used to form the object, while another is used to provide structural support during printing. The support elements are removed during a post-processing step. Parts printed using this process offer a wide range of mechanical and optical properties, including flexibility, translucency and transparency, and excellent surface finish. In addition, the smooth surface makes it possible to apply an additional coating for color and performance improvements.

Moreover, some resins have been medically certified and are biocompatible and sterilizable. These properties have made the technology indispensable for medical, anatomical modeling, and dental prototyping. Currently, the company Stratasys has commercialized the technology using the trade name PolyJet. Stratasys also markets a wide range of photopolymer resins.

An important extension of the material jetting technology is its ability to print composite materials. The company XJet has developed a technology called 'Nano Particle Jetting' (NPJ) [15]. The material used in the NPJ incorporates nanoparticles dispersed into the resin matrix. The nanoparticles, deposited in extremely thin layers and embedded in a resin matrix, provide new design options for fabricating components with very small feature sizes.

Multi Jet Fusion

In 2016, HP announced the commercialization of its Multi Jet Fusion 3DP technology. The Multi Jet Fusion (MJF) process can be considered a hybrid 3DP process, combining aspects of material jetting, drop-on-demand dispensing, and PBF [16]. The MJF process is illustrated in Figure 2.11.

The process begins by uniformly spreading polymer powder onto the powder bed. Once the layer is spread, the printer uses HP's thermal inkjet printheads to pattern the powder layer using an infrared (IR) absorbing fusing agent. Next, the printed areas are thermally fused using a high-intensity IR lamp. For some areas with fine or detailed features, a separate fluid controls the heat transfer from printed areas into the loose powder or adjacent areas. Once a layer has been patterned and fused, fresh powder is spread over the previous layer, and the process is repeated until the fabrication of the object has been completed. The process leverages HP's deep assets in imaging and printing to take the digital transformation of two-dimensional printed images into a 3D world of highly-functional, high-value manufactured items. The MJF process was initially designed to use Nylon 12 powder as feedstock. However, since its introduction, the MJF process has been tailored to be compatible with other polymers, including thermoplastics, elastomers, and thermosets. The only requirement for a compatible material is the morphology of the polymer. To ensure effective fusing, only semi-crystalline polymers, such as polyamides (PA12 and PA11), polyamides with dispersed glass beads, and polypropylene are used.

This section has provided a concise overview of 3DP technologies used in industry today. Some of these are already used for prototyping and fabricating specialized components and devices for radiation therapy applications and are discussed elsewhere

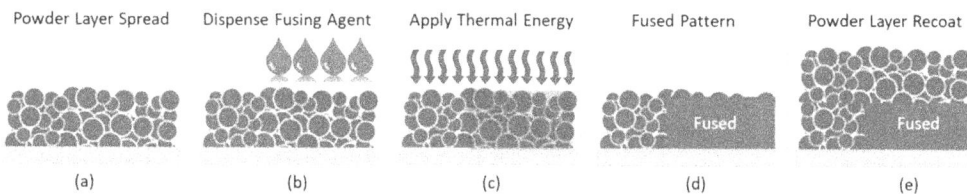

| Powder Layer Spread | Dispense Fusing Agent | Apply Thermal Energy | Fused Pattern | Powder Layer Recoat |
| (a) | (b) | (c) | (d) | (e) |

FIGURE 2.11   HP's Multi Jet Fusion 3D printing technology. Figure sourced with permission from: HP.

in this publication. References that provide additional information about each technology are provided at the chapter's end.

3DP MATERIALS

As discussed in previous sections, the types of materials used as 3DP feedstock are surprisingly large and varied and include polymers, metals, composites, and even biological materials. This section aims to provide a high-level overview of the most common types of materials used as feedstock for 3DP and AM technologies.

To begin, the choice of feedstock materials used for a 3DP application is guided by several factors. First, the properties and physical characteristics of the finished object must be considered. For example, properties such as thermal stability, hardness, tensile strength, flexibility, surface roughness, recyclability, and chemical inertness are defined by the application. Biocompatibility and sterilizability are other factors that are critically important for healthcare, medical, and therapeutic applications. Once the application requirements are established and the materials selected, the appropriate 3DP methods can be determined. The section is subdivided into four broad categories: polymers, metals and alloys, unconventional or engineered materials, and materials used for bioprinting and biofabrication applications. Figure 2.12 provides a simple taxonomy of the materials and lists the specific 3DP technologies associated with each raw material. The section begins with a review of polymer materials.

Polymers and Plastics

Currently, thermoplastics are the most commonly used 3DP materials, largely because of the increasing availability of desktop FDM printers. In addition, hobbyists and small, print-on-demand businesses are attracted to the technology because of the affordability, ease of use, and wide range of filament materials and suppliers. However, thermoplastics are also an important class of materials for many industrial and commercial applications.

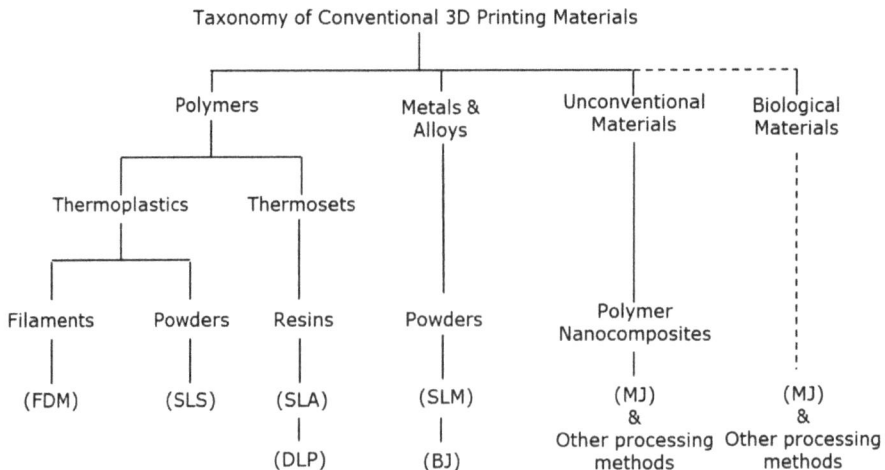

FIGURE 2.12   Taxonomy of conventional 3D printing materials.

In general, thermoplastic materials such as ABS, PLA, polyethylene terephthalate glycol (PETG), polyamides (PA), and thermoplastic polyurethane (TPU) provide strength, durability, flexibility, humidity and chemical resistance, and can be food-safe. Moreover, most thermoplastic materials are recyclable and reusable. In addition to FDM technologies, powders made from thermoplastic materials are used in SLS and other PBF technologies, such as HP's MJF printers. Typical costs for thermoplastic materials such as PLA are between US $15 and $20/kg.

Thermosetting plastic (thermosets) represents another important category of 3DP material. However, thermosetting materials cannot be remelted or reused, unlike thermoplastic materials. Thermosets are typically formulated into resins and used in SLA and DLP printing technology. During curing, polymer chains in the liquid resin cross-link in an irreversible physical process. As discussed in the previous section, the curing process involves exposing the resin to a radiation source, such as UV light. Since the chemical bonds formed during photopolymerization are irreversible, cured materials will remain solid permanently. Cured materials are typically very durable, with hard, smooth surface finishes, highly detailed geometries, and tight tolerances. The chemistry of photocurable resins is complex and often involves specialty solvents, and additional chemicals such as photoinitiators and adhesion promoters. Compared to other materials, photocurable resins are relatively expensive, with average costs between US $50 and $70/kg.

Metal and Alloy Powders

The fabrication of metal objects using 3DP methods involves the binding and joining of metal and metal alloy powders using DMLS, SLM methods, or HP's Metal Jet technology that involves the fabrication of a 'green body' using a binder fluid and sintering in a separate oven. The common factor for these methods is using micron-scale metal powders as the feedstock material. In theory, nearly any metal, such as aluminum, stainless steel, copper, and alloys such as Inconel and cobalt chromium, can produce 3D metal components. The challenge is to produce metal objects with solid densities that rival the densities achieved using MIM processes. Unsurprisingly, the cost of producing metal powders with uniform metallurgical properties, shapes, and sizes is high. For example, one of the more common materials, 316L stainless steel powders, can cost between US $400 and $500/kg, with less common metals and alloys costing significantly more.

Unconventional Materials

The materials discussed so far have been 'conventional,' meaning their physical properties and the properties of the finished component are largely determined by the macroscopic properties of the raw feedstock materials. However, this discussion uses the term 'unconventional' to identify materials with physical properties determined or 'tailored' before or during printing.

Developing new techniques that blend fundamental materials science with 3DP processes makes designing, engineering, and printing components with tailored or anisotropic physical properties possible. For example, several powder manufacturers already offer polymer powders that incorporate mesoscopic or microscopic glass beads to modify the overall strength of a component. Another example is the use of commercially available FDM filaments that contain strands of carbon fibers to print components with enhanced stiffness in one direction but maintain the intrinsic flexibility elsewhere. While it is outside the scope of this chapter to discuss this topic in more detail, it is safe to say that the prospects for materials-by-design manufacturing promise to revolutionize the world of AM.

Biological Materials

3DP using biological materials is an important and exciting area of research. While it will be many decades before we can fabricate functional human organs, research exploring tissue engineering is promising. It is outside the scope of this chapter to discuss tissue engineering and regenerative medicine. However, at the end of the chapter, there are references for readers who want to explore this subject in more detail [17].

SUMMARY

The objective of this chapter was to provide non-specialists with a short history describing the development of 3DP and AM technologies and familiarity with the technical operation of the five basic 3DP technologies. Table 2.1 below summarizes the different methods,

TABLE 2.1   The Methods, Materials, Formation Methods, and Selected Printer Manufacturers

Technologies and Methods	Feedstock Materials	Formation Methods	Selected Printer Manufacturers
Vat Polymerization			
Stereolithography (SLA)	Polymers	Cured with laser	3DSystems. Formlabs, DWS
Digital Light Processing (DLP)	Polymers	Cured with projector	Envisiontec,
Continuous Digital Light (CDLP)	Polymers	Cured with LED and O_2	Carbon, Envisiontec
Material Extrusion			
Fused Deposition Mod (FDM)	Polymers and Composites.	Fused with heat	Stratasys, MakerBot, Ultimaker
Powder Bed Fusion			
Selective Laser Sintering (SLS)	Polymers	Fused with laser	EOS. 3DSystems, Sinterit
Selective Laser Melting (SLM)	Metals	Fused with laser	EOS. 3DSystems. Renishaw
Multi Jet Fusion (MJF)	Polymers	Fused with radiant energy	HP
Electron Beam Melting (EBM)	Metals	Fused with electron beam	Arcam
Material Jetting			
Drop on Demand (DoD)	Fluid dispersions	Cured with heat	Solidscape (wax)
Nanoparticle Jetting (NPJ)	Fluid dispersions	Cured with heat	XJET
Polvjer	Polymers	Cured with UV light	Stratasys, 3DSystems
Binder Jetting			
Binder Jetting (BJM)	Metals. gypsum, and sand	Joined with binder	HP. ExOne. 3DSystems

processing details, and conventional printing materials that are used today. The table also provides a representative list of companies that have commercialized the technologies for industrial applications.

While there has been remarkable progress in the development of 3DP technology since the 1980s, it is clear that invention and progress will continue to accelerate. The motivation for continued innovation is the adoption rate of 3DP and AM in many new technical domains and application areas. For example, in medicine and healthcare, 3DP is currently used to fabricate patient-specific devices that range from the fabrication of dental implants to orthopedic and reconstructive components and surgical guides. In addition, as discussed in the following chapters, 3DP technologies are being adopted to improve the effectiveness of radiation therapy in treating different types of cancer. Specifically, information obtained from 3D imaging studies can be translated into data used by 3D printers to fabricate customized devices used in radiotherapy, such as bolus and brachytherapy applicators. These patient-specific devices help to minimize radiation damage to healthy tissue and organs while maximizing the effectiveness of the treatment. On the horizon, 3DP technology may be used for biofabrication applications. For example, inks formulated using a patient's cells to print tissue directly into wounds optimize skin grafts and minimize tissue rejection.

REFERENCES

[1] Grimm T. Users Guide to Rapid Prototyping. Society of Manufacturing Engineers; 2004.

[2] Wohlers T. Wohlers report 2014: 3D printing and additive manufacturing state of the industry annual worldwide progress report. Wohlers Associates; 2014.

[3] Wohlers T. Wohlers Report 2022: 3D Printing and additive manufacturing global state of the industry. Wohlers Associates; 2021.

[4] Swainson W. Method, medium, and apparatus for producing three-dimensional figure product. 1971. Available from: https://patents.google.com/patent/US4041476A/en

[5] Kodama H. Automatic method for fabricating a three-dimensional plastic model with photo-hardening polymer. *Rev Sci Instrum*. 1981;52:1770–1773.

[6] Hull C. Apparatus for production of three-dimensional object by stereolithography. 1986. Available from: https://patents.google.com/patent/US4575330A/en

[7] CNN. The night I invented 3D printing [Internet]. [cited 2014]. Available from: http://edition.cnn.com/2014/02/13/tech/innovation/the-night-i-invented-3d-printing-chuck-hall/.

[8] Deckard C. Apparatus for producing parts by selective sintering. 1997. Available from: https://patents.google.com/patent/US5597589A/en#

[9] Crump S. Apparatus and method for creating three-dimensional objects. 1989. Available from: https://patents.google.com/patent/US5121329A/en

[10] Foundation W. 3D Printing [Internet]. [cited 2023]. Available from: http://en.wikipedia.org/wiki/3D_printing.

[11] Whitaker M. The history of 3D printing in healthcare. *Bull R Coll Surg Engl*. 2014;96:228–229.

[12] Redwood B., Schoffeer, F, Garrent, B., *The 3D Printing Handbook: Technologies, Design and Applications*, 3D Hubs. 2017, ISBN-13 978-9082748505.

[13] HP. Technical whitepaper: HP Metal Jet Technology [Internet]. 2018. Available from: www8.hp.com/h20195/v2/GetPDF.aspx/4AA7-3333EEW

[14] Stasiak J, Champion D, Yadati U, et al. Chapter 61: HP's metal jet 3d printing technology in Inkjet printing in industry, in *Inkjet Printing in Industry*. Wiley, 2022;1391–1401.

[15] Oh Y, Bharambe V, Mummareddy B, et al. Microwave dielectric properties of zirconia fabricated using NanoParticle Jetting™. *Addit Manuf*. 2019;27:586–594.

[16] HP. Technical whitepaper: HP Multi Jet Fusion [Internet]. Available from: www.hp.com/us-en/printers/3d-printers/products/multi-jet-technology.html

[17] Stasiak JW. Industrial applications of 3D inkjet printing in the life sciences, in *Handbook of Industrial Inkjet Printing*. Wiley, 2017;661–680.

CHAPTER 3

Biocompatibility and Sterilization of 3D Printed Radiation Therapy Devices

Yuji Kamio and Stéphane Bedwani

INTRODUCTION

Several countries have legislation concerning medical devices to ensure public safety in relation to their use [1]. Government agencies, such as the U.S. Food and Drug Administration (FDA), Health Canada, and the European Medicines Agency (EMA) are generally responsible for ensuring the quality, performance, and safety of medical devices before authorizing their sale[1] within their jurisdictions. Despite a lack of global harmonization in the application of regulatory requirements [2], certain common principles have emerged, such as the adoption of a risk management system (RMS). An RMS assesses the risk toward patients and users at every stage in the life cycle of a medical device, including its design, manufacturing, distribution, use, and disposal. Although risk classification varies between countries, stricter regulations usually follow an increase in level of risk. Risk classification[2] criteria are typically defined according to whether the device is invasive or non-invasive, the duration of contact with the body tissues (i.e., limited, prolonged or permanent), and adverse biological effects (e.g., irritation, inflammation or other allergic reactions) that may occur during its specific use. Manufacturers seeking market clearance for new medical devices must usually undertake preclinical testing,[3] clinical trials, risk assessments, and post-market surveillance to ensure product safety in compliance with regulatory standards across distribution territories. In some cases, exemptions from certain regulatory requirements are granted, such as those for custom-made devices

---

1 The term *sale* may include rental and distribution, with or without compensation.
2 The FDA categorizes medical devices into three classes: Class I, II, and III; the EMA has four classes: Class I, IIa, IIb, and III; and Health Canada also employs four classes: Class I, II, III, and IV.
3 For conciseness, this chapter emphasizes fundamental concepts and risk assessment in preclinical testing.

DOI: 10.1201/9781003288404-3

[3–5]. However, these medical devices must still adhere to essential safety and performance requirements. By following international standards such as ISO 14971 [6] and ISO 13485 [7], manufacturers can implement a medical device-specific risk management and quality system, supporting the demonstration of their safety.

Additional measures must be taken when a medical device is intended to be in contact with the patient. First, the biocompatibility of the device must be demonstrated by the manufacturer. The manufacturer may hire a contract testing laboratory (CTL) [8] to carry out the biological and chemical tests required for biocompatibility based, for example, on ISO 10993 standards [9]. Second, the device in its final form must be free from all forms of chemicals (residues, leachables), pyrogens, and microbiological contamination resulting from the manufacturing process and should be restored to this state prior to each clinical use. The manufacturer must therefore specify a decontamination protocol based on the level of risk, often defined by the Spaulding classification [10–12]. This classification depends on the nature of the contact and includes three levels of risk: non-critical for intact skin, semi-critical for intact mucous membranes or non-intact skin, and critical for irritated mucous membrane or sterile tissue/bone/bloodstream. Table 3.1 presents an overview of medical devices in radiation oncology and their correspondence with the Spaulding classification. Decontamination is carried out progressively, starting with cleaning for all risk levels, followed by low-level disinfection for non-critical devices, high-level disinfection for semi-critical and critical devices, and sterilization for critical devices [13]. Cleaning generally involves scrubbing with a detergent to reduce the number of microorganisms, debris, and chemical residues. Disinfection aims to reduce residual viable microorganisms to a threshold deemed sufficient for use or sterilization. Sterilization is a validated process that inactivates virtually all viable microorganisms from a device. A manufacturer may hire a CTL to provide the documentation related to the validation of their decontamination process for presentation to regulatory agencies.

With the advent of 3D printing in the hospital environment, a healthcare facility (HF) can now fulfill the dual role of user and manufacturer of medical devices. Despite the numerous advantages that in-house production offers, a HF using its homemade medical devices should, in principle, strive to ensure its quality and safety on par with industry standards. However, this raises several issues for a HF taking on this new role, including training qualified personnel in 3D printing, monitoring the production chain, and ensuring a clear understanding of responsibilities at all stages of the device's life cycle. The FDA aligns with this perspective in an open discussion [14], questioning means to enable HFs to achieve a satisfactory level of safety. While establishing good practices[4] in 3D printing of medical devices could be one of these means [15–18], regulatory agencies have yet to implement concrete supportive measures.

In radiation oncology, several medical devices produced by 3D printing require special attention when it comes to their clinical use [19], especially when they are in contact with the patient. For example, boluses [20–22], superficial [23], intracavitary [24] brachytherapy

---

4 This may include: GMP – Good manufacturing practices; GLP – Good laboratory practices; and GCP – Good clinical practices.

TABLE 3.1 Categorization of Certain Examples of Medical Devices in Radiation Oncology and Their Correlation with the Spaulding Classification

	Body Contact	Spaulding Classification (Disinfection Level)[a]	Examples[b]
Non-contact device	None	N/A	• EBRT cutouts • BT transfer tubes • Anatomical models • DQA phantoms
Surface device	Intact skin	Non-critical (Low-level)	• Immobilization devices • Surface dosimeters • Transabdominal ultrasound probes
	Mucosal membrane	Semi-critical (High-level)	• Intraoral devices • Transrectal ultrasound probes
	Breached or compromised surface	[c] [d]	• Bolus materials • Orthovoltage cutouts • Surface BT applicators (Skin) • Intracavitary BT applicators (GYN, Rectum H&N)
Externally communicating device	Blood path, indirect	Critical (Sterilization)	• Vials/Syringes for contrast injection or RPT
	Tissue, bone or dentin		• Interstitial BT templates (Prostate, Breast, GYN, H&N) • Needles and sutures for BT • Combined intracavitary/interstitial BT applicators (GYN) • Balloon BT catheters (Breast) • Eye plaques for BT
	Circulating blood		• Intravascular BT catheter • Needles for contrast injection or RPT
Implant device	Tissue or bone		• Radioactive permanent BT seeds (prostate, breast) • Fiducial markers • Electromagnetic beacon transponders
	Blood		• Radioactive microspheres for SIRT • Radioactive stents for intravascular BT

Notes:

Abbreviations: DQA – Delivery quality assurance; EBRT – Electron beam radiation therapy; BT – Brachytherapy; GYN – Gynecology; H and N – Head and neck; RPT – Radiopharmaceutical therapy; SIRT – Selective internal radiation therapy.

[a] *Here is a list of infectious agents [29], organized in order of their resistance levels for disinfection:*
Low-level: Enveloped viruses, vegetative bacteria, fungi.
High-level: Fungal spore, naked viruses, mycobacteria, parasitic oocysts.
Sterilization: Bacterial spores, prions.

[b] *Examples offer a simplified overview; classifications may vary by intended use. Dashed lines indicate that a device can be in contact with multiple surfaces and consequently is assigned to the highest risk category.*

[c] *Breached or compromised skin.*

[d] *Irritated, breached or compromised mucosal membrane.*

applicators, and intraoral devices [25–27] fall into this category. While the production of a patient-specific device [28] can be conducted within the hospital, its design could be provided by a regulatory-approved commercial software application (e.g., 3D Bolus and 3D Brachy from Adaptiiv Medical Technologies). In this case, the FDA states that the provider of such software (which is regarded as a medical device production system) is also responsible for adhering to regulatory requirements [14]. The clinical use of any of these products should prompt consideration of safety issues, with special attention to decontamination and biocompatibility. However, a HF may not have the financial resources to hire a CTL, nor have access to testing facilities to assess thoroughly the safety of a medical device. One approach to address this situation is to collaborate with the industry, which can hire a CTL to perform the necessary tests, or to collaborate with a research laboratory with sufficient expertise to conduct these tests. Including these results in publications would provide relevant data to other device developers and potentially save them several costly tests. The rest of this chapter specifically focuses on biocompatibility testing and validation of sterilization processes related to 3D printed devices.

BIOCOMPATIBILITY OF RADIOTHERAPY DEVICES

The biocompatibility of a medical device indicates that it does not generate any undesirable biological effects for the patient[5] during normal use. This section discusses general concepts described in the international standard ISO 10993 [9], including its subparts [30–46], which are widely used as guidelines for biocompatibility testing by regulatory agencies such as the FDA [47]. A unique aspect of the ISO 10993 standard is that it is designed to be used within a RMS. There are other recognized standards, including those from the United States Pharmacopeia (USP) [48–50], which can also be used to validate a medical device.

Initial Assessment

The initial assessment is an important step in classifying a medical device to determine which tests are required to evaluate its biocompatibility. By defining the context in which the medical device will be used, this can help to determine the level of risk specific to its use and provide guidance for additional testing that may be required. A review of existing relevant data may help to reduce the number of tests required. In some circumstances, regulatory agencies may ask for additional testing beyond the ones described by ISO 10993.

Device Classification

The ISO 10993 standard applies only to medical devices designed for direct or indirect contact[6] with the patient. For example, if a brachytherapy needle/catheter passes through a 3D printed template before entering sterile interstitial tissues, there is an indirect contact between the 3D printed template and the interstitial tissue even though the template may not be in physical contact with it. The same principle would apply to a 3D

---

5 This also apply to the user in cases involving medical protection devices (e.g., medical gloves, surgical masks).

6 According to ISO 10993, a direct contact occurs when a medical device comes into physical contact with a body tissue, while an indirect contact occurs when a medical device doesn't come into physical contact with a body tissue but a fluid or gas passes thought it, before the fluid or gas comes into physical contact with body tissues.

printed template sutured through the skin. The classification of a medical device within ISO 10993 is determined by two key factors: the nature of contact and its duration. The nature of contact can be explained as follows.

- *Surface device:* A medical device that is in contact with one of the protective epithelial surfaces of the body (e.g., skin, mucosal membrane). This includes intact surfaces as well as breached/compromised surfaces (e.g., wound, burn, cancerous lesion) as long as the device doesn't penetrate through the surface. Biological tests should be conducted based on the scenario with the highest risk. For example, an orthovoltage X-ray therapy cutout could be placed over a cancerous skin lesion and an intracavitary brachytherapy applicator could be in contact with a vaginal tumor extension. In both cases, the device should be tested as if it is applied to a breached/compromised surface. On the other hand, a condom or transvaginal ultrasound can be considered as a semi-critical device using the Spaulding classification if the Manufacturer's instruction for use (IFU) specify it is only to be applied on intact mucosal surfaces [51].

- *Externally communicating device:* A medical device that penetrates through but not completely (i.e., located both inside and outside) one of the protective epithelial surfaces of the body (e.g., skin, mucosal membrane) resulting in a contact with either blood path (indirect contact; e.g., IV bag), tissue/bone/dentin (direct or indirect contact; e.g., arthroscope, dental filling) or circulating blood (direct contact; e.g., dialyzer). These devices can be partially or entirely located outside the patient. For example, a transvaginal oocyte retrieval needle is an externally communicating device (i.e., a critical device using the Spaulding classification) since the needle crosses the vaginal mucosa and sterile tissues to reach an ovarian follicle [51]. The needle guide attached to the transvaginal ultrasound probe is also an externally communicating device, even if it is entirely located outside the vaginal mucosal surface, since the needle passes through it before coming into contact with sterile tissues. On similar grounds, a combined intracavitary and interstitial (IC/IS) brachytherapy applicator would be considered an externally communicating device.

- *Implant:* A medical device that is entirely embedded beyond one of the protective epithelial surfaces of the body (e.g., skin, mucosal membrane) resulting in a contact with either circulating blood or tissue/bone. A radioactive stent used for intravascular brachytherapy is considered an implant within the circulating blood [52]. Its delivery system would qualify instead as an externally communicating device in contact with circulating blood [52].

Additional examples of devices used in radiation oncology, categorized by contact type, are given in Table 3.1. The contact duration is defined as the cumulative exposure between the medical device and the patient and is categorized as follows:

- *Limited:* The total exposure is up to 24 hours. Many radiation oncology devices, including immobilization accessories and boluses, could be classified in this category because the cumulative duration of all treatment fractions is typically less than 24 hours.

TABLE 3.2 Categorization of Medical Devices and Biocompatibility Test Matrix

	Body Contact	Duration of Contact[a]	USP Class	Biological Effects[b]				
				A – Cytotoxicity	B – Sensitization	C – Irritation or Intracutaneous reactivity	D – Acute systemic toxicity	E – Material mediated pyrogenicity
Surface device	Intact skin	Limited	I	•	•	•		
		Prolonged	I	•	•	•		
		Permanent	I	•	•	•		
	Mucosal membrane	Limited	I	•	•	•		
		Prolonged	III	•	•	•	•	•
		Permanent	V	•	•	•	•	•
	Breached or compromised surface	Limited	III	•	•	•	•	•
		Prolonged	V	•	•	•	•	•
		Permanent	VI	•	•	•	•	•
Externally communicating device	Blood path, indirect	Limited	IV	•	•	•	•	•
		Prolonged	V	•	•	•	•	•
		Permanent	VI	•	•	•	•	•
	Tissue, bone or dentin	Limited	IV	•	•	•	•	•
		Prolonged	VI	•	•	•	•	•
		Permanent	VI	•	•	•	•	•
	Circulating blood	Limited	IV	•	•	•	•	•
		Prolonged	VI	•	•	•	•	•
		Permanent	VI	•	•	•	•	•
Implant device	Tissue or bone	Limited	VI	•	•	•	•	•
		Prolonged	VI	•	•	•	•	•
		Permanent	VI	•	•	•	•	•
	Blood	Limited	VI	•	•	•	•	•
		Prolonged	VI	•	•	•	•	•
		Permanent	VI	•	•	•	•	•

Notes:

Abbreviation: USP – United States Pharmacopeia.

[a] *Duration of contact is defined as the cumulative sum of a single, multiple or repeated periods of contact between the medical device and the body region. It is categorized as follows:*
Limited: Up to 24 hours.
Prolonged: More than 24 hours but less than 30 days.
Permanent: Exceeds 30 days.

[b] *Although the correspondence between the USP classification system and ISO is reported in USP Chapter ⟨1031⟩ [50], there are currently no specific USP chapters for the following test requirements:* sensitization, subchronic toxicity, genotoxicity, chronic systemic toxicity, carcinogenicity, hemocompatibility, reproductive toxicity, and degradation. *Therefore, the list of biological tests required does not presently apply to the USP classification which is less restrictive than ISO 10993 for the same combination of body contact and duration of contact.*

- *Prolonged:* The total exposure is more than 24 hours but less than 30 days. An eye plaque used in brachytherapy typically remains in contact with the patient for a few days up to a week, which is considered a prolonged contact. For cervical cancer cases treated with MRI-based image-guided adaptive brachytherapy (IGABT), an intracavitary applicator could remain in the patient for more than 6 hours in a single day because of numerous time delays (e.g., imaging, planning, patient transport) even though the irradiation takes only a few minutes [53]. For a typical treatment of 5 fractions, the total contact time for such an applicator can potentially exceed 24 hours and be considered a prolonged contact.

F – Subacute/ Subchronic systemic toxicity	G – Genotoxicity	H – Implantation	I – Hemocompatibility	J – Chronic systemic toxicity	K – Carcinogenicity	L – Reproductive/ Developmental toxicity	M – Degradation
•		•					
•	•	•		•			
•		•					
•	•	•		•	•		
			•				
•	•	•	•	•	•		
•	•	•					
•	•	•		•	•		
	•		•				
•	•	•	•		•		
•	•	•					
•	•	•		•	•		
			•				
•	•	•	•				
•	•	•	•	•	•		

- *Permanent:* The total exposure is more than 30 days. Certain fiducial markers used in image-guided radiation therapy and most low dose rate brachytherapy radioactive sources remain in the patient indefinitely as permanent implants. It should be noted that a condom could be classified as a permanent mucosal surface device as a user could exceed an exposure of 30 days by using the same brand of condom over their lifetime [52].

Upon completion of the device classification, the biocompatibility test matrix outlined in ISO 10993 standard [9], or its FDA revised version [47], provides a list of all required biological tests for each device classification. A simplified version of this matrix is reproduced in Table 3.2, which also provides a correlation with the USP device classification [50]. According to ISO 10993, all medical devices that come into contact with a patient must minimally meet the criteria of being non-cytotoxic, non-irritating, and non-sensitizing, collectively known as the 'Big Three' in biocompatibility testing.

Review of Existing Data
A literature review can help to determine what biological test results are already available and whether they are applicable to the device being evaluated for biocompatibility. At the end of this exercise, a critical analysis of the existing data helps to determine if a reduction of the number of biological tests is possible. There are many biocompatible 3D printing materials on the market. In general, manufacturers of these products publish only a brief

TABLE 3.3   Thermal and Biocompatibility Properties of Common 3D Printed Materials [54–60]

Polymers		Material[a]	Manufacturer	Application[b]	T_g [°C]	HDT@1.8 MPa [°C]	T_m [°C]	Biocompatibility[c]
Thermoplastics	Amorphous	PMMA	–	Standard	63	51	N/A	–
		PETG	–	Engineering	81	63	N/A	–
		HIPS	–	Engineering	90	85	N/A	–
		ABS	–	Standard	105	89	N/A	–
		ASA	–	Engineering	104	98	N/A	–
		PC-ABS	–	Engineering	–	105	N/A	–
		PC	–	Engineering	147	160	N/A	–
		PSU/PSF	–	H. performance	–	167	N/A	–
		PEI	–	H. performance	–	195	N/A	–
	Semi-crystalline	Nylon 11, powder	Formlabs	Engineering	–	46	185	A to C
		PLA	–	Standard	63	51	155	–
		PVA	–	Engineering	70	53	200	–
		Polypropylene (PP)	–	Engineering	-20	64	131	–
		Polyamide/Nylon 12	–	Engineering	41	82	179	–
		Nylon 12, powder	Formlabs	Engineering	–	87	182	A to C
		Polyamide/Nylon 6	–	Engineering	47	93	218	–
		PEEK	–	H. performance	143	155	343	–

Thermosets	BioMed Durable	Formlabs	Engineering	–	40	N/A	A to E, H
	Tough 1500	Formlabs	Engineering	–	45	N/A	A to C
	BioMed Black	Formlabs	Engineering	–	49	N/A	A to C, H
	BioMed White	Formlabs	Engineering	–	52	N/A	A to E, H
	BioMed Clear	Formlabs	Engineering	–	54	N/A	A to H
	PU Rigid 650	Formlabs	Engineering	-19	59	N/A	A to C
	PU Rigid 1000	Formlabs	Engineering	-22	64	N/A	A to C
	BioMed Amber	Formlabs	Engineering	–	65	N/A	A to E
	High Temp	Formlabs	H. performance	–	101	N/A	–

Notes:

Values are not provided, multiple manufacturers may exist with varying technical specifications.

Abbreviations: T_g – Glass temperature; HDT – Heat deflection temperature; T_m – Melting temperature.

[a] Several materials listed in the table are generic, and manufacturers may offer a product branded as biocompatible. Consult the product's technical data sheet to determine which biocompatibility tests were conducted. Materials are sorted by ascending HDT.

[b] This column follows the format of polymer pyramids where polymers are organized according to their crystallinity and ranked according to their performance (standard, engineering, or high performance).

[c] A – Cytotoxicity, ISO 10993-5 or USP Class VI (87); B – Sensitization, ISO 10993-10; C – Irritation, ISO 10993-10 or USP Class VI (88); D – Acute systemic toxicity, ISO 10993-11 or USP Class VI (88); E – Pyrogenicity, ISO 10993-11 or USP Class VI (151); F – Subacute/subchronic systemic toxicity, ISO 10993-11; G – Genotoxicity, ISO 10993-3; H – Implantation, ISO 10993-6 or USP Class VI (88); I – Hemocompatibility, ISO 10993-4; J – Chronic systemic toxicity, ISO 10993-11; K – Carcinogenicity, ISO 10993-3.

summary of the biological tests performed and it is advisable to contact them for further information. Table 3.3 lists several 3D printing materials [54–60] and where applicable, indicates which biocompatibility tests have been successfully passed.[7] In particular, it is important to ensure that the manufacturing conditions of the published data are similar to those of the device being tested. The intended application of the device being tested should also be compatible with the published data.

Additional Testing

Even if the last two columns of Table 3.2 are not assigned to a device class (i.e., they are shown empty), these additional tests are dictated by the presence of a specific risk. Biological degradation tests are required if the device or any of its components are designed to be absorbed by the body or are likely to degrade upon contact with the body or its fluids. Part 9 of ISO 10993 describes the framework for identifying the risk of degradation [36]. Specific tests are detailed in Part 13 for polymers [40], Part 14 for ceramics, [41] and Part 15 for metals and alloys [42]. When a medical device contains chemicals that are carcinogenic, mutagenic, or reprotoxic, additional tests described in Part 3 are required [31]. In particular, biological tests for reproductive and/or developmental toxicity are indicated if a material contains leachable substances that may spread to the reproductive organs, a device is intended to come into contact with the reproductive organs, or a device is intended for a susceptible population (e.g., pregnant women, newborns).

The FDA, in its guidance for use of the ISO 10993 standard, describes that special consideration should be given when the addition of a protective layer could mask a biological interaction. This could include the application of a polymer coating that is susceptible to degrade over time or the application of a plastic membrane susceptible to rupture (e.g., friction causing a condom to tear). In these cases, biological testing with and without the barrier may be required [47].

There is a wide variety of intraoral devices used in dentistry. ISO 7405 is dedicated to the biocompatibility testing of these devices [61]. Some of these devices also have applications in radiation oncology, such as tongue retraction devices [25] in head-and-neck (H&N) radiotherapy and intraoral shields in brachytherapy and orthovoltage [27]. In principle, these devices should comply with both ISO 7405 and ISO 10993.

Material Characterization

Characterization of each component in a medical device is a mandatory step prior to biological testing [62]. These tests ensure that materials in the final product are suitable and safe for clinical use. The ISO 10993 standard dedicates two parts to this procedure: Part 18 for the chemical characterization [45] and Part 19 for the physical characterization [46]. These two approaches can also be used to establish equivalence between an established device and a prototype device and/or between a known material and new material.

Chemical characterization seeks to identify the possibility of finding leachable substances in the body that may be harmful to the patient's health. Leachables are

---

7 Biocompatibility tests that are not listed should not be interpreted as the device failing these tests. It is common for 3D printing manufacturers to increase the number of biocompatibility tests for a material over time.

substances that can potentially be in contact with the patient during normal clinical use. Extractables are substances that can be extracted in the laboratory using solvents [63] and contain additional entities. Simulated use extractables consider the intended application of a medical device (e.g., environment of the body), the contact duration as well as its packaging and sterilization. Polar (e.g., water, isopropyl alcohol) and nonpolar (e.g., hexane) solvents are used to create a fluid extract from a device sample [39]. The fluid extract is then incubated during shaking at a temperature and a duration used to simulate different clinical conditions. For example, limited contact devices could be extracted at 37°C for 24 hours while prolonged contact devices could be extracted at 50°C for 72 hours [63]. For permanent implants, regulatory agencies may require exhaustive extraction (i.e., creating a sequence of fluid extracts) instead of a simulated use extraction. The concentration and chemical composition of the leachable substances are then determined by a chromatography method.[8] For 3D printing, additives (e.g., stabilizers, fillers, plasticizers, adhesives, curing agents, coloring agents) can influence the extractable chromatography profile of extractables. Only compounds that have a concentration above an analytical evaluation threshold (AET) on the chromatogram are reported in a toxicity risk assessment (TRA) report. The AET threshold [µg/ml] is based on the threshold of toxicological concern (TTC) [µg/day] described in ISO 21726 that depends on the duration of contact [64]. The TRA is typically done by a professional toxicologist. Part 17 of ISO 10993 provides guidance to determine the appropriate or tolerable concentration of each leachable substances that would make the device safe to use [44].

Physical characterization is used to determine whether a medical device is both safe and functional by examining its physicochemical, morphological, and topographical properties. There is a wide range of properties that can be studied, but generally only those that are relevant to the application of interest should be considered. For example, some surface features could be conducive to bacterial colonization and growth. In general, brachytherapy applicators should be free of sharp edges and easy to clean (e.g., dead-end vs. open lumens). There are various methods and technologies available for material characterization. For example, infrared (IR) spectroscopy is commonly used to identify the chemical composition of a polymer from its spectral absorption signature. Alternatively, differential thermal analysis (DTA) or differential scanning calorimetry (DSC) are thermal approaches that can be used to evaluate the response of a polymer as a function of temperature. Other methods are available to evaluate the mechanical behavior of a polymer under various conditions including but not limited to tensile testing, hardness testing, and fatigue testing. Scanning electron microscopy (SEM) and atomic force microscopy (AFM) are examples of technologies that can be used to determine the morphology and topography of a material's surface. Again, expertise from a CTL may be required to perform these experiments. A CTL can provide a biological evaluation report (BER) for presentation to the regulatory agencies that includes analytical chemistry testing, toxicological risk assessment, and biocompatibility testing.

---

8 Analytical chemistry techniques used to analyse extractables from medical devices include inductively coupled plasma mass spectrometry (ICP-MS), liquid chromatography mass spectrometry (LC-MS), (headspace) gas chromatography mass spectrometry (GC-MS or GC-MS/HS), and graphite furnace atomic absorption spectrometry (GFAAS).

Biocompatibility Testing

The choice of a specific test or combination of tests depends on the nature of the medical device and its intended use. The biological tests described in the ISO 10993 standard include both *in vitro* assays (i.e., experiments on cell cultures conducted outside of a living organism) and *in vivo* assays (i.e., animal experiment closer to clinical conditions)[9] [39]. *In vitro* tests are simple, rapid, reproducible, and cost-effective but their results do not capture the intricate biological interactions that can happen in a living organism. In contrast, *in vivo* tests translate biological effects observed in animals to humans more accurately. By combining *in vivo* and *in vitro* tests, an ethically responsible approach can be taken to reduce the number of animals used [30]. The need for animal facility, specialized equipment, and highly trained personnel to perform these tests generally requires the support of a CTL.

Cytotoxicity

Cytotoxicity is assessed qualitatively and quantitatively using *in vitro* tests to determine whether contact with a medical device can cause damage to human cells. Part 5 of ISO 10993 [33] describes these tests, which involve exposing cultured cells (e.g., L929 murine fibroblast cells) at an incubation temperature of 37°C for 24 hours. Qualitative tests include direct contact assays for low density materials, agar overlay assays commonly used for elastomeric closures, and elution assays for polymers. In a direct contact assay, a sample material is placed directly over a monolayer of cultured cells and leachable compounds diffuse into the culture medium. In an agar overlay assay, a thin layer of nutrient agar acts as a cushion between the sample material and the cultured cells. Leachable compounds diffuse to the cell layer via the agar layer. In an elution assay, cells are exposed to the medical device's extraction fluid (e.g., using simulated use extraction conditions with a serum-supplemented culture medium like MEM or DMEM).[10] Shafiee *et al.* provide a review of these cytotoxicity tests [65]. The effects on cell morphology, viability, growth, and/or colony formation are examined to determine cytotoxicity. Quantitative evaluation can be performed with fluorescence microscopy using specific dyes such as MTT, neutral red, or Calcein-AM. Told *et al.* included a cytotoxicity evaluation of A549 lung carcinoma cells seeded directly on 3D printed inserts made of PLA, PETG, ABS, HIPS, Polyamide, and Polyjet and stereolithography (SLA) photoresins that were incubated for 48 hours [66]. For these materials, they didn't find a decrease in cell viability using flow cytometry with an Annexin V assay. Kozakiewicz *et al.* used spectrophotometry with an XTT cell viability assay to show higher cytotoxicity in adult human dermal fibroblast cells exposed to compounds from a paper-based 3D printer relative to a control [67]. They showed that a protective coating of 2-octyl-cyanoacrylate could be used to significantly reduce this cytotoxicity. Gruber and Nickel reported large differences in cytotoxicity results in an interlaboratory comparison study ($n = 52$) where each laboratory was asked to analyze the same PE and PVC samples using an elution test [68].

---

9 Sample preparation must comply with ISO 10993 Part 12.
10 Minimum essential media and Dulbecco's modified eagle medium.

Sensitization and Irritation

Contact with a medical device should not cause the patient to develop redness and swelling from an allergic reaction with prolonged or repeated exposures (i.e., sensitization) or even a more acute and immediate inflammatory response (i.e., irritation). The procedure described in Part 10 of ISO 10993 is used for the evaluation of biological effects attributed to sensitization and irritation [37]. This procedure suggests screening with *in vitro* tests to minimize the number of *in vivo* tests conducted on animals. Sensitization is commonly assessed using animal tests such as the murine local lymph node assay (LLNA), the guinea pig maximization test (GPMT), and the guinea pig closed patch test (i.e., Buehler test). Coleman *et al.* validated that the *in vitro* SenCeeTox® assay could be used with an EpiDerm™ skin model to detect the presence of known sensitizers in the extraction fluids of silicone medical devices [69]. Svobodová *et al.* conducted a pilot study to compare an *in vitro* sensitization test (LuSens assay) with an *in vivo* approach (LLNA assay) [70]. Irritation is usually evaluated *in vivo* using rabbits. These tests can include irritation (e.g., dermal skin and mucosa) and intracutaneous reactivity tests for implants. Pellevoisin *et al.* developed an *in vitro* test for irritation using the SkinEthic™ reconstructed human epidermis (RHE) model and tested it on extraction fluids from PVC and silicone samples with and without known irritants [71]. Irritation tests on human volunteers may also be conducted if *in vitro* and *in vivo* tests result in non-sensitization and non-irritation.

Systemic Toxicity and Pyrogenicity

Systemic toxicity refers to a situation in which contact with a medical device causes the patient to experience an adverse effect at a site distant from the point of contact. This usually occurs when chemical compounds of the device are absorbed and then diffused throughout the body. According to Part 11 of ISO 10993 [38], systemic toxicity tests are typically performed in rodents and are categorized according to the duration of exposure as follows:

- *Acute systemic toxicity:* An adverse effect occurs at any time within 72 hours after a single, repeated or continuous exposure of less than 24 hours in total.
- *Subacute systemic toxicity:* An adverse effect occurs after repeated or continuous exposure of more than 24 hours but less than 28 days.
- *Subchronic systemic toxicity:* An adverse effect occurs after repeated or continuous exposure for up to 90 days (or 14 days for intravenous studies).
- *Chronic systemic toxicity:* An adverse effect occurs after repeated or continuous exposure of typically 6 to 12 months.

Depending on the intended clinical use of the device, exposure of the device sample within rodents' bodies is generally realized by injection (e.g., intravenous or intraperitoneal) or implantation.[11] Animal studies are used to establish a relationship

---

11 The implanted specimen often provides enough tissues to evaluate the local effects of implantation as described in Part 6 of ISO 10993 in addition to the systemic toxicity described in Part 11 of ISO 10993.

between the amount of sample administered and the biological effects observed in an individual or in a population. These effects are determined on the basis of parameters that may include but are not limited to: observation of clinical signs, body weight, food and water consumption, hematological and clinical chemistry findings, organ weights, gross pathology, histopathological changes, specific organ toxicity, microbiological evaluations, biochemical markers, and neurological evaluations.

Material-mediated pyrogenicity refers to a situation where the chemical compounds of a medical device induce a febrile response (i.e., fever). This aspect is covered briefly in Part 11 of ISO 10993 [38] and in more details in ISO 21582 [72]. Three tests are currently available to assess material-mediated pyrogenicity in medical devices: the *in vivo* rabbit pyrogen test (RPT), the *in vitro* bacterial endotoxin test (BET), and the *in vitro* human cell-based pyrogen test (HCPT).

Implantation
Part 6 of ISO 10993 outlines testing requirements for the evaluation of local effects after implantation [34]. *In vivo* testing typically involves implanting a first sample of the device in animal tissue and a second sample of a control material in a similar animal. The site and duration should be representative of the intended use of the implant device. A comparison between the test and control experiments is used to assess a biological response based on differences in macroscopic and histopathologic observations in the implanted region.

Hemocompatibility
Part 4 of ISO 10993 specifies requirements for the evaluation of hemocompatibility [32]. Hemocompatibility refers to the ability of a medical device to interact with blood without causing harm (e.g., infection, thrombosis). There are five categories of hemocompatibility tests: thrombosis, coagulation, platelets, hematology, and complement system. The number of test categories that need to be evaluated depends both on the intended use of the medical device and the type of contact. *In vivo* tests in dogs, pigs, and sheep are generally preferred when thrombosis risk assessment is required. These animal models provide a vasculature that approaches those of humans in terms of geometric complexity and dimensions. *In vitro* tests using human blood are usually preferred to evaluate the other hemocompatibility test categories.

Genotoxicity and Carcinogenicity
The evaluation of a medical device's potential to cause genetic damage or mutations when it comes into contact with living organisms is detailed in Part 3 of ISO 10993 [31]. For example, genotoxicity may be assessed by a series of *in vitro* tests including: an Ames bacterial reverse mutation assay, a genetic mutation test in mammalian cells (e.g., mouse lymphoma TK assay), and a final clastogenicity[12] test in mammalian cells (e.g., CHO/

---

12 In general, a clastogen is a mutagenic agent (e.g., bleomycin) that causes breaks in DNA resulting in a gain, loss, or rearrangement of chromosomal material.

HGPRT[13] assay on Chinese Hamster Ovary (CHO) cells). If a positive result is obtained from any of these tests, regulatory agencies can require further investigation using *in vivo* animal models (e.g., mouse or rat micronucleus[14] test). Otherwise, the device is presumed to contain mutagenic compounds.

To assess whether a medical device has a long-term risk of causing cancer, Part 3 of ISO 10993 suggests a series of *in vivo* tests. These tests are generally costly because they require monitoring a population of mice for 18 months or rats for 24 months to detect evidence of cancer. Alternatively, transgenic mice predisposed to develop cancer can be used for a shorter period of 6 months.

STERILIZATION OF RADIOTHERAPY DEVICES

Bacteria are microorganisms that are ubiquitous in our environment and within our own bodies. While most bacteria are non-pathogenic (e.g., those making the gut micro-biota) some are responsible each year for the spread of hospital-acquired nosocomial infections [73]. The bioburden is defined as the population (i.e., number and type) of viable microorganisms present on or in a medical device. Sterilization is defined as any process that removes, kills, or deactivates all forms of life [74]. In its strictest sense, ster-ility is defined as the complete absence of microorganisms. Device manufacturers are responsible to provide safe sterile products by validating and controlling their manu-facturing processes that can be accomplished through either aseptic manufacturing or terminal sterilization. For fused deposition modeling (FDM) 3D printing, it should be noted that while extrusion temperatures (>200°C) are likely high enough to ensure those medical devices are printed sterile, manipulations of the device between printing and the operating room introduce some level of contamination (i.e., bioburden) requiring terminal sterilization [58, 75–77]. Perez *et al.* found that 44 out of 45 of their control test bar samples were positive for growth due to contamination during manufacturing and transport [78]. While protective covers (e.g., probe cover, condoms) are used to pre-vent cross-contamination, they should not be used to reduce the level of decontamin-ation required for the device underneath as these sheaths have a high rate of perforations [73]. Regulatory agencies like the FDA require medical device manufacturers to identify and validate at least one method of sterilization (including a cleaning and disinfection protocol) in their IFU [79]. For regulatory purposes, sterility is defined by an acceptable probability of contamination. There must be a compromise between the risk of having a non-sterile device and the risk of having a medical device that fails during a medical procedure due to material damage from an overly aggressive sterilization process [80]. An acceptable level of risk for most medical devices and sterilization processes is one contaminated device per million manufactured. Validation of a sterilization process is done under worst-case conditions using microorganisms having a higher resistance to the sterilization process than the ones found in the natural product bioburden. Bacteria

---

13 Hypoxanthine-guanine phosphoribosyltransferase (HPRT).
14 A micronucleus (MN) is a broken fragment of chromosome.

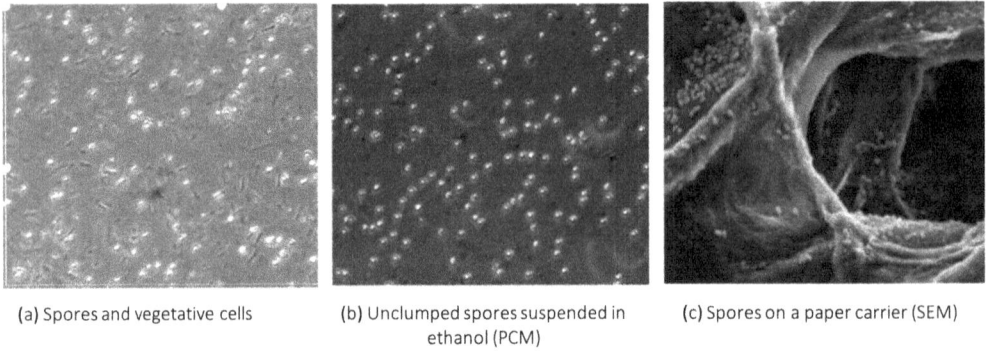

| (a) Spores and vegetative cells | (b) Unclumped spores suspended in ethanol (PCM) | (c) Spores on a paper carrier (SEM) |

FIGURE 3.1   Bacillus spores in different conditions imaged by phase-contrast microscopy (PCM) and scanning electron microscopy (SEM). Figure sourced with permission from McCauley et al. [82–84].

of the *Bacillaceae* family[15] have the ability to undergo sporulation as a survival mechanism when exposed to an adverse environment unconducive to growth [81]. Spores (i.e., endospores) are stripped-down (0.5–1 μm) versions of these bacteria that enables them to lie dormant for extended periods (some have been reported to be viable after millions of years) [82]. When conditions favorable for growth are reestablished, these spores germinate back into their vegetative cells for reproduction. These thick-walled spores are also particularly resistant to most sterilization processes making them the ideal challenge microorganism for their validation. Figure 3.1 shows microscopy images of *Bacillus* spores in various conditions.

Overview of Sterilization Methods

Various sterilization processes [73, 85] are depicted in Figure 3.2 and their properties compared in Table 3.4. It should be noted that not all sterilization methods are destructive.

Sterilization by Filtration

Sterilization by filtration is a non-destructive method that works by physically separating microorganisms present within a liquid or gas by size using specially designed filters [86]. These filters work in a similar way as some common everyday items like tap water purification filters, HEPA vacuum filters, and N95 masks. There are two types of sterilization filters, namely depth filters, which trap microorganisms in their internal structure (e.g., diatomaceous earth) and membrane filters[16] that retain all particles of a given size at their surface [87]. Membrane filters are appropriate for use in the pharmaceutical industry to sterilize parenteral injection drugs (e.g., those involving biologics). Microorganisms are separated through a combination of sieving/screening, entrapment (i.e., lodged in the

---

15 Bacterias of the *Bacillaceae* family are Gram-positive and rod-shaped (0.5 – 1 μm × 1 – 4 μm). It should be noted that most are non-pathogenic to humans and not a biological safety risk for laboratory personnel.

16 Common membrane filter materials include cellulose (nitrate, ester, acetate), nylon polycarbonate and polyester (for track-etched filters). Polysulfone and polyvinvylidene difluoride filters are recommended for drugs containing proteins. Viscous liquids require positive pressure to achieve an acceptable flow rate.

pores) or adsorption (e.g., by electrostatic attraction) [88]. Pore sizes are rated according to the size of the microorganism they can remove, typically 0.2 μm (appropriate for bacteria removal) but smaller pore size are also available (e.g., 0.03 μm for mycoplasma removal) [89]. While not applicable to solid medical devices, sterilization by filtration can be used to sterilize water used to clean them aseptically. After use, membrane filters themselves are sterilized using steam sterilization.

Steam Sterilization

Steam (i.e., moist heat) sterilization has been used for over a century as the most standard, cost-effective and reliable way to sterilize critical medical devices (e.g., surgical tools) on-site [90, 91]. Autoclaves (i.e., pressurized vessels) specialize in replacing air by saturated steam under pressure. In the chamber, saturated steam increases the temperature of cooler surfaces by releasing energy stored[17] in the steam during its condensation from gas to liquid [92]. This temperature inactivates microorganisms through irreversible protein denaturation of vital enzymes [93]. It should be noted that superheated steam (like air) is a poor thermal conductor. Therefore, there is only one pressure that is used by autoclaves to provide steam for every one temperature[18] [94, 95]. For brachytherapy applicators containing long and narrow lumens, the presence of residual air and condensate can become barriers preventing a good contact between steam and their surfaces. There are some moisture-sensitive devices that should not be steam sterilized. These include medical devices with embedded electronics due to corrosion, immiscible anhydrous oils, and dry powders that would be compromised by moisture.

Dry Heat Sterilization

Dry heat sterilizers can be used for moisture-sensitive items and other materials able to sustain very high temperatures (e.g., glassware, metals, dry powders compromised by moisture or chemicals). Dry heat sterilization is performed either using cabinet ovens or industrial conveyor tunnel systems that operate continuously [110]. Most dry heat sterilizers use a forced-air system (as opposed to static-air) involving the use of air blower fans to distribute HEPA-filtered heated air uniformly within the sterilizer. Absorption of heat by the medical device's exterior surface is transferred to its interior (including long and narrow lumens) by thermal conduction [111]. Relative to steam sterilization, dry heat sterilization is a slower process (i.e., 1–2 hours)[19] where cellular components are incinerated by oxidation [93]. It should be noted that the higher temperatures (e.g., 160°C–170°C)[20] involved in dry heat sterilization are not compatible with many 3D printed polymers [112].

---

17 Saturated steam at 100°C contains seven times more energy than water at the same temperature.
18 The relationship between pressure and temperature is given in saturated steam tables.
19 Air at 121.1°C contains seven times less energy than saturated steam at the same temperature.
20 Dry heat is commonly used for depyrogenation of glass and metal devices at 250°C (and a cycle time of 30 minutes) allowing to destroy bacterial endotoxins.

TABLE 3.4 Comparison Chart for the Main Types of Sterilization Processes

Sterilization Type	Steam	Dry Heat	Filtration	Ethylene Oxide	Hydrogen Peroxide Gas Plasma	Vaporized Hydrogen Peroxide	Peracetic Acid	Radiation
Prevalence in hospitals	Standard method	Not common	Only for liquid and gas	Common (downtrend)	Common (uptrend)	Common but less than HPGP	Common (for endoscopes)	Not common (outsource)
Sterilant	Saturated steam	Heated air	Pore size	$C_2H_4O_2$ gas	H_2O_2 vapor	H_2O_2 vapor	CH_3CO_3H liquid	Gamma [96] (10 kCi Co-60)
Dosage	4 min at 132°C or 30 min at 121°C [97]	120–60 min at 160°C–170°C [73]	0.01–0.2 μm [98]	12h (EtO) + 2h ventilation (35% RH) [99]	24–60 min cycles [100]	16–52 min cycles [101]	6 minutes (23 min total with two rinses)	20–50 kGy [102] (several hours and shipping)
Temperature	121°C–132°C	160°C–170°C or 250°C	20°C–25°C	20°C–32°C [99] /50°C–60°C (degassing)	47°C–56°C [100]	~50°C [101]	45°C–60°C [103]	30°C–60°C [104–106]
Materials Incompatibility	Heat- and moisture-sensitive materials	Heat-sensitive materials	All solid materials	Almost none, no liquids, aerate soft plastics and elastomers 24h	Few, no liquids, medical paper pouch or mated nylon	Few, no liquids, medical paper pouch or mated nylon	Devices that cannot be fully immersed	Very few but PFA, PTFE, Delrin have Tolerance ~5 kGy [102]
Lumen penetration	Good for dynamic air removal cycles	Excellent	N/A	Excellent. 24h lumen cycle if L > 90 cm [99]	Stainless steel: D > 0.7 mm and L < 50 cm [100]	52 min cycle: D > 1.8 mm and L < 31 cm [101]	Excellent	Excellent
Environmental exposure/waste	None	None	None	5 ppm/15 min emissions [107] 0.1% (EG, ECH)	0.3 ppm peak emissions [108] (H_2O and O_2)	7–20 ppm peak emissions [108] (H_2O and O_2)	Chemical waste (acetic acid and H_2O_2)	Radioactive waste (Co-60)

Advantages	Standard, robust, cost-effective, fast, reliable, non-toxic, glass, metal, rubber	Depyrogenate at 250°C (30 min), glass, metal, oil, and powders, non-toxic.	Suited for biologics (liquids), non-toxic, heat-sensitive liquids	Most materials, reliable, long narrow and dead-end lumens [109] electronics	Suited for most materials, fast, low moisture, no ventilation, no catalytic conversion	Suited for most materials, fast, low moisture, no ventilation	Suited for endoscopes, cameras, surgical tools, non-toxic byproducts	Suited for most materials, non-toxic, reliable, penetrates surfaces, reduces pyrogens
Disadvantages	Heat-sensitive devices (e.g., endoscopes), moisture corrosion (e.g., electronics)	Heat transfer is slow, Heat-sensitive devices	Not for medical devices, expensive filters, not lethal	Long cycles, off-gassing, EtO is flammable, explosive carcinogenic, toxic byproducts	Low penetration affected by insufficient cleaning and lumens ($\propto$ material), limited load weights.	Low penetration affected by insufficient cleaning and lumens, higher H_2O_2 emissions than HPGP.	One device at a time, need to use critical devices immediately, corrosion	Few centers, large volumes, not for biologics, radiolytic products, ventilation of toxic ozone gas.

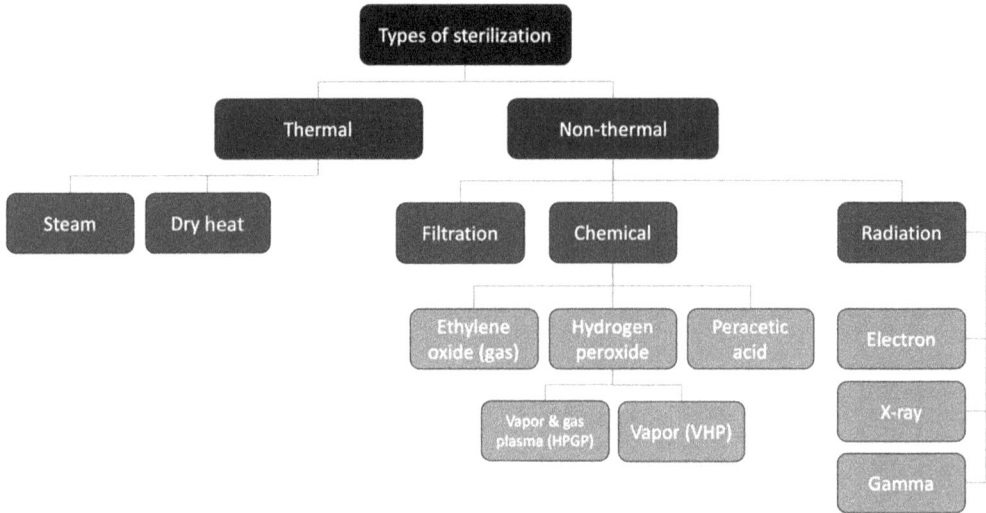

FIGURE 3.2   Overview of different types of sterilization methods.

Ethylene Oxide Gas Chemical Sterilization

Since the 1950s there has been in increase in the use of medical devices made of heat-sensitive (i.e., thermolabile) materials (e.g., plastics). Ethylene oxide (EtO) gas sterilization is the oldest and most commonly used[21] low-temperature chemical sterilization process used in hospitals and also accounts for 50% of the industrial terminal sterilization market [80]. EtO ($C_2H_4O_2$) is a volatile gas at room temperature (boiling point of 10.7°C), is colorless, heavier than air, and both highly flammable and explosive[22] [73, 80]. Moreover, EtO is a known carcinogen with a perceptible sweet odor of ether at levels that are already toxic (~500 ppm). EtO inactivates microorganisms by alkylation of vital cellular proteins and DNA where hydrogen atoms are replaced by hydroxyethyl groups [80, 93]. EtO cycle times are greatly reduced in a high relative humidity environment (i.e., 35%–80% RH). It is thought that bacterial spores swell up with humidity allowing EtO to penetrate more easily through pores on their surfaces [81]. During conditioning, a chamber/liner bag is loaded, humidified and air is removed with a vacuum. EtO gas is then injected or released from a glass ampoule at concentrations of 400–1200 mg/L and items are exposed for 12–24 hours [113]. Following sterilization, EtO is purged (e.g., to an exhaust ventilation system) and active aeration is performed for 24 hours to allow degassing of EtO absorbed by the materials[23] [73]. Besides EtO, toxic residues such as ethylene glycol (EG) and ethylene chlorohydrin (ECH) can remain on sterilized materials. EtO is reported to have very good lumen penetration. For example, a Line-Pickerill helix with a long (1 m) and

---

21 Other chemical gas sterilization methods include ozone, chlorine dioxide, and nitrogen dioxide.

22 As a deterrent to explosions, some systems mix EtO with a diluent (e.g., 8.5% EtO and 91.5% CO_2) requiring a pressurized vessel or use nitrogen blanketing. Electronic batteries need to be completely sealed off.

23 Aeration time can be reduced to 8–12 hours in systems that heat the chamber to 50–60°C. Small abator technology can also reduce EtO emissions to 0.1% using a catalyst resin that converts EtO into biodegradable organic compounds.

narrow (2 mm) dead-end lumen is claimed to be sterilizable using EtO [109]. However, it is rarely used to reprocess endoscopes as some failures have been reported [73].

Vaporized Hydrogen Peroxide Chemical Sterilization

Since the 1990s vaporized hydrogen peroxide (VHP) has been used increasingly as a less toxic and more environmentally friendly alternative to EtO. Liquid hydrogen peroxide (H_2O_2) is a common high-level disinfectant at 7.5% concentration for 30 minutes and eventually breaks down into water (H_2O) and oxygen (O_2). During conditioning, the chamber is heated to ~50°C and a vacuum is used to remove air. During sterilization, 59%[24] H_2O_2 is pulled from a disposable cartridge and injected into the chamber at a concentration of 6–24 mg/L after passing through a heated vaporizer [73, 104, 114, 115]. This vapor diffuses throughout the chamber and penetrates the packaging of medical devices. After a cycle-specific time, air is reintroduced to bring the chamber back to atmospheric pressure and after a second cycle-specific time, a vacuum is used to evacuate the chamber to prepare it for another injection of VHP (with two or more injections per cycle). STERRAD® sterilizers use a variation of this technology named hydrogen peroxide gas plasma (HPGP) where a low-temperature gas plasma is ignited using an RF-generated electrical field between injections (when the chamber is at low pressure) [73, 114, 116]. As a result of this plasma, H_2O_2 splits into free radicals that recombine as O_2 and H_2O when the electric field is switched off [117]. HPGP gas plasma itself has little antimicrobial effect [118]. However, it has been reported that the gas plasma allows HPGP to reduce H_2O_2 emissions by a factor of 27 to 67 relative to VHP that uses a catalytic converter [108]. In both VHP and HPGP, cells are inactivated by the oxidation of proteins, lipids, and surface membrane from interactions with hydroxyl (-OH) radicals [93, 118]. During aeration, residual H_2O_2 is purged using a vacuum for VHP and plasma for a set time in HPGP. Relative to EtO, cycle times for VHP and HPGP are much shorter (i.e., <60 minutes) but lumen penetration[25] and the number of lumens allowed per load are more limited [100, 101, 119]. It should be noted that items must be thoroughly dried before sterilization since any residual water will cause cold spots that condenses H_2O_2 making it unavailable for the sterilization process. HPGP and VHP load weights are also more limited than steam autoclaves [114].

Liquid Chemical Sterilization

Some high-level chemical disinfectant can be used for liquid chemical sterilization of medical devices that can be fully immersed (e.g., endoscope, camera). For instance, glutaraldehyde has long been used to disinfect flexible endoscopes in automated endoscope reprocessor (AER). There are concerning health effects related to the use of glutaraldehyde that prompted manufacturers to develop glutaraldehyde-free disinfectant

---

24 In some STERRAD® cycles, sterilant is concentrated from 59% to 84–94% before injection into the chamber.

25 Lumen penetration for VHP/HPGP depends on the cycle time, the lumen dimensions, and the type of material. User manuals only specify values for a few validated materials (i.e. mainly stainless steel, Teflon and polyethylene).

like ortho-phthalaldehyde (OPA) and peracetic acid [120]. For example, the Steris System 1E® reprocessor is a portable tabletop system meant to be used with proprietary mix (i.e., Steris S40®) of 35% peracetic acid and an anti-corrosion formulation [104]. After dilution (>1820 mg/l), the liquid sterilant is circulated for 6 minutes at 45°C–60°C on the interior and exterior surfaces of an endoscope [121]. Two rinse cycles with filtered water (e.g., 0.1 μm) bring the total cycle time to 23 minutes [103]. Peracetic acid (CH_3CO_3H) is an acetic acid (CH_3COOH) with an additional oxygen atom that inactivates cells through the oxidation of proteins, lipids, and surface membranes [73, 104]. Peracetic acid[26] eventually breaks down into acetic acid (i.e., vinegar) and H_2O_2. It should be noted that only one medical device can be sterilized at a time and critical medical devices must be used immediately following sterilization [103, 104]. Some healthcare institutions have successfully replaced their use of EtO with a combination of VHP or HPGP and peracetic acid [120].

Sterilization by Radiation

Gamma radiation[27] sterilization accounts for 40% of the industrial terminal sterilization market [80]. A category IV industrial gamma sterilizer is an extensive facility (119×46 ft^2) that can process large quantities of products in aluminum containers called totes ($2 \times 3 \times 6$ ft^3 weighting ~1022 lbs) [122]. Multiple double-encapsulated Co-60 sources are arranged in source racks (tens of kCi to several MCi) stored in a 20-ft deep pool of water when not in use [80, 123]. High doses[28] of 20 to 50 kGy (25 kGy being the most common) are required to sterilize bacterial spores. Some facilities operate at low temperatures as the radiation doses are high enough to heat up products to 30°C–40°C (for a few hours) [124]. After clearing the room, source racks are raised from the pool to irradiate fully packed totes on a conveyor system with dwell times of several hours [80, 104]. Products are released after the minimum and maximum dose received are confirmed with dosimeters[29] [125, 126]. Gamma radiation inactivates bacterial spores by DNA scission from secondary electrons and to a lesser extent by radiation-induced oxidation from free radicals (e.g., hydroxyl radicals and peroxides) [93]. It should be noted that outsourcing low volumes of 3D printed radiotherapy devices to a gamma sterilization facility would not be financially viable. Moreover, conventional radiotherapy sources have limitations that are not compatible with the very high radiation dose levels required for sterilization.

---

26 In the United Stated, OSHA (Occupational Safety and Health Administration) limits both EtO and H_2O_2 exposures to 1 ppm measured as an 8-hour TWA (time-weighted average). OSHA also limits the short-term (i.e., 15 minutes) excursion limit for EtO and peracetic acid to 5 ppm and 0.4 ppm respectively.

27 Electron beam facilities (5–10 MeV) account for the remaining 10% of the terminal sterilization industrial market. Their main advantage relative to gamma sterilization is a quicker cycle time (a few minutes) but totes have to be thinner, the dose is less homogenous and materials can heat up to ~50°C (for a few minutes). Some X-ray facilities combine advantages of gamma and electron sterilization facilities but these account for a small fraction of the industrial sterilization market.

28 At lower doses (0.1–10 kGy) gamma radiation is used in food irradiation to extend the shelf-life of products.

29 Dosimeters for radiation sterilizers include alanine pellets, radiochromic film dosimeters (using an aminotriphenylmethane dye), and radiation-sensitive PMMA (Perspex).

Material Compatibility and Prototype Testing

The selection of an appropriate material for a 3D printed radiotherapy device depends both on the 3D printing technology and the type of sterilization process available to the user. While steam sterilization is usually the preferred method, the thermal properties of available 3D printed polymers may require a low-temperature sterilization method (i.e., HPGP/VHP, EtO, or Gamma). Polymers can be broadly categorized as thermoplastics, thermosets, or elastomers (e.g., natural latex, synthetic silicone, thermoplastic elastomer (TPE), thermoplastic polyurethane (TPU)). Thermoplastics used in FDM 3D printing become pliable at high temperatures and resolidify upon cooling. Thermoplastics are further categorized according to their crystalline structure as either amorphous or semi-crystalline. Thermosets used in SLA 3D printing are irreversibly cured[30] (solidified) from a viscous polymer resin using UV light.

The glass transition temperature (T_g) is the temperature at which a polymer changes from a hard solid (i.e., glassy) state to a soft pliable (i.e., leathery) state [127]. Figure 3.3 illustrates the thermomechanical behavior of different polymer types as a function of their modulus (i.e., structural rigidity). Polymer chains of thermoplastic amorphous polymers are random and disordered, commonly giving these materials a transparent appearance. Amorphous polymers gradually soften at temperatures higher than T_g until becoming a viscous fluid (i.e., they do not melt). On the other hand, semi-crystalline thermoplastics have regions of stable and ordered tightly packed crystalline lamellae, commonly giving these materials an opaque appearance.[31] At temperatures higher

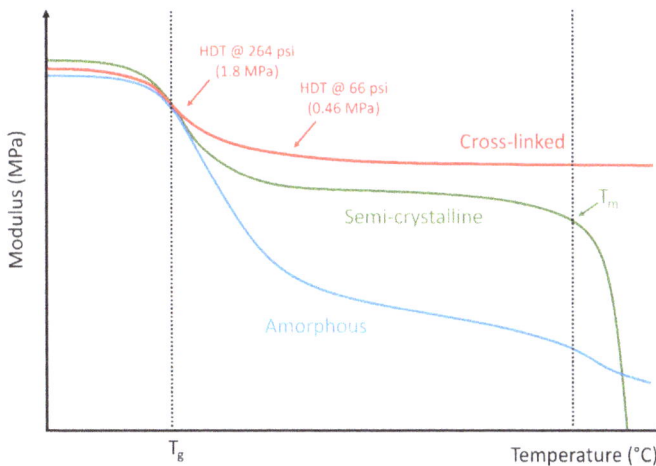

FIGURE 3.3 Changes in the modulus (i.e., structural rigidity) of polymers having different chain structures (but the same T_g values) as a function of temperature. Key thermal properties (i.e., T_g, HDT, T_m) are illustrated. Figure is schematic and produced by authors to illustrate trends.

---

30 Curing involves cross-linking small polymer chains together with covalent bonds giving a very stable structure. Other curing methods involve the use of heat, radiation, moisture, or activators.

31 Several lamellae plates merge to form larger spherulites structures having different index of refraction relative to the amorphous regions.

TABLE 3.5   Polymer Properties Based on Their Chain Structures

| | Polymers (Plastic) | | |
| | Thermoplastics | | |
Properties	Amorphous	Semi-crystalline	Thermosets
Chain structure	Random and disordered	Stable and ordered	Cross-linked
Appearance	Transparent	Opaque	Varies (clear to opaque)
Melting point (T_m)	None (softens)	Yes	None (combustion)
Thermal expansion[a]	Low	High	Low
Chemical resistance	Low	High	High

Note:
[a] *Thermal expansion is listed in Manufacturer's material datasheets as the coefficient of thermal expansion*
[μm/m°C].

than T_g, amorphous regions gradually soften but the crystalline regions remain highly ordered giving structure to the bulk of the material [127]. While these materials can be used at temperatures higher than T_g, their specific heat dramatically increases around their melting temperature (T_m) at which point they become fully liquid. For this reason, semi-crystalline polymers tend to shrink and warp more than amorphous polymers[32] when they are cooled after printing. This effect can be reduced by keeping the printing bed temperature around T_g [58]. Thermoset polymers are the most dimensionally stable as a result of their isotropic cross-linked chain structure. The curing process increases their T_g values [128]. Once cured, these materials will undergo combustion at very high temperatures instead of melting [127]. Table 3.5 lists some properties of polymers based on their chain structures.

While the T_g temperature is a property of the polymer making the bulk of the material, the rigidity of a material can be reinforced with the addition of fillers and stabilizers or reduced with plasticizers [128]. The heat deflection temperature (HDT) is defined as the temperature at which a standard test bar (e.g., ASTM D648) similar to the one shown in Figure 3.4(a) and (b), deflects (i.e., bends) a specified distance (e.g., 0.25 mm) under a specified load. The two most common loads used for HDT testing are 0.46 MPa (i.e., 66 psi) and 1.8 MPa (i.e., 264 psi). 3D printing manufacturers usually recommend using their materials at temperatures below HDT.[33] Table 3.3 lists T_g and HDT values at 1.8 MPa for several common 3D printed materials.

In the literature, several studies aimed to characterize differences in 3D printed polymers before and after sterilization. These differences can be mechanical, thermal, structural, and morphological [66, 132]. Moreover, sterilization compatibility often depends more on the design of the device than its materials. For example, long and thin printed parts are more likely to show deformations after steam sterilization than short and thick printed parts. Similarly, low infill percentages in FDM 3D printed parts are more likely to show deformations after steam sterilization [133]. Even if there are deformations,

---

32 A well-known exception is ABS that is known for warping despite its amorphous chain structure.

33 A load of 1.8 MPa gives the more conservative HDT value. Some manufacturers also list the Vicat softening point (VSP) which is used for similar purposes. The VSP is the temperature at which a flat-pointed needle penetrates a plastic a specified distance (e.g., 1 mm) under a specified load (e.g., 10 or 50 N).

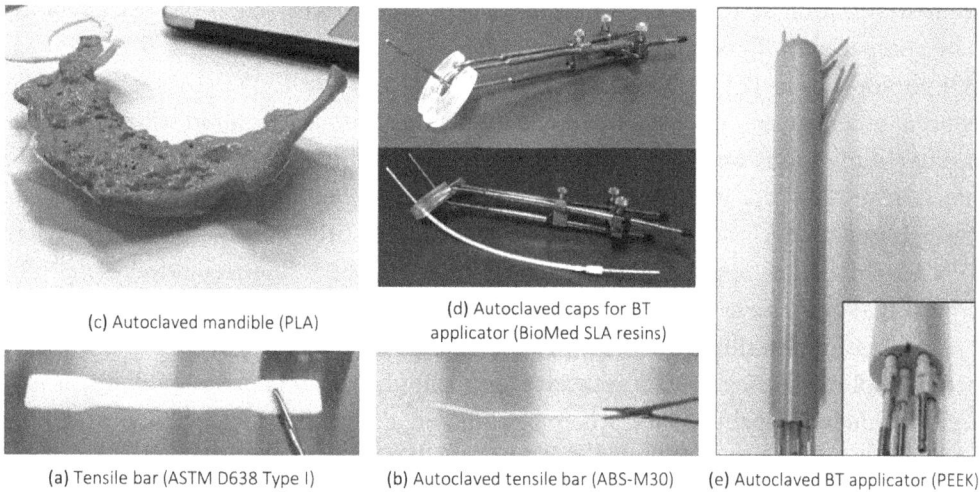

(c) Autoclaved mandible (PLA)

(d) Autoclaved caps for BT applicator (BioMed SLA resins)

(a) Tensile bar (ASTM D638 Type I)

(b) Autoclaved tensile bar (ABS-M30)

(e) Autoclaved BT applicator (PEEK)

FIGURE 3.4   Tensile bar showing deflection (a and b, Perez et al.). 3D printed devices after steam sterilization: (c) mandible (Wiseman et al), (d) Montreal split-ring applicator (Kamio et al.), and (e) patient-specific cylindrical template (PSCT) (Kudla et al.). Figures sourced with permission from [78, 129–131].

prototype testing after sterilization can be successful if dimensional inaccuracies do not compromise the overall functionality of the device. Another important consideration is whether the 3D printed device is intended for single-use sterilization (i.e., disposable) or for repeated sterilization (i.e., reusable) [134]. While many engineering polymers in Table 3.3 can be validated for single-use applications (e.g., SLA photoresins), high performance polymers (with an HDT higher than the temperature of sterilization) may be preferred for repeated sterilization applications.

Most authors do not recommend steam sterilization with heat-sensitive amorphous thermoplastics like PETG [66, 132, 135], HIPS [66], ABS [66, 78], and PC-ABS [78] as their T_g temperatures are below the sterilization temperature of 121°C. Figure 3.4(a) and (b) show an ABS tensile test bar with visible bending and indentation following steam sterilization. However, more performant amorphous thermoplastics like PC [78], PC-ISO [78], PPSU [78], and PEI [78] have been found to be sterilizable at 121°C. Several authors reported significant deformations using steam sterilization with heat-sensitive semi-crystalline thermoplastics like PLA [66, 133, 135] and polypropylene (PP) [135]. Figure 3.4(c) shows a PLA 3D printed mandible with visible signs of melting after steam sterilization [129]. However, Boursier et al. reported good results for a PLA tibia model following steam sterilization at 121°C for 20 minutes [136]. Neijhoft et al. reported that 2.5-cm long PLA cylinders did not bend significantly when their diameters were larger than 5 mm but bended significantly when they were thinner [77]. Rynio et al. reported successful sterilization of PLA, PETG, and PP aortic arch templates using a nonstandard low-temperature steam cycle at 105°C for 3 hours [135]. Furthermore, more performant semi-crystalline thermoplastics like polyamide/nylon [66, 135] and PEEK [130] have been found to be steam sterilizable. Figure 3.4(e) shows a PEEK patient-specific cylindrical template (PSCT) made of PEEK for GYN brachytherapy that was validated for steam sterilization at 132°C for 4 minutes [130]. Steam sterilization has been reported to be compatible with several thermoset polyjet [66, 137, 138] and SLA [131, 135, 138, 139] photoresins at 121°C [135, 138], 132°C [131, 139], and 134°C [137]. Sharma *et al.* reported an expansion of cured materials following steam sterilization with an increase in outer dimensions and a decrease in inner lumen dimensions [138]. Figure 3.4(d) shows 3D printed caps in BioMed Clear and BioMed Amber SLA photoresins (Formlabs, Massachusetts, USA) that allow the attachment of interstitial needles to an intracavitary GYN brachytherapy applicator [131]. These caps include a fine resolution 3D printed screw thread that can be sterilized at 132°C for single-use applications [131]. Lindegaard *et al.* successfully sterilized their 3D printed Vienna-style intravaginal template brachytherapy applicator using a steam autoclave [140]. Similarly, Mohammadi *et al.* successfully sterilized their 3D printed multichannel cylinder applicator (MCA) made of a high-temperature SLA photoresin using a steam sterilization cycle at 134°C for 35 minutes [141]. Told *et al.* do not recommend dry heat sterilization at 180°C for PLA, PETG, ABS, HIPS but found it compatible with a polyjet photoresin [66]. Fuentes *et al.* found that PLA and PETG materials can be sterilized using a nonstandard dry heat sterilization cycle at a low-temperature of 140°C for 3 hours since dry air does not cause hydrolytic degradation [132].

Low-temperature chemical sterilization with EtO gas is compatible with almost all materials. More specifically, EtO has been validated for sterilization of ABS [78, 142], PETG [135], PC-ABS [78], PC [78], PC-ISO [78], PPSU [78], PEI [78], PLA [133, 135], PP [135], nylon [135], and SLA photoresins [135]. Some authors recommend the use of EtO for sterilization of their 3D printed brachytherapy applicator [143, 144]. Similarly, low-temperature chemical sterilization using VHP is compatible with most materials. However, Tyvek® peel pouches must be used instead of medical paper pouches as cellulose absorbs H_2O_2 and nylon materials can become brittle with oxidation [73]. HPGP has been validated for sterilization of ABS [66, 78, 135, 142, 145], PETG [66, 76, 135], HIPS [66], PC-ABS [78], PC [78], PC-ISO [78], PPSU [78], PEI [78], PLA [66, 76, 142], PP [135], polyamide/nylon [66, 135, 142], and SLA and polyjet photoresins [66, 135]. Cunha *et al.* and Sethi *et al.* successfully sterilized their 3D printed PC-ISO cylinder applicators for GYN brachytherapy using HPGP [24, 146]. Similarly, Toro *et al.* successfully sterilized an ABS mandibular anatomic model using VHP [147]. While low-temperature radiation sterilization is compatible with most materials, it can induce chain scission or cross-linking in polymers[34] [80, 124, 148]. Cracking of polyethylene knee bearing due to cross-linking has been reported [73]. Electrons trapped in contact lenses made of glassy polymers like PMMA can cause a yellow discoloration [80]. Gamma sterilization of test bar samples in ABS, PC, PC-ABS, PC, PC-ISO, PPSU, and PEI has been validated by Perez *et al.* [78]. Kozakiewicz *et al.* successfully sterilized cuboids from a paper-based 3D printer using gamma sterilization [67].

---

34 In particular, polytetrafluoroethylene (PTFE), fluorinated ethylene propylene (FEP), polyacetals (e.g., Delrin), and natural polypropylene are mechanically degraded through chain scission that can be accelerated by radiation-induced oxidation in the presence of air.

Microbiological Inactivation Principles

Inactivation of spores by a sterilization process usually[35] [82, 118, 119] follows a log-linear kinetic behavior as shown by equation (3.1):

$$N = N_0 \cdot 10^{-(t-t_0)/D} \tag{3.1}$$

Where N_0 is the initial spore population (i.e., bioburden) at a time/dose t_0, N is the viable spore population after a sterilization time/dose t, and D is the D-value [149]. The D-value (i.e., decimal reduction value) represents the sterilization dose required to reduce a spore population by 90% (i.e., a factor of 10) [149–151]. It is a measure of the resistance of the spore population to the sterilization process. For steam sterilization, D-values are conventionally specified at a reference temperature of 121.1°C (i.e., 250°F). D-values depend on the spore type, the process condition (e.g., temperature and steam contact), and the material substrate[36] [83, 150]. It should be noted that inactivation kinetics describes an exponential decrease that asymptotically trends to but never reaches a zero viable spore population, therefore there is always a statistical probability that a spore may survive a sterilization process [150]. From equation (3.1) with $t_0 = 0$ we can infer the following:

$$F_{bio} \equiv F_0 \equiv t_f = D_{121.1} \cdot \left[\log\left(N_0\right) - \log\left(N_f\right)\right] = D_{121.1} \cdot \text{SLR} \tag{3.2}$$

Equation (3.2) is illustrated on the log-linear survival curve shown in Figure 3.8. By definition, the D-value is −1/slope of the spore population line. The D-value can also be expressed as a function of the spore log reduction (SLR) which describes the decrease in spore population and the F_0-value. The F_0-value[37] represents the lethality of a steam sterilization process and is expressed in equivalent time in minutes at 121.1°C. For example, sterilization processes usually aim for a lethality of $12 \cdot D_{121.1}$. It should be noted that equation (3.2) is only valid at a specific temperature (e.g., 121.1°C) that does not represent the wide range of temperatures involved in a steam sterilization cycle [152]. The relationship between the D-value and the temperature also follows a log-linear kinetic behavior as follows:

$$D = D_0 \cdot 10^{-(T-T_0)/z} \tag{3.3}$$

Where the Z-value represents the temperature increase T required to reduce a spore resistance (i.e., D-value) by 90%. By definition, the Z-value[38] [153] is −1/slope of the D-value vs. temperature line on a log-linear plot. From equations (3.2) and (3.3) we can

---

35 Low-penetration sterilization processes like VHP and HPHP can exhibit a non-linear (biphasic) survival curve due to spore clumping or insufficient cleaning that may not be extrapolated in the same way.

36 For example, McCauley and Gillis reported a wide range of $D_{121.1}$ values (i.e. from 1.2 minutes to 6.1 minutes) for G. Stearothermophilus inoculated on 10 rubber stoppers.

37 F_h for dry heat sterilization.

38 In practice, the Z-values are determined from a linear regression using two or three D-values measured at different temperatures.

calculate the total lethality F_0 of a steam sterilization cycle at a reference temperature of $T_0 = 121.1°C$ from successive T_i measurements as follows:

$$F_{phys} \equiv F_{(T=121.1,Z)} = \sum_{i=1}^{n} \Delta t \cdot 10^{(T_i - 121.1)/z} \qquad (3.4)$$

where ($\Delta t = t_{i+1} - t_i$) is suitably short interval of time (e.g., 1 minute) between two temperature measurements[39] of the product using thermocouple sensors [150–152]. It should be noted that while Δt represent an actual clock time interval, F_{phys} represents a fictitious equivalent time at 121.1°C. It is also common to use 10°C as a reference Z-value.[40] Using equation (3.4) with a single time interval and a Z-value of 10°C, we can deduce that a cycle of 30 minutes at 121.1°C would result in about the same reduction in spore population as a cycle of 2.4 minutes at 132°C. Lethality is therefore a lot more sensitive to temperature increases than time. Spores having larger Z-values are less sensitive to temperature changes than spores with low Z-values [152]. The lethality can either be determined using physical thermocouple data (F_{phys}) with equation (3.4) or biologically (F_{bio}) using equation (3.2).[41] If sterilization is successful, the final spore population becomes the probability of having a non-sterile unit (PNSU) [150]. An equivalent concept is the sterility assurance level (SAL), which is the probability of having a single viable microorganism on a product after sterilization [150]. The SAL can be calculated using equation (3.5) as follows:

$$SAL = 10^{\left[\log(N_0) - SLR\right]} \qquad (3.5)$$

where the SLR can be determined from the F-value using equation (3.2). For regulation purposes, sterilization processes are often validated to achieve an SAL $\leq 10^{-6}$. Table 3.6 lists D-values and Z-values for common spores used in the validation of sterilization processes as well as reference values recommended by ISO 11138 for F-value calculations.

Steam Autoclave Parameters

There are two important types of steam autoclave vessels: Biological Indicator Evaluation Resistometer (BIER) vessels[42] [82, 165, 166] and process vessels. Figure 3.5(a) shows a BIER (i.e., resistometer) vessel typically used by Biological Indicator (BI) manufacturers and CTLs. Performance requirements for resistometers are specified in ISO 18472 [167]. Their main function is to evaluate D-values using either a survivor curve (SC) as

---

39 Lethality at temperatures <100°C are considered negligible.

40 The proper definition of F_0 is $F_0 \equiv F_{(T=121.1°C, \ Z=10°C)}$.

41 If the final spore population is a countable number ($N_f > 1$ CFU or colony forming unit) as determined by plate counting.

42 BIER vessels have smaller chambers and are able to deliver lethality in a precise, repeatable and concise square-wave cycle where the sterilization temperature is reached quickly (i.e., with rapid charge and exhaust) and controlled within a very tight tolerance of ±0.5°C.

TABLE 3.6   Inactivation Properties of Bacterial Spores Used in BI

Spores	Incubation T.	Heat shock T.	Steam		Dry Heat		EtO	H$_2$O$_2$	Gamma
			D-value (121°C)	Z-value	D-value (160°C)	Z-value	D-value (600 mg/ L)	D-value (1.5 mg/ L)	D-value
ISO 11138 (ref)	–	–	1.5 min	10°C	2.0 min	20°C	2.0 min	–	–
G. Stearother.	55°C–60°C	98°C	2.0 min	6°C	–	–	–	0.72 min	–
B. Atrophaeus	30°C–35°C	83°C	0.5 min	10°C	6.6 min	20°C	6.5 min	–	–
B. Subtilis	30°C–35°C	83°C	0.5 min	10°C	5.0 min	20°C	3.9 min	0.32 min	0.6 kGy
B. Pumilus	30°C–35°C	68°C	–	–	–	–	–	–	1.9 kGy

Source: Data compiled from [154–161].

Notes:

Abbreviations: Geobacillus Stearothermophilus, Bacillus Atrophaeus, Bacillus subtilis, Bacillus Pumilus.

[a] Heat shock activation time is 10 min for B. Atrophaeus and B. Subtilis and 15 min for G. Stearothermophilus and B. Pumilus.

[b] The D-values listed are only examples since they also depend on the substrate material that was used [83].

[c] The EtO D-values listed are at a T = 54°C and 60% RH.

[d] Minimum BI population specified by ISO 11138 is 10^5 for Steam and H$_2$O$_2$ and 10^6 for dry heat and EtO [161].

[e] The reference Z-value for F-value calculations involving dry heat depyrogenation processes is 46.4°C.

[f] Membrane filters used in sterilization by filtration are validated using small vegetative bacteria like Brevundimonas diminuta (0.2 µm) and Acholeplasma laidlawii (0.1 µm).

illustrated Figure 3.8 (if spore populations are countable) or a fraction negative method[43] [149] like Holcomb-Spearman-Karber (HSK) or Stumbo-Murphy-Cochran (SMC) [149, 151]. On the other hand, process vessels as shown in Figure 3.5(b) are typically found in healthcare facilities and have larger chambers used for routine sterilization. They allow more variation in conditions as BIER vessels with sterilization temperatures controlled within a broad −1/+2°C band [168]. Briefly, a process vessel is made of an inner chamber and an outer jacket that fills with steam that enters the chamber through a steam inlet as shown in Figure 3.5(b) [92]. There is a drain at the bottom of the chamber where air and condensate are evacuated by gravity or a vacuum system. Products are placed on a loading car containing shelves as shown in Figure 3.5(c).

Important factors that influence a steam sterilization process include time, temperature, steam quality (i.e., saturated steam as opposed to wet or superheated steam), direct steam contact, air removal, and drying [170]. The curves in Figure 3.6 show example gauge pressure [inHg][44] [95] over time in steam sterilization cycle, and the associated numerical data are available, typically as printouts from the sterilization unit. These printouts are invaluable when investigating sterilization failures. It should be noted that the temperature curve indicated on the printout (i.e., chamber temperature) cannot be

---

43 Fraction negative methods derive conclusions from information contained in the quantal zone where some samples are positive for growth (i.e. non-sterile) and some negative for growth (i.e. sterile).

44 Gauge pressure [psig] excludes the ambient pressure (i.e. 14.7 psi at sea level) as opposed to the absolute pressure [psi].

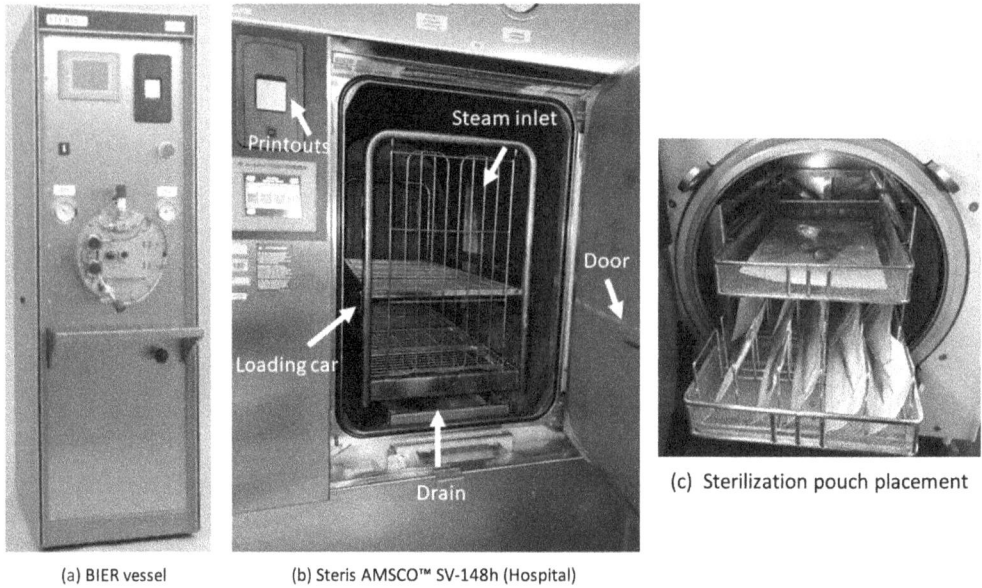

FIGURE 3.5   Autoclaves for steam sterilization: BIER/resistometer vessel (a, courtesy of sterilizers. com), process vessel used by healthcare facilities (b), sterilization pouch placement (c, courtesy of Astell Scientific) [162–164]. Sterilization pouches in (c) are shown vertical on a rack with one inch distance between them.

used to calculate F-values with equation (3.4) as the product temperature measured with thermocouples increases more slowly [152]. There are three phases to a steam sterilization cycle: conditioning (i.e., pre-conditioning), sterilization, and exhaust (i.e., drying). In a gravity cycle[45] [170, 171], steam slowly displaces air to the drain since it is lighter. These cycles should only be used with unwrapped non-porous (i.e., glossy) loads (e.g., glassware and metal) and loads unable to withstand a vacuum [170]. On the other hand, porous (i.e., matted) loads and loads wrapped in sterilization pouches should be sterilized with a dynamic air removal cycle[46] (e.g., a pre-vacuum cycle) [79, 170]. The conditioning phase of a pre-vacuum cycle typically includes three to four alternating pressure and vacuum pulses both to purge the air out of the chamber and product and gradually humidify and heat up the product to reduce the risk of damage [79, 170]. Vacuum pulses are specified in inches of mercury [inHg][47] and are used to evaporate any condensate during conditioning and exhaust. This is important as any air or condensate will prevent a good contact with steam that may result in sterilization failures. For brachytherapy devices, proper air removal is particularly important for sterilization of long and narrow lumens. Sterile barrier systems like disposable self-sealing sterilization pouches[48] have

---

45 Liquids and gels also use a gravity cycle with the exception of a slow exhaust without vacuum when returning the chamber to atmospheric pressure to avoid liquid loss from boil-overs (or purging the load into the drain).

46 Steam flush pressure pulse (SFPP) is another type of dynamic air removal cycle that is considered equivalent to a pre-vacuum cycle for the same exposure (e.g., 4 minutes at 132°C).

47 A perfect vacuum at sea level is 29.92 inHg.

48 Traditional load wrappings consist of used reusable woven textiles, requiring laundering. Modern disposable blue SMS polypropylene unwoven sheets are composed of Meltblown PP (sterile barrier) sandwiched between two layers of Spunbond PP for strength and durability.

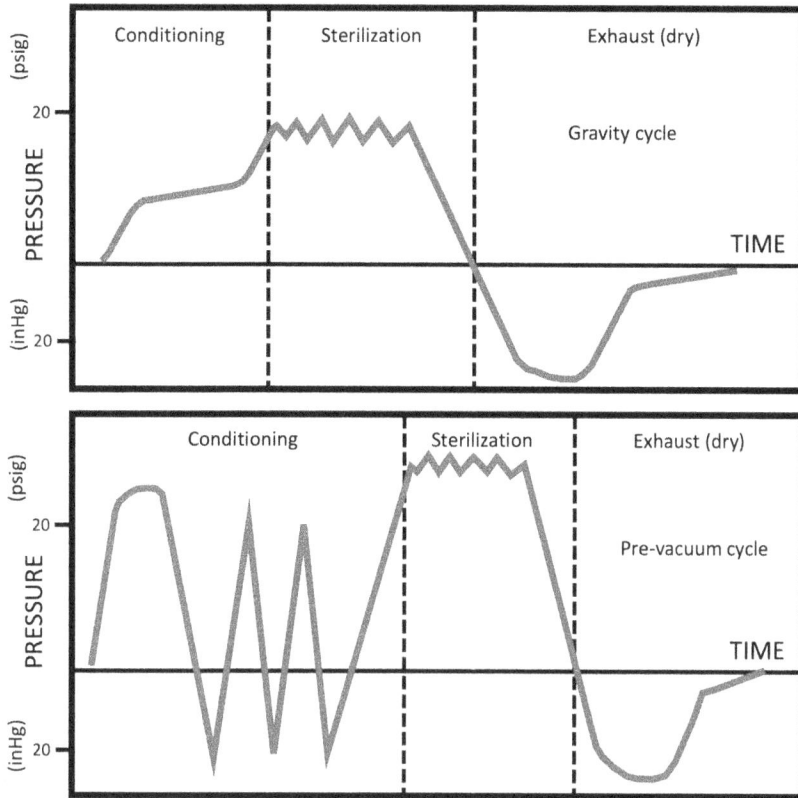

FIGURE 3.6   Comparison of gravity and pre-vacuum steam autoclave cycles. Figure based on data compiled from [97, 169].

a medical grade paper side with pores that expand to allow steam to enter during sterilization and a waterproof plastic side that is used to visually confirm that the vacuum successfully dried the product during the exhaust phase. Figure 3.5(c) shows a load configuration that allows good steam contact and the evacuation of condensate to the drain. Brachytherapy devices with dead-end lumens should be in a position that allows condensate to be properly drained. Loads that are too crowded using a bad configuration can create wet loads and wet packs. Brachytherapy devices with dead-end lumens should be in a position that allows condensate to be properly drained. Wet packs on sterilization pouches compromises their sterile barrier that leads to contamination of products [170, 172]. Chemical indicators, for example, type 5[49] integrating indicators, can be placed inside the load and will react to all known critical process variables (pressure, temperature, and the presence of steam) [82, 163]. General requirements for chemical indicators are specified in Part 1 of ISO 11140 [173]. Autoclave QA for proper air removal should include periodic testing with a vacuum leak test[50] and a Bowie-Dick air removal challenge

---

49 Sterilization pouches also include a type I CI which uses an ink that changes color with heat to indicate that the product has been exposed to the sterilization process.

50 In a vacuum leak test, the chamber is under vacuum for a specified time (e.g., 15 minutes) and a pressure differential (leak rate) of <1 mmHg/min is maintained from start to finish.

[171]. A Bowie-Dick test pack consists of an indicator sheet (e.g., Type 2 CI) between dense layers of porous substrate and reticulated foam [171]. This test produces a change of color (e.g., from yellow to purple) on the CI sheet after running a Bowie-Dick cycle at 132°C–134°C, a result that is required to pass the challenge [174]. The Association for the Advancement of Medical Instrumentation (AAMI) and regulatory agencies recommend the use of industry standard cycles whenever possible. Industry standard cycles for steam sterilization include 30 minutes at 121°C and 4 minutes at 132°C followed by 20–30 minutes drying time.

Validation of a Sterilization Process

Biological indicators (BIs) are test systems that contain a calibrated population of microorganisms (e.g., spores) with a specified resistance (e.g., D-value, Z-value) to a sterilization process [82]. D-values on a BI's Certificate of Analysis (CoA) are usually specified within ± 20% using a resistometer [165]. The purpose of a BI is to provide a biological validation of the physical lethality delivered by a sterilization process [152]. As opposed to CIs, BIs reacts to all known and unknown critical process variables but require additional time to be cultured. General and specific requirements for BIs are specified in the ISO 11138 series [175–178], the USP chapter ⟨55⟩ [179] and the European Pharmacopoeia (EP) [180]. Figure 3.7(a) and Figure 3.7(b) show a spore suspension[51] used for the direct inoculation of a product or custom BI [82]. Figure 3.7(c) shows a basic spore strip[52] (i.e., piece of paper with 10^5 or 10^6 spores) in a sterile envelope [82]. As shown in Figure 3.7(c) some custom BIs come in a variety of geometries (e.g., microstrips, threads, metal wires). These are used to create process challenge devices (PCD) as shown in Figure 3.7(e) where custom BIs and/or CIs are embedded in the most challenging locations to sterilize in a product. Figure 3.7(d) shows self-contained BIs (SCBIs) that combine a spore carrier with a glass ampoule of culture medium. After sterilization, the ampoule is crushed by compressing the sides of the plastic vial and a color change (e.g., purple to yellow) indicates growth. SCBI[53] [82] are more reliable since their results are not affected by uncertainties in D-values related to the culture medium as well as removing the risk of accidental contamination during handling and culturing [181]. Most SCBIs can usually be used with a reduced incubation time (RIT) (e.g., 24 hours). In general, spores from BIs or PCDs are cultivated during shaking in an incubator for 7 days in Trypsic soy broth (TSB) (i.e., Soybean-Casein Digest) culture medium at a temperature conducive to spore growth. A heat shock treatment can also be useful to promote germination of spores before culture [119, 182]. Sonication in an ultrasonic tank and the use of surfactant (e.g., USP fluid D) can help to recover (i.e., detach) spores/bacteria from 3D printed objects for culture in TSB or agar plates [82, 119, 145]. Figure 3.7(f) shows both a sample of TSB medium after culture positive for growth (i.e., turbid TSB) and one negative for growth (i.e., clear TSB). Turbidity can also be assessed using a spectrophotometer by comparing

---

51 Spores are usually suspended as shown in Figure 3.1(b) in an ethanol solution unconducive to growth.
52 For VHP/HPGP sterilization, these strips are made of glass fiber or stainless steel in a Tyvek envelope.
53 For liquid products, liquid submersible BIs (LSBIs) are SCBIs designed to be submerged in the liquid.

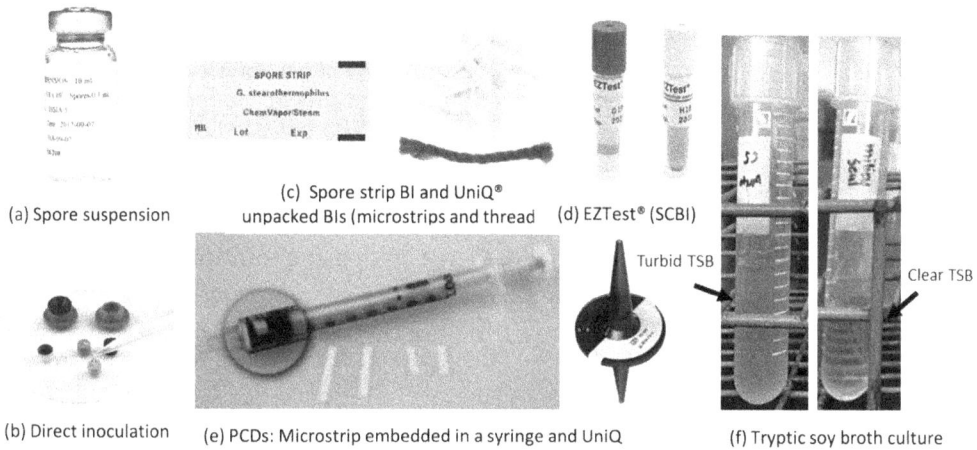

(a) Spore suspension

(b) Direct inoculation

(c) Spore strip BI and UniQ® unpacked BIs (microstrips and thread

(d) EZTest® (SCBI)

(e) PCDs: Microstrip embedded in a syringe and UniQ

Turbid TSB

Clear TSB

(f) Tryptic soy broth culture

FIGURE 3.7   Direct inoculation of products using spore suspension (a and b) or unpacked biological indicators (BI). Examples of spore strips (c, d, and e) BI and self-containing BIs (SCBI) (courtesy of Mesa Laboratories) [183, 184]. Results from the validation of a sterilization process (f, courtesy of the Grandvaux Lab at CRCHUM, Montreal, Canada). Figures sourced with permission.

a sterilized sample with a non-sterilized control. Table 3.6 lists incubation and heat shock temperatures for common spores used in sterilization challenge: *G. Stearothermophilus* (for steam and VHP/HPGP), *B. Atrophaeus* (for dry heat and EtO), *B. subtilis* (an easier challenge option for most methods), and *B. Pumilus* (for radiation). It should be noted that dosimetry data are more often used than biological data for validation of radiation sterilization processes [181].

BIs are an essential tool for sterilization cycle development, cycle validation and routine monitoring [82, 181]. Guidance on the development and validation of sterilization processes can be found in several ISO documents: Part 1 of ISO 17665 (Steam) [185], ISO 20857 (Dry heat) [186], Part 1 of ISO 11135 (EtO) [187], ISO 22441 (VHP/HPGP) [188], Part 1 of ISO 11137 (Radiation) [189] as well as USP chapter 1229 [190]. Cycle development and validation are commonly performed by a CTL using custom BIs to provide the necessary documentation for regulatory agencies. At the point of use, cycle validation of the sterilization process recommended in the medical device's IFU and routine monitoring could be done using a combination of an SCBI and sterilizer QA (e.g., Bowie-Dick challenge). Steam cycle development and validation for heat-stable materials are usually done with an overkill method that has the advantage of not requiring any knowledge of the natural bioburden occurring on a product [184, 191]. Overkill validation may therefore require precursor studies such as a product *D*-value study and/or location mapping studies. A product *D*-value study is usually performed by a CTL using a resistometer. Relative to the *D*-value of the BI, the product may reduce its resistance (e.g., leaching of a sporicidal toxin) or increase it (e.g., if spores are coated or get clumped together by porous surfaces) [118, 184]. A BI can be selected as a surrogate of the product for validation of a sterilization process only if its *D*-value (as stated on the CoA) is greater than or equal to the *D*-value of the product [192]. Otherwise, a PCD of equivalent resistance to the product or a direct inoculation technique should be used [184]. Load mapping studies involve using physical sensors (e.g., thermocouples for steam, chemical/humidity sensors for EtO) to identify the most challenging location to sterilize within the chamber (i.e., cold spots) [184, 191]. Product mapping studies involve using small sensors (e.g., custom BIs) to identify the most challenging location to sterilize within the product itself [184, 191]. For brachytherapy devices, this could be in the middle of a long narrow open lumen or at the end of a dead-end lumen. When comparing multiple locations within a PCD, each having multiple replicate BIs, equation (3.6) can be used to calculate the most probable number (MPN) of spores from fraction negative results at that location [149, 193, 194].

$$\mathrm{MPN} = \ln\left(\frac{n}{r}\right) \tag{3.6}$$

where *n* is the number of replicate BIs and *r* is the number of growth negative BIs. For example, if 1/3 BIs is growth negative at a location, the MPN is 1.1 spores at that location.

There are three overkill approaches described in the ISO standards: a half-cycle approach, a partial cycle calculation approach, and a full cycle approach[54] [184, 185, 191, 196, 197]. The half-cycle overkill approach is illustrated in Figure 3.8 and is the most common and conservative validation method. In this method, an initial population of 10^6 spores/BI is inactivated using the half-cycle time. Since an SLR of 6 is required to show negative growth at the half-cycle, we can deduce that the full cycle would have an additional 6 SLR as margin of safety. This results in an SLR of 12 that guarantees an SAL of 10^{-6} or better on the natural product bioburden (as long as its *D*-value is less than or equal to the one of the BI). In cycle development, the half-cycle time is often reduced until some BIs are positive for growth and this time is increased slightly until all BIs are negative for growth (i.e., half-cycle window) to find the shortest cycle time that can be validated. The overkill partial cycle calculation approach requires either direct spore counts or fraction negative data and is covered elsewhere [184, 191]. It should be noted that all overkill methods assume extrapolation of a log-linear survival curve. The common practice is to repeat the sterilization validation three times to show repeatability with a first-time pass rate of 100%. This is not always easy to achieve in practice and it is possible to improve these results by reducing the spore population within the limits recommended by ISO standards[55] [177, 185, 196]. Overkill methods can lead to sterilization cycles that are too aggressive for heat-sensitive devices. In this case, it is possible to validate a softer cycle by

---

54 A full cycle overkill approach can be developed by calculating the BI population required to achieve a lethality F_{bio} of 12 minutes and adding $0.5 \cdot$ SLR as a margin of safety (i.e. the sterilization process is validated if it can sterilize a BI with a population $\geq 1 \cdot 10^{6+0.5}$ spores/BI).

55 Most ISO standards recommend a reference *D*-value of 1–1.5 minutes for sterilization validation that provides some flexibility. For example, for *G. Stearothermophilus* spores with a *D*-value of 2.5 minutes, a BI population of $1 \cdot 10^{3.6}$ will give an equivalent challenge to a spore population with a *D*-value of 1.5 minutes. However, 10^5 is usually the smallest population used in practice to satisfy Part 3 of ISO 11138-3.

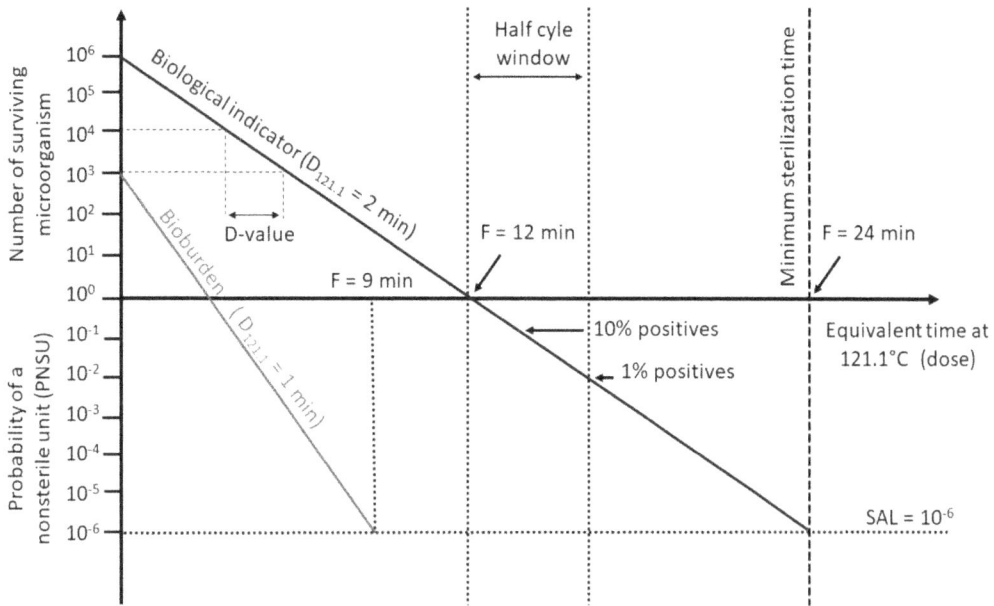

FIGURE 3.8   Overkill half-cycle method. Figure based on [124, 195] with permission. Process time (i.e., clock time) could be used instead of equivalent time but the F-values stated would have to be corrected for temperature differences relative to 121.1°C.

using the BI/BB (biological indicator/bioburden[56]) method [193, 198]. The BI/BB method requires an additional precursor study to identify the most resistant spore formers naturally found on the product (e.g., using boil/heat shock treatment). Guidance on the characterization of bioburden is provided in ISO 11737 [199]. It is then possible to use knowledge of the natural bioburden to select a BI with a much smaller resistance (e.g., *B. Subtilis* instead of *G. Stearothermophilus*) and population to validate a SAL of 10^{-6} for the product.

In the literature, a few studies included a biological validation of sterilization processes for their 3D printed devices. However, the methodology used often differs from ISO standard testing. For example, some authors included a bacteriological validation using non-spore-forming bacteria that likely provide an easier challenge than bacterial spores [66, 133, 145]. McFarland standards can help to adjust the turbidity of a bacterial suspension to a given concentration used to contaminate a 3D printed device [133, 145]. Perez *et al.* found that most (i.e., 221/225) of their test bar samples made of ABS, PC-ABS, PC, PPSU, and PEI contaminated during manufacturing and transport were negative for growth following steam, EtO, HPGP, and gamma radiation sterilization [78]. Aguado-Maestro *et al.* inoculated the inside of PLA cylinders and found that they could be sterilized with steam at 134°C for 35 minutes and EtO but not HPGP [133]. Rynio *et al.* successfully validated a steam sterilization cycle at 121°C for 30 minutes as well as

---

56 Cycle development based solely on the bioburden is possible but the BB method is rarely used as it does not establish an SAL for the sterilization process.

EtO and HPGP sterilization processes for an aortic arch template made of PLA, PETG, Nylon, PP, and SLA photoresins using *G. Stearothermophilus* and *B. Atrophaeus* [135]. Grandjean-Lapierre *et al.* validated a steam sterilization process at 132°C for 4 minutes using a direct inoculation of *G. Stearothermophilus* on 3D printed nasopharyngeal swabs made of SLA photoresin [139]. Kudla *et al.* contracted a CTL to validate a SAL of 10^{-6} using a BI overkill approach for their PSCT brachytherapy applicator made of PEEK using a steam sterilization cycle at 132°C for 4 minutes [130]. Diab-Elschahawi *et al.* validated an HPGP sterilization process with an overkill half-cycle method using PCDs made of 5-cm stainless steel BIs [119]. These custom BIs were embedded in the middle of 50-cm single channel stainless steel lumens with an inner diameter of 0.7 mm [119]. They found that insufficient cleaning that was simulated using an inorganic and organic challenge considerably affected the percentage of BIs negative for growth (i.e., from 80% to 8.3%) [119].

SUMMARY

While 3D printing offers new possibilities to make novel devices for adaptive radiotherapy, biocompatibility and sterilization of these devices are important safety aspects and often overlooked. This is especially important for critical brachytherapy devices that are in prolonged contact with mucosal surfaces and/or interstitial catheters. For these applications, while selecting materials already tested by the manufacturer for biocompatibility (e.g., using ISO 10993 standards) is a good starting point, additional testing specific to the device and application may be needed. Publications reporting the development of these devices should correctly specify the level of biocompatibility of these materials (e.g., short-term vs. long-term mucosal contact). Similarly for these devices, prototype testing after sterilization and a validation of the recommended sterilization process using a biological spore challenge should be performed prior to patient use. This may require contracting a CTL or collaborating with a research laboratory having sufficient expertise to conduct these tests. As compatibility with a sterilization process depends both on the materials used and the geometry and function of the device, including these tests in scientific publication would help to provide guidance for the wider radiation oncology community. It should be noted that documented transmissions of pathogens in commercial medical devices are rarely reported, which may be attributed to the wide margin of safety required by industry standards [73]. Overall, this chapter includes useful information for the 3D printing user striving to achieve a similar standard for patient safety.

REFERENCES

[1] *Medical device regulations: Global overview and guiding principles*, World Health Organization, 2003.

[2] *Principles of Medical Devices Classification*, Global Harmonization Task Force, 2012.

[3] *Guidance for health care professionals on special access and custom-made medical devices*, Health Canada, 2016.

[4] *Questions and answers on custom-made devices and considerations on adaptable medical devices and patient-matched medical devices*, Medical Device Coordination Group, 2021.

[5] *Custom device exemption—Guidance for industry and food and drug administration staff*, U.S. Food and Drug Administration, 2014.

[6] *ISO 14971:2019 Medical devices—Application of risk management to medical devices*, International Organization for Standardization, 2019.

[7] *ISO 13485:2016 Medical devices—Quality management systems—Requirements for regulatory purposes*, International Organization for Standardization, 2016.

[8] *ISO/IEC 17025:2017 General requirements for the competence of testing and calibration laboratories*, International Organization for Standardization, 2017.

[9] *ISO 10993-1:2018 Biological evaluation of medical devices—Part 1: Evaluation and testing within a risk management process*, International Organization for Standardization, 2018.

[10] E. Spaulding, "The role of chemical disinfection in the prevention of nosocomial infections," in *Proceedings of the international conference on nosocomial infections*, 1970, vol. 1971: American Hospital Association Chicago, pp. 254–274.

[11] *Decontamination and reprocessing of medical devices for health-care facilities*, World Health Organization, 2016.

[12] *Guidelines for environmental infection control in health-care facilities; recommendations of CDC and the Healthcare Infection Control Practices Advisory Committee (HICPAC)*, Healthcare Infection Control Practices Advisory Committee (U.S.), 2017.

[13] *ISO 11139:2018 Sterilization of health care products—Vocabulary of terms used in sterilization and related equipment and process standards*, International Organization for Standardization, 2018.

[14] *Discussion paper: 3D printing medical devices at the point of care*, U.S. Food and Drug Administration, 2021.

[15] *3D printing of medical devices*, Alberta Health Services, 2020.

[16] *ISO 14155:2020 Clinical investigation of medical devices for human subjects—Good clinical practice*, International Organization for Standardization, 2020.

[17] *Quality System (QS) regulation/medical device good manufacturing practices*, U.S. Food and Drug Administration, 2022.

[18] *Good laboratory practice for nonclinical laboratory studies (21 CFR 58), §58.3*, U.S. Food and Drug Administration, 2022.

[19] M. Ashenafi, S. Jeong, J. N. Wancura, L. Gou, M. J. Webster, and D. Zheng, "A quick guide on implementing and quality assuring 3D printing in radiation oncology," *Journal of Applied Clinical Medical Physics*, p. e14102, 2023. https://aapm.onlinelibrary.wiley.com/doi/epdf/10.1002/acm2.14102

[20] J. M. Park, J. Son, H. J. An, J. H. Kim, H.-G. Wu, and J.-i. Kim, "Bio-compatible patient-specific elastic bolus for clinical implementation," *Physics in Medicine and Biology*, vol. 64, no. 10, p. 105006, 2019.

[21] S. Su, K. Moran, and J. L. Robar, "Design and production of 3D printed bolus for electron radiation therapy," *Journal of Applied Clinical Medical Physics*, vol. 15, no. 4, pp. 194–211, 2014.

[22] M. A. Astrahan *et al.*, "An interactive treatment planning system for ophthalmic plaque radiotherapy," *International Journal of Radiation Oncology* Biology* Physics*, vol. 18, no. 3, pp. 679–687, 1990.

[23] R. Bellis, A. Rembielak, E. A. Barnes, M. Paudel, and A. Ravi, "Additive manufacturing (3D printing) in superficial brachytherapy," *Journal of contemporary brachytherapy*, vol. 13, no. 4, pp. 468–482, 2021.

[24] J. A. M. Cunha *et al.*, "Evaluation of PC-ISO for customized, 3D printed, gynecologic HDR brachytherapy applicators," *Journal of Applied Clinical Medical Physics*, vol. 16, no. 1, pp. 246–253, 2015.

[25] C. Herpel *et al.*, "Individualized 3D-printed tissue retraction devices for head and neck radiotherapy," *Frontiers in Oncology*, vol. 11, p. 628743, 2021.

[26] S. Cleland *et al.*, "Dosimetric evaluation of a patient-specific 3D-printed oral positioning stent for head-and-neck radiotherapy," *Physical and Engineering Sciences in Medicine*, vol. 44, no. 3, pp. 887–899, 2021.

[27] R. X. Larouche, C. Martel, M. Lebeau, A. Jutras, D. Roberge, and S. Bedwani, "A digital workflow to create patient-specific radiation oral shields for orthovoltage," *Cureus Journal of Medical Science*, 2023. www.cureus.com/posters/2541-a-digital-workflow-to-create-patient-specific-radiation-oral-shields-for-orthovoltage

[28] *Definitions for personalized medical devices*, International Medical Device Regulators Forum, 2018.

[29] N. J. Rowan, T. Kremer, and G. McDonnell, "A review of Spaulding's classification system for effective cleaning, disinfection and sterilization of reusable medical devices: Viewed through a modern-day lens that will inform and enable future sustainability," *Science of The Total Environment*, vol. 878, p. 162976, 2023.

[30] *ISO 10993-2:2006 Biological evaluation of medical devices—Part 2: Animal welfare requirements*, International Organization for Standardization, 2006.

[31] *ISO 10993-3:2014 Biological evaluation of medical devices—Part 3: Tests for genotoxicity, carcinogenicity and reproductive toxicity*, International Organization for Standardization, 2014.

[32] *ISO 10993-4:2017 Biological evaluation of medical devices—Part 4: Selection of tests for interactions with blood*, International Organization for Standardization, 2017.

[33] *ISO 10993-5:2009 Biological evaluation of medical devices—Part 5: Tests for in vitro cytotoxicity*, International Organization for Standardization, 2009.

[34] *ISO 10993-6:2016 Biological evaluation of medical devices—Part 6: Tests for local effects after implantation*, International Organization for Standardization, 2016.

[35] *ISO 10993-7:2008 Biological evaluation of medical devices—Part 7: Ethylene oxide sterilization residuals*, International Organization for Standardization, 2008.

[36] *ISO 10993-9:2019 Biological evaluation of medical devices—Part 9: Framework for identification and quantification of potential degradation products*, International Organization for Standardization, 2019.

[37] *ISO 10993-10:2021 Biological evaluation of medical devices—Part 10: Tests for skin sensitization*, International Organization for Standardization, 2021.

[38] *ISO 10993-11:2017 Biological evaluation of medical devices—Part 11: Tests for systemic toxicity*, International Organization for Standardization, 2017.

[39] *ISO 10993-12:2021 Biological evaluation of medical devices—Part 12: Sample preparation and reference materials*, International Organization for Standardization, 2012.

[40] *ISO 10993-13:2010 Biological evaluation of medical devices—Part 13: Identification and quantification of degradation products from polymeric medical devices*, International Organization for Standardization, 2010.

[41] *ISO 10993-14:2001 Biological evaluation of medical devices—Part 14: Identification and quantification of degradation products from ceramics*, International Organization for Standardization, 2001.

[42] *ISO 10993-15:2019 Biological evaluation of medical devices—Part 15: Identification and quantification of degradation products from metals and alloys*, international Organization for Standardization, 2019.

[43] *ISO 10993-16:2017 Biological evaluation of medical devices—Part 16: Toxicokinetic study design for degradation products and leachables*, International Organization for Standardization, 2017.

[44] *ISO 10993-17:2023 Biological evaluation of medical devices—Part 17: Toxicological risk assessment of medical device constituents*, International Organization for Standardization, 2023.

[45] *ISO 10993-18:2020 Biological evaluation of medical devices—Part 18: Chemical characterization of medical device materials within a risk management process*, International Organization for Standardization, 2020.

[46] *ISO/TS 10993-19:2020 Biological evaluation of medical devices—Part 19: Physico-chemical, morphological and topographical characterization of materials*, International Organization for Standardization, 2020.

[47] *Use of International Standard ISO 10993-1, "Biological evaluation of medical devices— Part 1: Evaluation and testing within a risk management process"*, U.S. Food and Drug Administration, 2020.

[48] *General Chapter, ⟨87⟩ Biological Reactivity Tests, In Vitro*, United States Pharmacopeia, 2015.

[49] *General Chapter, ⟨88⟩ Biological Reactivity Tests, In Vivo*, United States Pharmacopeia, 2023.

[50] *General Chapter, ⟨1031⟩ The Biocompatibility of Materials Used in Drug Containers*, United States Pharmacopeia, 2023.

[51] L. Moshkanbaryans, C. Meyers, A. Ngu, and J. Burdach, "The importance of infection prevention and control in medical ultrasound," *Australasian Journal of Ultrasound in Medicine*, vol. 18, no. 3, pp. 96–99, 2015.

[52] T. Rollins, "How to categorize a medical device per ISO 10993-1, Nelson Labs," 2015. www.nelsonlabs.com/videos-gallery/how-to-categorize-a-medical-device-per-iso-10993-1

[53] *Imaging strategies for definitive intracavitary brachytherapy of cervical cancer*, Cancer Care Ontario, 2014.

[54] Facundo Arceo. "3D filament glass transition temperatures." https://3dsolved.com/3d-filament-glass-transition-temperatures/ (accessed 2023).

[55] Stratasys Ltd. "Product datasheets." www.stratasys.com/en/materials/materials-catalog/ (accessed 2023).

[56] Formlabs Inc., "Technical Datasheets." https://formlabs.com/materials/medical/ (accessed 2023).

[57] Omnexus the materiel selection platform. "Heat deflection temperature of plastics." https://omnexus.specialchem.com/polymer-properties/properties/heat-deflection-temperature-of-plastics (accessed 2023).

[58] Matterhackers Inc., "What material should I use in a high temperature environment?" https://help.matterhackers.com/article/109-what-material-should-i-use-in-a-high-temperature-environment

[59] 3D Systems Inc., "Accura ClearVue Datasheet." www.3dsystems.com/materials/accura-clearvue (accessed 2023).

[60] "All About PP 3D Printing Filament: Materials, Properties, Definition." www.xometry.com/resources/3d-printing/pp-3d-printing-filament/ (accessed 2023).

[61] *ISO 7405:2018 Dentistry—Evaluation of biocompatibility of medical devices used in dentistry*, International Organization for Standardization, 2018.

[62] D. E. Albert, "Material and chemical characterization for the biological evaluation of medical device biocompatibility," in *Biocompatibility and performance of medical devices*, J.-P. Boutrand Ed.: Woodhead, 2012, pp. 65–94.

[63] M. Turner, "How to apply extractables and leachables to medical devices. Medical Engineering Technologies." https://met.uk.com/uploads/images/pdfs/How-To-Apply-Extractables-And-Leachables-To-Medical-Devices.pdf

[64] *ISO/TS 21726:2019 Biological evaluation of medical devices—Application of the threshold of toxicological concern (TTC) for assessing biocompatibility of medical device constituents*, International Organization for Standardization, 2019.

[65] M. A. M. Shafiee, M. A. M. Asri, and S. S. S. Alwi, "Review on the in vitro cytotoxicity assessment in accordance to the International Organization for Standardization (ISO)," *Malaysian Journal of Medicine and Health Sciences*, vol. 17, no. 2, pp. 261–269, 2021.

[66] R. Told *et al.*, "A state-of-the-art guide to the sterilization of thermoplastic polymers and resin materials used in the additive manufacturing of medical devices," *Materials and Design*, vol. 223, p. 111119, 2022.

[67] M. Kozakiewicz, P. Szymor, and R. Olszewski, "Cytotoxicity of three-dimensional paper-based models from a three-dimensional paper-based printer," *NEMESIS Negative Effects in Medical Science: Oral and Maxillofacial Surgery*, vol. 3, no. 1, pp. 1–15, 2018.

[68] S. Gruber and A. Nickel, "Toxic or not toxic? The specifications of the standard ISO 10993-5 are not explicit enough to yield comparable results in the cytotoxicity assessment of an identical medical device," *Frontiers in Medical Technology*, vol. 5, p. 1195529, 2023.

[69] K. P. Coleman *et al.*, "Evaluation of an in vitro human dermal sensitization test for use with medical device extracts," *Applied In Vitro Toxicology*, vol. 1, no. 2, pp. 118–130, 2015.

[70] L. Svobodová *et al.*, "Sensitization potential of medical devices detected by in vitro and in vivo methods," *ALTEX*, vol. 38, no. 3, pp. 419–430, 2021. doi: 10.14573/altex.2008142. Epub 2021 Jan 26. https://pubmed.ncbi.nlm.nih.gov/33497461/

[71] C. Pellevoisin *et al.*, "SkinEthic™ RHE for in vitro evaluation of skin irritation of medical device extracts," *Toxicology in Vitro*, vol. 50, pp. 418–425, 2018.

[72] *ISO/TR 21582:2021 Pyrogenicity—Principles and methods for pyrogen testing of medical devices*, International Organization for Standardization, 2021.

[73] W. A. Rutala and D. J. Weber, "Guideline for disinfection and sterilization in healthcare facilities, 2008," 2008. www.cdc.gov/infectioncontrol/pdf/guidelines/disinfection-guidelines-H.pdf

[74] Ethide Laboratories Inc., "How to validate sterility in autoclaves vs. radiation sterilized medical products." https://ethidelabs.com/how-to-validate-sterility-in-autoclaves-vs-radiation-sterilized-medical-products

[75] S. K. Bhatia and K. W. Ramadurai, *3D Printing and Bio-Based Materials in Global Health*, Springer, 2017. https://link.springer.com/book/10.1007/978-3-319-58277-1#about-this-book

[76] O. Oth, C. Dauchot, M. Orellana, and R. Glineur, "How to sterilize 3D printed objects for surgical use? An evaluation of the volumetric deformation of 3D-printed genioplasty

guide in PLA and PETG after sterilization by low-temperature hydrogen peroxide gas plasma," *The Open Dentistry Journal*, vol. 13, no. 1, 2019.

[77] J. Neijhoft, D. Henrich, A. Kammerer, M. Janko, J. Frank, and I. Marzi, "Sterilization of PLA after fused filament fabrication 3D printing: Evaluation on inherent sterility and the impossibility of autoclavation," *Polymers,* vol. 15, no. 2, p. 369, 2023.

[78] M. Perez *et al.*, "Sterilization of FDM-manufactured parts," in *2012 International Solid Freeform Fabrication Symposium*, 2012. University of Texas at Austin.

[79] Steris, "Guide to Steam Sterilization Cycles – Steam Flush Pressure Pulse."

[80] B. Lambert and J. Martin III, "Chapter III. 1.2: Sterilization of Implants and Devices," in *Biomaterials Science: An Introduction to Materials in Medicine*, Third Edition, B.D. Ratner, A.S. Hoffman, F.J. Schoen, and J.E. Lemons Eds.: Academic Press, pp. 1339–53, 2013.

[81] Andersen Sterilizers Inc., "How does Ethylene Oxide Sterilize?" www.anderseneurope. com/sterilisations.php?id=5#:~:text=At%20the%20start%20of%20the,to%20reduce%20 EtO%20residual%20levels

[82] K. McCauley, N. Robichaud, K. Gardner, and C. Hostler, "Biological indicators for sterilization," in *Handbook of Validation in Pharmaceutical Processes*, Fourth Edition, J. Agalloco, P. DeSantis, A. Grilli, and A. Pavell Eds.: CRC Press, 2021, pp. 205–216. www. taylorfrancis.com/books/edit/10.1201/9781003163138/handbook-validation-pharmac eutical-processes-fourth-edition-james-agalloco-phil-desantis-anthony-grilli-anthony-pavell?refId=6d767a83-1306-4f79-bfc3-b52585ed796b&context=ubx

[83] K. McCauley and J. R. Gillis, "The effect of carrier material on the measured resistance of spores," *Pharmaceutical Technology*, Vol. 2007 no. 2 (Suppl.), May 1, 2007.

[84] Kurt McCauley, "Product D-value studies: A critical tool when developing a sterilization process". www.expresspharma.in/product-d-value-studies-a-critical-tool-when-develop ing-a-sterilisation-process

[85] General Chapter, ⟨1211⟩ Sterilization and Sterility Assurance of Compendial Articles, United States Pharmacopeia, 2011.

[86] S. E. Walsh and S. P. Denyer, "Filtration sterilization," in *Russell, Hugo and Ayliffe's: Principles and Practice of Disinfection, Preservation and Sterilization*, A.P. Fraise, J.-Y. Maillard, S.A. Sattar Eds.: Wiley, 2013, pp. 343–370.

[87] W. A. Eudailey, "Membrane filters and membrane-filtration processes for health care," *American Journal of Hospital Pharmacy*, vol. 40, no. 11, pp. 1921–1923, Nov. 1983. [Online]. Available: www.ncbi.nlm.nih.gov/pubmed/6650520.

[88] Ethide Laboratories Inc., "Sterilization by filtration for parenteral and biologic products." https://ethidelabs.com/sterilization-by-filtration-for-parenteral-and-biologic-products

[89] Critical Filtration Process Inc., "How to choose the best sterilizing filter for your applica-tion?" www.criticalprocess.com/blog/how-to-choose-the-best-sterilizing-filter-for-your-application

[90] C. O. Hancock, "Heat sterilization," in *Russell, Hugo and Ayliffe's: Principles and Practice of Disinfection, Preservation and Sterilization*, A. P. Fraise, J.-Y. Maillard, and S. Sattar Eds., Wiley, 2013, pp. 277–293.

[91] P. DeSantis, "Steam sterilization in autoclaves," in *Handbook of Validation in Pharmaceutical Processes,* Fourth Edition, J. Agalloco, P. DeSantis, A. Grilli, and A. Pavell Eds.: CRC Press, 2021, pp. 217–230.

[92] Consolidated Sterilizer Systems, "Sterilization 101: How does a laboratory autoclave work?" https://consteril.com/search/how+does+a+laboratory+autoclave+work/

[93] H. Shintani, "Validation of sterilization procedures and usage of biological indicators in the manufacture of healthcare products," *Biocontrol Science*, vol. 16, no. 3, pp. 85–94, 2011.

[94] Ethide Laboratories Inc., "How do autoclaves sterilize medical devices?" https://ethidelabs.com/how-do-autoclaves-sterilize-medical-devices/#:~:text=As%20mentioned%20earlier%2C%20autoclaves%20operate,known%20as%20a%20biphasic%20mixture

[95] L. Clement and J. Biley, "Understanding steam sterilizer physical parameters," *Infection Control Today*. https://rwjms.rutgers.edu/research/core_facilities/ses/documents/SterilizerParameters.pdf

[96] Nordion Inc., "C-188 Colbalt-60 sources," 2014. www.nordion.com/products/c-188-cobalt-60-sources

[97] Steris Plc., "Operator manual for Amsco® Century™ Medium Steam Sterilizers," 2004. https://physiology.case.edu/media/eq_manuals/eq_manual_century_medium_prevacuum_sterilizer_manual.pdf

[98] it4ip. "ipPORE™ track-etched membrane filters polycarbonate (PC) and polyester (PET)." www.it4ip-iontracktechnology.com/product-portfolio/ippore/ (accessed 2023).

[99] Andersen Sterilizers Inc., "Key operators study guide for Anprolene gas sterilization". www.eqmisa.com/articulos/PN4740_030509-Anprolene-Study-Guide9.pdf

[100] Advanced Sterilization Products (ASP), "STERRAD® 100 NX® Sterilization System User's Guide," 2020. https://eifu.asp.com

[101] Steris Plc., "V-PRO® maX 2 operator's manual," 2021. https://ww1.steris.com/onbDocs/V550/0/4553041.pdf

[102] Nordion Inc., "Reference guide for gamma compatible materials," 2011. www.nordion.com/wp-content/uploads/2014/10/GT_Gamma_Compatible_Materials.pdf

[103] Steris Plc., "Operator manual for the system 1E® liquid chemical sterilant processing system". https://ww1.steris.com/onbDocs/V533/1/4256646.pdf

[104] M. Patel, "Medical sterilization methods," Lemo USA Inc., 2003.

[105] C. Beerlage, B. Wiese, A. R. Kausch, and M. Arsenijevic, "Change in radiation sterilization process from gamma ray to X-ray," *Biomedical Instrumentation and Technology*, vol. 55, no. s3, pp. 78–84, 2021.

[106] Kruse Training Inc., "Common polymer materials specific heat capacity ranges". https://krusetraining.com/wp-content/uploads/2017/12/List-Of-Materials-Specific-Heat-Capacity-Ranges.pdf

[107] Andersen Sterilizers Inc., "Zero Emissions." www.sterility.com/zero-emissions/ (accessed 2023).

[108] Advanced Sterilization Products (ASP), "Comparison Study of Environmental Hydrogen Peroxide Levels of STERRAD® Systems and STERIS V-PRO® Low Temperature Sterilizers Reveals Striking Differences," 2016. https://krusetraining.com/wp-content/uploads/2017/12/List-Of-Materials-Specific-Heat-Capacity-Ranges.pdf

[109] Andersen sterilizers Inc., "Ethylene Oxide (EtO or EO) – The Future Of Gas Sterilization." www.anderseneurope.com/assets/files/library/1633460361.pdf

[110] G. Sheaffer and K. Warrier, "Validation of dry heat sterilization and depyrogenation," in *Handbook of Validation in Pharmaceutical Processes,* Fourth Edition, J. Agalloco, P. DeSantis, A. Grilli, and A. Pavell Eds.: CRC Press, 2021, pp. 271–299.

[111] Ethide Laboratories Inc., "Steam sterilization vs. dry heat sterilization for medical devices and products." https://ethidelabs.com/steam-sterilization-vs-dry-heat-sterilization-for-medical-devices-and-products/#:~:text=Dry%20heat%20sterilization%20uses%20exceptionally,minimizing%20material%20degradation%20following%20sterilization

[112] Ethide Laboratories Inc., "Dry heat depyrogenation vs. sterilization for sterile products." https://ethidelabs.com/dry-heat-depyrogenation-vs-sterilization-for-sterile-products/#:~:text=Sterilization%20is%20any%20process%20that%20removes%2C%20kills%2C%20or%20deactivates%20microbes,walls%20of%20gram%2Dnegative%20bacteria

[113] Andersen Sterilizers Inc., "Owner's manual for Anprolene® AN74i gas sterilization." www.scribd.com/document/476184691/andersen-products-anprolene-an74i-owners-manual

[114] N. A. Robinson and R. W. Eveland, "Using HPG sterlization for heat-sensitive devices," 2015. www.google.com/url?sa=t&rct=j&q=&esrc=s&source=web&cd=&ved=2ahUKEwiGp_r0ioiEAxVJF1kFHfhMCPMQFnoECBIQAQ&url=https%3A%2F%2Fwww.steris.com%2F-%2Fmedia%2Fdocuments%2Fpdfs%2Fendoscope-reprocessing%2F1501cetest.ashx&usg=AOvVaw2yRI9O4WO7S2ueMid-ETOg&opi=89978449

[115] 3M Co., "3M™ Attest™ Rapid Readout Biological Indicator System Designed for STERRAD® 100NX® System, STERRAD® NX® System, and STERRAD® 100S System Vaporized Hydrogen Peroxide Sterilizers." https://multimedia.3m.com/mws/media/1306253O/3m-attest-for-vaporized-hydrogen-peroxide-biological-indicator-comparison.pdf

[116] G. McDonnell, "Gas plasma sterilization," in *Russell, Hugo and Ayliffe's: Principles and Practice of Disinfection, Preservation and Sterilization*, A. P. Fraise, J.-Y. Maillard, and S. Sattar Eds.: Wiley, 2013, pp. 333–342.

[117] Advanced Sterilization Products (ASP), "Vaporized hydrogen peroxide gas plasma technology." www.asp.com/en-us/articles-and-white-papers/vaporized-hydrogen-peroxide-gas-plasma-technology-explained

[118] H. Shintani, A. Sakudo, P. Burke, and G. McDonnell, "Gas plasma sterilization of microorganisms and mechanisms of action," *Experimental and Therapeutic Medicine*, vol. 1, no. 5, pp. 731–738, 2010.

[119] M. Diab-Elschahawi, A. Blacky, N. Bachhofner, and W. Koller, "Lumen claims of the STERRAD 100NX sterilizer: Testing performance limits when processing equipment containing long, narrow lumens," *American Journal of Infection Control*, vol. 39, no. 9, pp. 770–4, Nov 2011, doi: 10.1016/j.ajic.2011.01.010

[120] United States Environmental Protection Agency, "Reducing ethylene oxide and glutaraldehyde use," 2002. https://19january2017snapshot.epa.gov/www3/region9/waste/archive/p2/projects/hospital/glutareth.pdf

[121] Steris, "Operator manual for the System 1E® liquid chemical sterilant processing system". https://ww1.steris.com/onbDocs/V537/0/4366282.pdf

[122] Nordion Inc., "JS-10000 hanging tote irradiator," 2011. www.nordion.com/wp-content/uploads/2014/10/GT_JS10000_Irradiator_datasheet.pdf

[123] Gamma Industry Processing Alliance, "A comparison of gamma, e-beam, x-ray and ethylene oxide technologies for the industrial sterilization of medical devices and healthcare products," 2017. https://gipalliance.net/wp-content/uploads/2013/01/GIPA-WP-GIPA-iia-Sterilization-Modalities-FINAL-Version-2017-October-308772.pdf

[124] R. E. Harrington, T. Guda, B. Lambert, and J. Martin, "Sterilization and disinfection of biomaterials for medical devices," in *Biomaterials Science*, W. R. Wagner, S. E. Sakiyama-Elbert, and M. J. Yaszemski Eds.: Elsevier, 2020, pp. 1431–1446.

[125] Far West Technology Inc. www.fwt.com/index.htm (accessed 2023).

[126] Harwell dosimeters Ltd. www.harwell-dosimeters.co.uk/ (accessed 2023).

[127] Proto Labs Inc., "Glass Transition Temperature of Polymers: the importance of glass transition temperatures (Tg) in plastic injection molding." www.protolabs.com/resources/design-tips/glass-transition-temperature-of-polymers

[128] 3Dresyns, "Tg, HDT, and mechanical properties depend on printing specifications." www.3dresyns.com/pages/tg-hdt-and-mechanical-properties-depend-on-printing-specifications#:~:text=Light%20power%2C%20wavelength%2C%20and%20energy,printing%20and%20post%20processing%20specifications

[129] J. Wiseman, T. Rawther, M. Langbart, M. Kernohan, and Q. Ngo, "Sterilization of bedside 3D-printed devices for use in the operating room," *Annals of 3D Printed Medicine*, vol. 5, p. 100045, 2022.

[130] M. Kudla, F. Bachand, J. Moore, and D. Batchelar, "Patient-specific cylinder templates for hybrid interstitial vaginal brachytherapy: Feasibility of automated 3-D design, 3D printing, and dosimetric outlook," *Brachytherapy*, vol. 22, no. 4, pp. 468–476, Jul–Aug 2023, doi: 10.1016/j.brachy.2023.03.002

[131] Y. Kamio *et al.*, "Prototype testing the 3D-printed Montreal split-ring applicator (GYN) using biocompatible materials," *Radiotherapy and Oncology*, vol. 158, pp. S152–S153, 2021.

[132] J. M. Fuentes, M. P. Arrieta, T. Boronat, and S. Ferrándiz, "Effects of steam heat and dry heat sterilization processes on 3D printed commercial polymers printed by fused deposition modeling," *Polymers*, vol. 14, no. 5, p. 855, 2022.

[133] I. Aguado-Maestro, M. De Frutos-Serna, A. González-Nava, A. Merino-De Santos, and M. García-Alonso, "Are the common sterilization methods completely effective for our in-house 3D printed biomodels and surgical guides?," *Injury*, vol. 52, no. 6, pp. 1341–1345, 2021.

[134] B. Segedin, M. Kobav, and H. B. Zobec Logar, "The use of 3D printing technology in gynaecological brachytherapy—A narrative review," *Cancers*, vol. 15, no. 16, p. 4165, 2023.

[135] P. Rynio *et al.*, "Effects of sterilization methods on different 3D printable materials for templates of physician-modified aortic stent grafts used in vascular surgery—A preliminary study," *International Journal of Molecular Sciences*, vol. 23, no. 7, p. 3539, 2022.

[136] J.-F. Boursier, A. Fournet, J. Bassanino, M. Manassero, A.-S. Bedu, and D. Leperlier, "Reproducibility, accuracy and effect of autoclave sterilization on a thermoplastic three-dimensional model printed by a desktop fused deposition modelling three-dimensional printer," *Veterinary and Comparative Orthopaedics and Traumatology*, vol. 31, no. 6, pp. 422–430, 2018.

[137] E. Shaheen, A. Alhelwani, E. Van De Casteele, C. Politis, and R. Jacobs, "Evaluation of dimensional changes of 3D printed models after sterilization: a pilot study," *The Open Dentistry Journal*, vol. 12, pp. 72–79, 2018.

[138] N. Sharma *et al.*, "Effects of steam sterilization on 3D printed biocompatible resin materials for surgical guides—An accuracy assessment study," *Journal of Clinical Medicine*, vol. 9, no. 5, p. 1506, 2020.

[139] S. Grandjean Lapierre *et al.*, "Clinical evaluation of in-house-produced 3D-printed nasopharyngeal swabs for COVID-19 testing," *Viruses*, vol. 13, no. 9, p. 1752, 2021.

[140] J. C. Lindegaard *et al.*, "Individualised 3D printed vaginal template for MRI guided brachytherapy in locally advanced cervical cancer," *Radiotherapy and Oncology*, vol. 118, no. 1, pp. 173–175, 2016.

[141] R. Mohammadi, Z. Siavashpour, S. R. H. Aghdam, S. Fazli, T. Major, and A. A. Rohani, "Manufacturing and evaluation of multi-channel cylinder applicator with 3D printing technology," *Journal of Contemporary Brachytherapy*, vol. 13, no. 1, pp. 80–90, 2021.

[142] W. Zhang, X. Lin, and J. Jiang, "Dimensional accuracy of 3D printing navigation templates of chemical-based sterilisation," *Scientific Reports*, vol. 12, no. 1, p. 1253, 2022.

[143] F. Biltekin, H. Akyol, M. Gültekin, and F. Yildiz, "3D printer-based novel intensity-modulated vaginal brachytherapy applicator: feasibility study," *Journal of Contemporary Brachytherapy*, vol. 12, no. 1, pp. 17–26, 2020.

[144] S. Sekii *et al.*, "Inversely designed, 3D-printed personalized template-guided interstitial brachytherapy for vaginal tumors," *Journal of Contemporary Brachytherapy*, vol. 10, no. 5, pp. 470–477, 2018.

[145] R. Bosc *et al.*, "Bacteriological and mechanical impact of the Sterrad sterilization method on personalized 3D printed guides for mandibular reconstruction," *Scientific Reports*, vol. 11, no. 1, p. 581, 2021.

[146] R. Sethi *et al.*, "Clinical applications of custom-made vaginal cylinders constructed using three-dimensional printing technology," *Journal of Contemporary Brachytherapy*, vol. 8, no. 3, pp. 208–214, 2016.

[147] M. Toro, A. Cardona, D. Restrepo, and L. Buitrago, "Does vaporized hydrogen peroxide sterilization affect the geometrical properties of anatomic models and guides 3D printed from computed tomography images?," *3D Printing in Medicine*, vol. 7, no. 1, pp. 1–10, 2021.

[148] G. Grams, "Sterilization, packaging, and materials: critical considerations (Medical Design Briefs)," 2017. www.medicaldesignbriefs.com/component/content/article/27480-sterilization-packaging-and-materials-critical-considerations

[149] G. Moruzzi, Y. Lou, and R. D. Fritz, "Decimal reduction value (D) from fraction negative experiments via maximum likelihood estimation: An enabling spreadsheet and its implications on methodology and current standards," *Journal of Food Process Engineering*, vol. 45, no. 12, p. e14164, 2022.

[150] M. L. Bernuzzi, "Moist heat sterilization principles." Parenteral Drug Association. www.pda.org.

[151] Mesa Laboratories Inc., "Webinar series: Validation of a Sterilization Process. Part 1 Microorganisms, Sterilization Standards and Definitions." https://info.mesalabs.com/en/sterilization-validation-webinar-series-0?_gl=1*e9nj5v*_gcl_aw*R0NMLjE3MDY3MjQwMjkuQ2p3S0NBaUFfT2V0QmhBdEVpd0FQVGVRWjA1bDRfdGGxQNzZyNWRWTkdZZHp5RE9nZ2FmZ21hY0VWcDFubC1KRVRsUTdYd3p3TXV0YWWx4b0NvV2dRQXZEX0J3RQ..*_gcl_au*MTYxNTgyNjQ5MS4xNzA2NzI0MDI5

[152] J. R. G. Garret Krushefski, "The most important letter in SteriliZation is Z," *Spore News*, vol. 5, no. 5, pp. 1–8, 2008.

[153] B. Larson, "Z-value Calculation," *Spore News*, vol. 3, no. 2, 2006. https://mesalabs.com/spore-news-white-papers/z-value-calculation

[154] Mesa Laboratories Inc., "Population assay instructions for spore suspensions." https://info.mesalabs.com/hubfs/1.%20Sterilization%20and%20Disinfection%20Control/Website/Population%20Assays/TS-405%20v3.pdf

[155] G. McDonnell, "Amsco V-PRO 1 A new sterilization method " presented at the CSC Annual Scientific Conference University of Cambridge, England, 2010.

[156] P.C. Das, "Sterilization mathematics," 2020. https://pres.net.in/wp-content/uploads/2022/11/Sterilization-Mathematics_Palash-Das.pdf

[157] T. Miorini, "Sterilization of medical devices," *World Federation For Hospital Sterilisation Sciences Education*, pp. 1–35, 2008.

[158] S. R. B. Sella *et al.*, "Development of a low-cost sterilization biological indicator using Bacillus atrophaeus by solid-state fermentation," *Applied Microbiology and Biotechnology*, vol. 93, pp. 151–158, 2012.

[159] Ethide Laboratories Inc., "D value vs. Z value calculations for medical devices and product sterilization". https://ethidelabs.com/d-value-vs-z-value-calculations-for-medical-devices-and-product-sterilization/#:~:text=Z%20values%20are%20calculated%20based,reduction%20in%20the%20D%20value

[160] H. N. Prince, "D-values of Bacillus pumilus spores on irradiated devices (inoculated product)," *Applied and Environmental Microbiology*, vol. 36, no. 2, pp. 392–393, 1978.

[161] Terragene Inc., "Biological indicators quality parameters." https://terragene.com/wp-content/uploads/Archivos/productflyers/Biological%20Indicators%20Quality%20Parameters.pdf

[162] sterilizers.com. https://store.sterilizers.com/Chamber-Assy-steam-Bier (accessed 2023).

[163] 3M Co., "Technical information for 3M™ Attest™ Steam Chemical Integrator." www.3m.com/3M/en_US/p/d/b5005158062

[164] Astell Scientific Ltd. "The Astell 33 – 63 Liter Closed Door Drying Steam Sterilizer Range." https://astellautoclaves.com/steam-sterilizers/ (accessed 2023).

[165] Mesa Laboratories Inc., "What is the D-ifference in D-value?," *Spore News*. https://mesalabs.com/spore-news-white-papers/what-is-the-d-ifference-in-d-value

[166] J. R. Gillis, "How much variation should you allow when you specify a D-value?," vol. 2, no. 1. https://mesalabs.com/spore-news-white-papers/d-value-variation

[167] *ISO 18472:2018 Sterilization of Health Care Products—Biological and Chemical Indicators—Test Equipment*, International Organization for Standardization, 2018.

[168] R. Lewis, "Practical guide to autoclave validation," *Pharmaceutical Engineering*, vol. 22, no. 4, pp. 78–88, 2002.

[169] Steris Plc., "Operator manual for AMSCO 600® medium steam sterilizer," 2023. www.manualslib.com/manual/3050288/Steris-Amsco-600-Medium-639v-3.html?page=34

[170] M. Dion and W. Parker, "Steam sterilization principles," *Pharmaceutical Engineering*, vol. 33, no. 6, pp. 1–8, 2013.

[171] Consolidated Sterilizer Systems, "The definitive guide to steam sterilization cycles". https://consteril.com/steam-sterilization-cycles-guide

[172] R. Seavey, "Troubleshooting failed sterilization loads: Process failures and wet packs/loads," *American Journal of Infection Control*, vol. 44, no. 5, pp. e29–e34, 2016.

[173] *ISO 11140-1:2014 Sterilization of health care products—Chemical indicators—Part 1: General requirements*, International Organization for Standardization, 2014.

[174] Steris, "Technical data for VERIFY® Bowie-dick test pack". https://ww1.steris.com/onbDocs/V419/1298/688105.pdf

[175] *ISO 11138-1:2017 Sterilization of health care products: Biological indicators. Part 1: General requirements*, International Organization for Standardization, 2017.

[176] *ISO 11138-2:2017 Sterilization of health care products—Biological indicators—Part 2: Biological indicators for ethylene oxide sterilization processes*, International Organization for Standardization, 2017.

[177] *ISO 11138-3:2017 Sterilization of health care products — Biological indicators—Part 3: Biological indicators for moist heat sterilization processes*, International Organization for Standardization, 2017.

[178] *ISO 11138-4:2017 Sterilization of health care products—Biological indicators—Part 4: Biological indicators for dry heat sterilization processes*, International Organization for Standardization, 2017.

[179] *General Chapter, ⟨55⟩ Biological indicator resistance performance tests*, United States Pharmacopeia, 2005.

[180] European Pharmacopoeia, "5.1.2 Biological indicators and related microbial preparations. European Pharmacopoeia 9.2," ed: EDQM Strasbourg, 2017.

[181] R. Bancroft, "Sterility assurance: Concepts, methods and problems," in *Russell, Hugo and Ayliffe's: Principles and Practice of Disinfection, Preservation and Sterilization*, A. P. Fraise, J.-Y. Maillard, and S. Sattar Eds., 2013, pp. 408–417.

[182] K. McCauley, "Heat shock/heat activation " *Spore News*, vol. 5, no. 3, pp. 1–5. https://mesalabs.com/spore-news-white-papers/heat-shock-heat-activation#:~:text=From%20a%20microbiological%20stand%20point,spores%20inducing%20them%20to%20germinate

[183] Mesa Laboratories Inc. https://mesalabs.com/products/sterilization-cleaning-monitoring (accessed 2023).

[184] Mesa Laboratories Inc., "Webinar Series: Validation of a Sterilization Process. Part 2 Overkill method".

[185] *ISO 17665-1:2006. Sterilization of health care products—Moist heat—Part 1: Requirements for the development, validation and routine control of a sterilization process for medical devices*, International Organization for Standardization, 2006.

[186] *ISO 20857:2010 Sterilization of health care products — Dry heat — Requirements for the development, validation and routine control of a sterilization process for medical devices*, International Organization for Standardization, 2010.

[187] *ISO 11135:2014 Sterilization of health-care products — Ethylene oxide — Requirements for the development, validation and routine control of a sterilization process for medical devices*, International Organization for Standardization, 2014.

[188] *ISO 22441:2022 Sterilization of health care products — Low temperature vaporized hydrogen peroxide — Requirements for the development, validation and routine control of a sterilization process for medical devices*, International Organization for Standardization, 2022.

[189] *ISO 11137-1:2006 Sterilization of health care products—radiation—part 1: Requirements for development, validation and routine control of a sterilization process for medical devices*, International Organization for Standardization, 2006.

[190] *General Chapter, ⟨1229⟩ Sterilization of Compendial Articles*, United States Pharmacopeia, 2020.

[191] K. M. Laurent Berliet, "How to prove a sterility assurance level of 10-6 part 1: the overkill method(s)," *Spore News*. https://mesalabs.com/spore-news-white-papers/the-overkill-methods

[192] S. R. Laurent Berliet, "Why perform a product D-value study? part 1," *Spore News*, vol. 15, no. 1, pp. 1–6. https://info.mesalabs.com/hubfs/1.%20Sterilization%20and%20Disin fection%20Control/Literature%20and%20Campaign%20Material/Spore%20News/21-Literature-Spore-News-Why-Perform-a-Product-D-value-Study-R02.pdf

[193] L. B. Kurt McCauley, "How to prove a sterility assurance level of 10-6 part 2: the biological indicator/bioburden method " *Spore News*. https://mesalabs.com/spore-news-white-papers/how-to-prove-a-sterility-assurance-level-of-10-part-2-the-biological-indicator/bioburden-method

[194] G. Krushefski, "Selecting a biological indicator with appropriate resistance performance to monitor a validated sterilization cycle," *Spore News*, vol. 2, no. 2. https://mesalabs.com/spore-news-white-papers/selecting-bis-for-sterilization-cycle

[195] B. McEvoy and N. J. Rowan, "Terminal sterilization of medical devices using vaporized hydrogen peroxide: A review of current methods and emerging opportunities," *Journal of Applied Microbiology*, vol. 127, no. 5, pp. 1403–1420, Nov. 2019, doi: 10.1111/jam.14412

[196] R. Mueller, "Reusable medical devices: BI selection, overkill validation approaches, and first-time validation pass rates in common healthcare steam sterilization cycles (Medical Design Briefs)," 2018. www.medicaldesignbriefs.com/component/content/article/32817-reusable-medical-devices-bi-selection-overkill-validation-approaches-and-first-time-validation-pass-rates-in-common-healthcare-steam-sterilization-cycles

[197] Ethide Laboratories Inc., "Overkill method for sterilization validation". https://ethidel abs.com/overkill-method-for-sterilization-validation/#:~:text=This%20method%20is%20used%20to,microorganism%20burden%20during%20cleaning%20procedures

[198] Mesa Laboratories Inc., "Webinar Series: Validation of a Sterilization Process. Part 3 Biological Indicator/Bioburden method". https://info.mesalabs.com/en/en/sterilization-validation-webinar-series-bioburden

[199] *ISO 11737-1:2018 Sterilization of health care products—Microbiological methods—Part 1: Determination of a population of microorganisms on products*, International Organization for Standardization, 2018.

CHAPTER 4

3D Printing for External Beam Photon Therapy

Daniel Craft

INTRODUCTION

This chapter introduces readers to the various applications, advantages, and potential limitations of using 3D printing in photon beam radiation therapy. The rationale for using 3D printing is discussed with emphasis on relative benefits of 3D printing compared to conventional manufacturing techniques. A brief summary of various 3D printing technologies is included. Due to the requirements for external beam photon therapy, a brief section addressing printable media analysis is provided. Illustrative clinical case studies are summarized to demonstrate successful applications of 3D printing. These case studies build upon foundational medical physics development and demonstrate practical use in the clinic, with benefits including improvement of treatment accuracy or efficiency, or both.

RATIONALE BEHIND 3D PRINTING TECHNOLOGY

The rationale for implementing a 3D printing program in the radiation oncology clinic for photon beam therapy is multifaceted. The applications of 3D printing may depend on a department's particular processes, personnel, and patient population. A general motivation for 3D printing, however, is the personalization of patient devices through automated and digital processes.

There are several areas in photon beam therapy to which 3D printing can be expected to add significant value. First, if patient-specific devices, such as shields, molds, or bolus are being produced by some manual process in the clinic, 3D printing can eliminate previously unavoidable human imprecision, error, and uncertainty in the manufacturing process, to offer improved geometric accuracy and fit. Second, 3D printing can often improve the efficiency of producing patient specific devices relative to manual methods. Third, 3D printing can equip a department with the tools to create entirely novel devices that were previously impossible or unfeasible. Finally, 3D printed devices can improve

DOI: 10.1201/9781003288404-4

the patient experience significantly by making devices more comfortable, in offering a personalized approach.

Improved Accuracy

One of the most common uses for 3D printing in photon radiation therapy is in creating patient-specific bolus. Conventional solutions for photon bolus include use of uniform thickness standard gel sheet bolus or hand fabrication of a wax or gauze-based bolus. Using 3D printing allows a clinic to design and fabricate a uniform or variable thickness bolus that is much more conformal to a patient's surface without introducing air gaps that are encountered with sheet bolus, or the thickness and density variations that are likely with wax and gauze. While bolus is not the only 3D printable device that can benefit from improved manufacturing accuracy, it provides a compelling case study in the advantages of 3D printing.

It is well known that using standard sheet bolus can cause air gaps between the skin and the bolus. These air gaps introduce undesirable and unpredictable dose distributions by reducing the dose to the skin. Furthermore, these gaps are not reproducible, increasing the overall uncertainty of the radiation plan delivery. Several studies have shown the deleterious effects of unintended air gaps. For example, Lobo et al. [1] showed that the magnitude of underdosing increases with decreasing field size, bolus thickness, and air gap size. Butson et al. [2] reported that, using a 6-MV beam, the skin can be underdosed by as much as 10% with a 1-cm air gap, depending on field size and angle of incidence. A study by Khan et al. [3] showed that surface dose reductions will become clinically significant for air gaps greater than 5 mm. The clinical consequences of these air gaps have also been demonstrated. For one study of 85 post-mastectomy radiotherapy (PMRT) patients, it has been shown that a custom fit bolus was associated with significantly lower incidences of complications relative to the group that received traditional sheet bolus [4].

Using 3D printed bolus can dramatically improve the accuracy and fit of bolus, thereby decreasing air gaps and reducing the uncertainty in the dose received by the patient. The advantages of 3D printed bolus over standard bolus have been demonstrated in various body sites and by numerous groups. Wang et al. [5] compared a custom 3D printed bolus to standard Superflab vinyl sheet bolus for the pelvic region of an anthropomorphic phantom as well as in treating a patient for squamous cell carcinoma of the penile shaft. For both the phantom and the patient, the mean volume of air gap was reduced significantly by using 3D printed bolus. For the phantom study, the air gap volume decreased from 314 cm^3 to 4.56 cm^3. The patient's air gap volume was reduced from 169 cm^3 with the standard bolus to 46.1 cm^3 with a custom bolus. The improved conformality is clearly demonstrated in Figure 4.1. This figure shows the difference in fit between standard and 3D printed bolus, demonstrating the superiority of 3D printed bolus to fit complex patient surfaces. The improved accuracy of fit provided dosimetric advantages with the error in delivered dose reduced from 5.69% with standard bolus to 1.91% with custom bolus.

Other groups have had similar success with custom 3D printed bolus. Robar et al. [6] studied 3D printed bolus versus conventional bolus for a group of 16 patients undergoing chest wall radiotherapy. Among other improvements, the frequency of air gaps greater

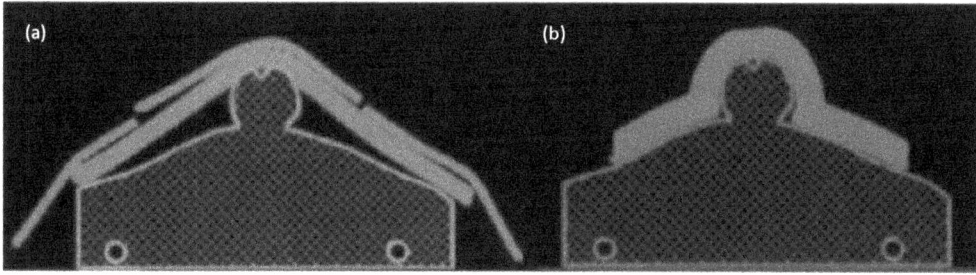

FIGURE 4.1 Axial CT images showing the difference in conformity between (a) standard sheet bolus and (b) 3D printed custom bolus when placed on an anthropomorphic pelvis phantom. Figure sourced with permission from [5].

than 5 mm was reduced from 30% to 13% with custom bolus. Baltz *et al.* [7] developed a technique to produce patient-specific 3D printed bolus for patients undergoing total scalp irradiation. This custom bolus was used to reduce maximum air gaps for treated patients from 1.5 cm with standard sheet bolus to 0.7 cm with 3D printed bolus.

Improved Process Efficiency

The studies cited in the previous section demonstrate clearly that 3D printed bolus improves the accuracy of conforming to the patient surface, compared to generic bolus, a key benefit of personalization of the device. At the same time, the automation of the design and fabrication steps offered by 3D printing can allow improvements in efficiency of workflow.

Given that most radiotherapy courses are fractionated, one important efficiency to be realized is decreasing daily setup time for patients. Because the 3D printed bolus is so much more conformal and fits better, it is much easier to accurately locate on the patient. In the study of Robar *et al.* [6] the mean setup time for their 16 patients was reduced from 104 to 76 seconds. While Wang *et al.* [5] only analyzed a single patient case, they observed that setting up the 3D bolus took them less than one minute, compared to their standard set up which generally takes four to five minutes. They concluded that their 'custom workflow also has the potential to substantially reduce treatment set-up time.'

Using a 3D printing workflow can be more operationally efficient and potentially safer during upstream steps of the radiation therapy process, as well. Designing a 3D printed object for a treatment site can be at least partially automated. An automated or semi-automated 3D printing process offers safety advantages over manual processes, as emphasized in the report of AAPM Task Group 100 on *application of risk analysis methods to radiation therapy quality management* that ranks various methods for reducing risk [8]. The report underlines that automation and computerization of processes is superior to merely following a set protocol or standard policy, and much safer than relying solely on education and training. In the context of adoption of 3D printing, even if a clinic has a clearly defined policy or protocol on producing a device manually, the systematic approach and automation and removal of steps subject to human error should reduce failure modes.

A relevant aspect of introducing 3D printing processes to a clinic are the initial and ongoing costs of the technology and its operation. On one hand, most commercially available 3D printing plastics are relatively inexpensive. Considering only the material costs of fused deposition modeling (FDM) printing, for example, a chest wall bolus printed with polylactic acid (PLA) is 4–6 times less expensive than purchasing generic sheet bolus. However, the cost of the 3D printer must be considered, as well as any repairs and ongoing maintenance. There are many types of 3D printers, some inexpensive and others introducing a significant capital cost. Each introduces operational and material expenses specific to the technology selected. Depending on a clinic's needs and plans for use, that cost could be recovered as custom phantoms and custom patient-specific devices can cost several thousand dollars each, for example. Alternatives to 3D printing at the point-of-care (PoC) exist, for example, currently some institutions opt to design the patient device in-house and outsource the 3D printing itself using an on-demand (OD) service. Chapter 11 of this book provides detail on the decision between printing at the PoC and OD services for obtaining 3D printed devices.

Improvements to Patient Devices Enabled by 3D Printing

The example of 3D printing of bolus provides a use case in the clinic with advantages of improving quality of treatment and efficiency. However, another potential advantage is the incorporation of entirely novel features. An example of this is shown in Figure 4.2, which is taken from Robar *et al.* [6]. This figure illustrates new functionality by incorporating a recess to house an optically stimulated luminescent dosimeters (OSLD) within 3D printed bolus. The design allows the dosimeters to be placed reproducibly between fractions, which is essential to comparing measurement to expected planned dose values. In concept, this approach could be used with any type of *in vivo* dosimeter with knowledge of its dimensions. Commercial, regulatory-approved software (e.g., 3DBolus, Adaptiiv Medical) now includes features like these, allowing known points in the dose distribution to be used for the creation of dosimeter pockets.

Various other enhancements to patient devices are possible. The digital design of bolus, or any patient-specific device, may include patient identifiers or device orientation markings. For example, a bolus could be printed to include the patient's medical record number imprinted on the surface, along with orientation labels to ensure correct placement on the patient. Printing technologies such as Multi Jet Fusion (MJF) support printing in color on any surface of the device, allowing inclusion of identifiers, QR, or bar codes, as well as images chosen by the patient, e.g., in the context of pediatric treatment. Illustrative examples of this are given in Chapter 8 of this book, with a discussion of developments in 3D printed patient immobilization.

Beyond treatment devices, patient-specific anthropomorphic phantoms can be created to test beam delivery in unusual anatomical scenarios, and for end-to-end testing of new clinical techniques. Like the previously mentioned bolus, these devices can be designed with custom dosimeter cavities to enable measurement at predefined locations of interest. Patient-specific tumor models can also be used in staff or patient education.

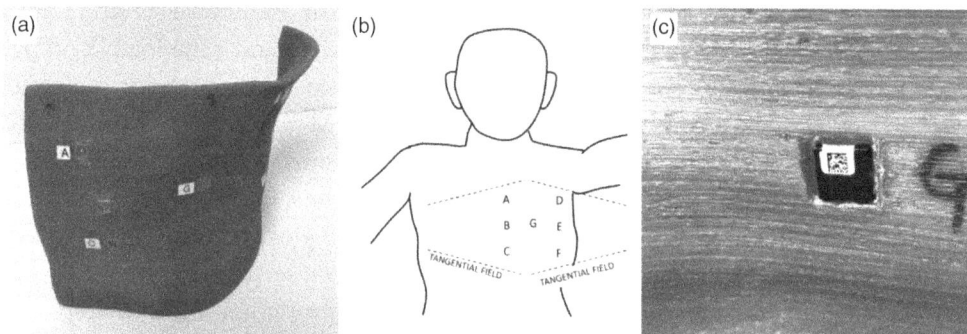

FIGURE 4.2   An example of a helpful modification to an existing device that is possible with 3D printing. A patient-specific bolus (a) can be designed to include specific dosimeter locations (b), with the model designed to contain those dosimeters (c) reproducibly each fraction. Figure sourced with permission from [6].

Effect of 3D Printing on Patient Outcomes

A true metric of success for any new medical technology is the degree of value added in the care of patients. This value can take many forms, from direct improvements on the efficacy of treatment, to improving the patient experience during the medical intervention. Relative to historic manual fabrication methods, 3D printing has proven to increase accuracy of fit of a range of devices and to potentially reduce costs; certainly these advantages serve to benefit patients. To date, however, research into specific clinical outcomes, e.g., tumor control, normal tissue complication, quality of life, or experience during treatment with implementation of 3D printing workflows has been sparse. A review of 3D printing in radiation oncology was conducted in 2020 by Rooney *et al.* [9] that analyzed 103 published studies. According to this report, 50.5% of published studies focused on a dosimetric evaluation of 3D printed materials and devices, while only 5.8% reported on patient comfort outcomes. Only 1.9% reported clinical outcomes, while 19.4% evaluated patient positional accuracy, 10.7% evaluated the cost of printing, and 9.7% reported on workflow efficiencies. The paucity of clinical outcome data likely reflects the recent introduction of 3D printing technologies into radiation oncology departments. Despite most studies being focused on dosimetry, most articles included in this review described potential benefits, including workflow improvements, lowering of costs, and improving patient comfort. Clearly, most research into implementing 3D printing in radiation oncology has been preclinical, focused on feasibility and dosimetry. The underlying value has been discussed primarily qualitatively, with most studies indicating significant value.

COMMON 3D PRINTING TECHNOLOGIES FOR PHOTON BEAM THERAPY

3D printing encompasses a range of disparate technologies with the common characteristic of fabrication with an additive, and usually layer-based process, distinct from subtractive or formative manufacturing techniques. Each individual printing technology will support certain materials with varying physical and radiological properties. 3D printing technology is currently subdivided into seven primary categories, as defined by the joint international standard ISO/ASTM 52900:2021. This standard organizes 3D printing into the following categories: binder jetting, directed energy deposition, material extrusion, material jetting, powder bed fusion, sheet lamination, and vat photopolymerization. Various 3D printing technologies and materials have been described in detail, in Chapter 2.

In planning for integration of 3D printing methods into photon beam therapy, one must make decisions regarding the approach to fabrication, for example, whether the device will be printed directly, or, e.g., whether the printing will produce a mold into which the device will be poured. A clinical department may choose to 3D print devices at the point of care using lower-cost 3D printers, or may outsource this step to an OD service, potentially leveraging more complex printing technologies that support a different range of materials. Finally, various technologies to acquire the digital source data for device design are available.

Options for Printing Devices for Photon Beam Therapy

3D printing can be used to produce patient devices for various applications in photon beam radiation therapy. A survey of common practices in the clinics today will illustrate two main approaches: the final product may be 3D printed directly or may employ 3D printing as just one of several steps in the fabrication process, but may not produce the device directly. Patient-specific bolus can be directly 3D printed, employing material extrusion or MJF technologies, for example, using polyamide 12 (PA12) or thermoplastic polyurethane (TPU) polymers with known radiation qualities. Alternatively, a mold can be 3D printed, which can then be filled with, e.g., a skin-safe silicone material. These various options will produce bolus that will be geometrically similar, but with different material compositions, e.g., differing in electron density, uniformity, and potentially involving different failure modes that can result during fabrication. Examples of bolus that is directly printed and generated with a mold are shown in Figure 4.3.

In additional to technical characteristics of the final product, workflow considerations must be part of this decision-making. PoC printing, e.g., with FDM or stereolithography (SLA) printers in the clinic will allow the practitioner to control the fabrication process as well as the timing, and give access to a range of filament or resin media that offer appropriate material and radiological characteristics. If the device is printed directly, post-processing steps may be required prior to use, including removal of supports, surface preparation, and appropriate cleaning. 3D printing of a mold may be faster than printing a device directly because the mold itself does not require uniformity in its composition and a near-tissue density. This approach is capable of producing devices with mechanical flexibility that is difficult to achieve with most printing technologies, but adds steps of, e.g., silicone pouring, curing, and removal. OD services provide a range of material options, allow design of the device in the clinic, while reducing operational costs and

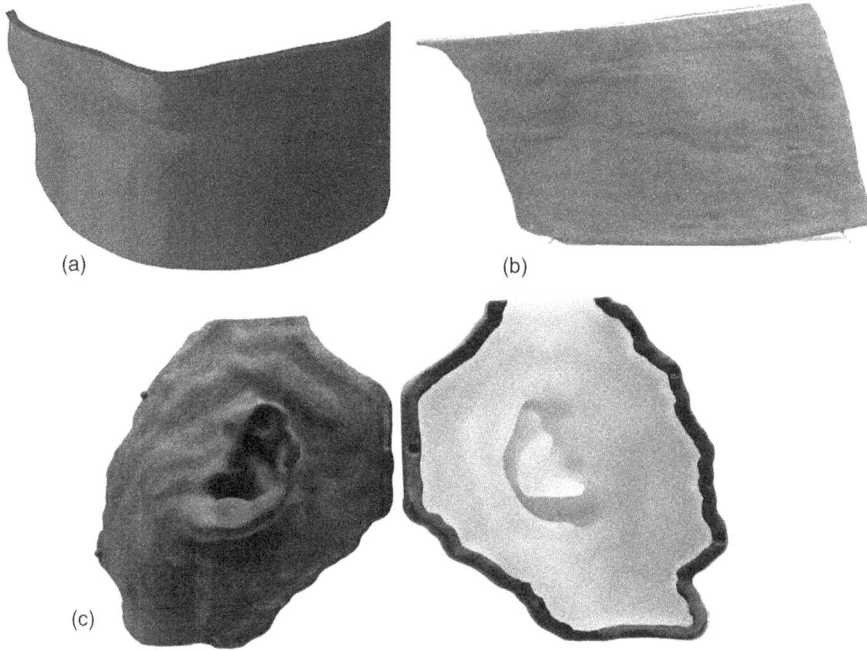

FIGURE 4.3 Examples of options for 3D printed photon bolus including (a) a fused deposition modeling (FDM) printed bolus fabricated using rigid polylactic acid (PLA), (b) a Multi Jet Fusion (MJF) printed bolus using flexible thermoplastic polyurethane (TPU), and (c) a bolus produced by printing a mold using MJF using polyamide 12 (PA12) and filling with highly flexible skin-safe silicone.

needs for equipment and space. Today, OD services may be used to source either directly printed or poured mold options with a time frame that is appropriate to most photon radiotherapy workflows.

Source Data for Patient-Specific Designs

Every 3D printed part originates as a 3D digital model, and the input data for the modeling process can be obtained in various ways. For example, if a medical physicist were to design a new quality assurance (QA) phantom, computer aided design (CAD) tools may be used to define the desired geometry. If the desired product is patient-specific, such as a bolus or an anthropomorphic phantom, the source data must be volumetric or result from surface imaging of the patient. These image data are most often acquired using computed tomography (CT) imaging, magnetic resonance imaging (MRI), or 3D optical surface scanning. For the majority of cases in external beam photon therapy, a planning CT image has already been acquired for treatment planning purposes, and thus it is also used in the design of the device, so long as it offers appropriate spatial resolution and field of view. MRI can be used if it is available and sufficiently free of spatial distortion. Although CT data can be acquired with a slice thickness on the order of 1 mm or less, which is sufficient for most designs, some studies have shown that using an optical surface scanner may be an excellent alternative due to its improved surface resolution.

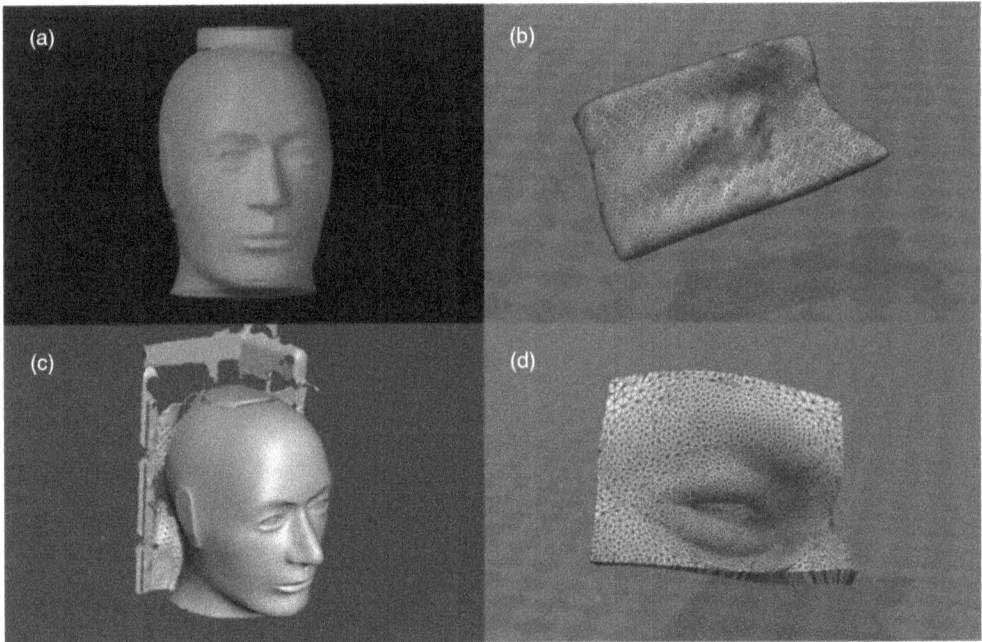

FIGURE 4.4 (a) A volumetric rendering of an anthropomorphic phantom using CT data, compared to a volumetric rendering of the same phantom in (c) derived from surface-scanner data. The resulting custom bolus design for the CT volume is shown in (b), and the bolus shown for the surface-scanner volume is shown in (d). This demonstrates the high level of surface fidelity that is attainable with surface-scanning based imaging compared to CT. Figure sourced with permission from [10].

Figure 4.4 from Dipasquale *et al.* [10] shows the relative accuracy and detail of a CT image of an anthropomorphic phantom versus a surface scan. This approach may provide improved surface sampling and improved fit to the patient.

Compared to a typical minimum CT slice thickness of 0.7 to 1.0 mm, a surface scanner can provide a resolution on the order of tens of micrometers. Additionally, a surface scan can be done very quickly in the simulation position or even during a consultation appointment, allowing for a custom bolus to be ready at the time of CT or MRI simulation. Surface scanning does not use any ionizing radiation and is therefore safe, and various scanning technologies are available including structured light imaging or photogrammetry, even on smartphones [11]. Despite these advantages of a surface scanning, the CT scan may be used given that it is 'free' information, i.e., it is performed as part of the normal radiotherapy planning workflow and doesn't require procuring and installing an additional new piece of equipment.

SPECIAL CONSIDERATIONS OF 3D PRINTED MATERIALS FOR CLINICAL USE

A wide range of material options is available for most 3D printing technologies, e.g., filaments for FDM printing, resins for SLA, and polymer powders for MJF. Whenever a new material is considered for clinical use, it is important to thoroughly commission it with a focus on material suitability, physical and radiological properties.

3D Printing Material Selection in Photon Radiotherapy

Before any dosimetric analysis is conducted, a thorough evaluation of candidate materials should be conducted. Given the range of 3D printing applications in radiation oncology to date, multiple references citing materials for FDM, SLA, MJF, and other technologies exist, providing guidance to new clinical users [9]. After selecting a material, if printing is to be done at the PoC, one must assess environmental requirements, e.g., the provision of sufficient ventilation, depending on the material used. It is advisable to acquire a limited quantity of the selected media, to print a few small test objects as well as objects that are typical of the planned application. For example, first tests may include small geometric objects with directly measurable dimensions. Additional test prints may include typical boluses or applicator geometries, depending on the intended use. Initial testing should assess the reliability and consistency of printing, i.e., quantifying the 'success rate' in achieving a viable print. Most 3D printers require configuration of various settings controlling the fabrication. For FDM printing, for example, these include the travel speed during printing and translating without printing, layer height, extruder flow rate, nozzle temperature, infill percentage, infill pattern, and details of the substrate of the printed object, i.e., whether a raft or a brim is used in the first printed layers to ensure adhesion to the build plate. These settings are printer-specific but have been included in many publications for common printers [9]. Necessary post-processing steps, e.g., removal of supports or finishing of the surface, should be assessed. After determining printing parameters and post-processing requirements, an estimate of the total time required can be made to determine whether these methods will be feasible for meeting the anticipated timelines and demand in the clinic. Once this assessment is completed, the radiological properties of 3D printed materials and devices may be evaluated.

3D Printing Material Radiological Evaluation

The next step in commissioning a new material and 3D printing process is to evaluate the radiological properties of the material for the applicable use case. For external beam photon therapy, this is an essential exercise, with requirements extending well beyond those that would be relevant, e.g., to printing anatomical models or geometric phantoms. It is important to note that the results of radiological characterization of a material will be specific to the material as well as to the settings of the 3D printer used, and thus changing those settings would likely warrant recommissioning. With fixed material and printer settings, some variability in the fabricated product can still occur, e.g., in terms of dimensional stability or material uniformity, and these should be assessed by printing a sufficient sample of parts and measuring these parameters.

A vital step during material/printer radiological evaluation is to determine the relationship between the measured Hounsfield Unit (HU) and physical density. This can be done by printing a set of test parts and by imaging with CT. Slab-type geometries can be useful since their dimensions can be measured directly, and following a

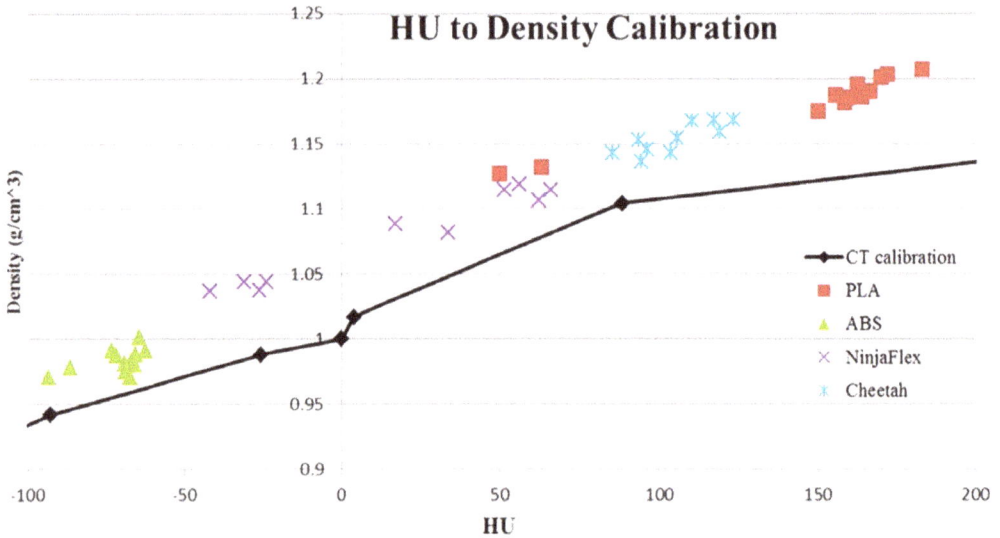

FIGURE 4.5   A standard CT calibration curve may fail to model a selection of plastics commonly used in material extrusion 3D printing. Additionally, it can be seen that the exact properties of 3D printed objects can vary, even when composed of the same material. Figure sourced with permission from [12].

measurement of mass, physical density can be determined. By calculating a mean HU value within a selected region of interest in CT image data, one may plot density versus HU, as shown in Figure 4.5. This example demonstrates an attribute exhibited by some available FDM-printed plastics: since they differ in elemental composition from human tissues, measurements may deviate somewhat from expected values on a standard CT calibration curve. This measurement would inform the medical physicist in determining whether density overrides need to be performed in the treatment planning system to ensure accurate dose calculations in that material. It is important to note this behavior is material dependent, and some materials have been shown to occur as expected on a CT calibration curve [12].

It is important to validate treatment planning system calculations within, or immediately below the material (e.g., in the case of patient bolus) to verify the actual HU/density assigned in the treatment planning system. For example, Burleson [13] showed measured electron and mass density ratios occurring on the CT calibration curve, corresponding to an HU of 260 (Figure 4.6). When this value is used in calculation of a percent depth dose (PDD) in the treatment planning system and compared to measurement, agreement to within approximately 0.5% is obtained (Figure 4.7).

In addition to the controlled measurements described above, end-to-end testing can be performed during the commissioning process, e.g., using *in vivo* dosimeters contained in printed pockets in bolus, with comparison of measurement to planned dose values at predetermined locations [6]. This allows for measurements with more complex and realistic geometries compared to slab-type setups.

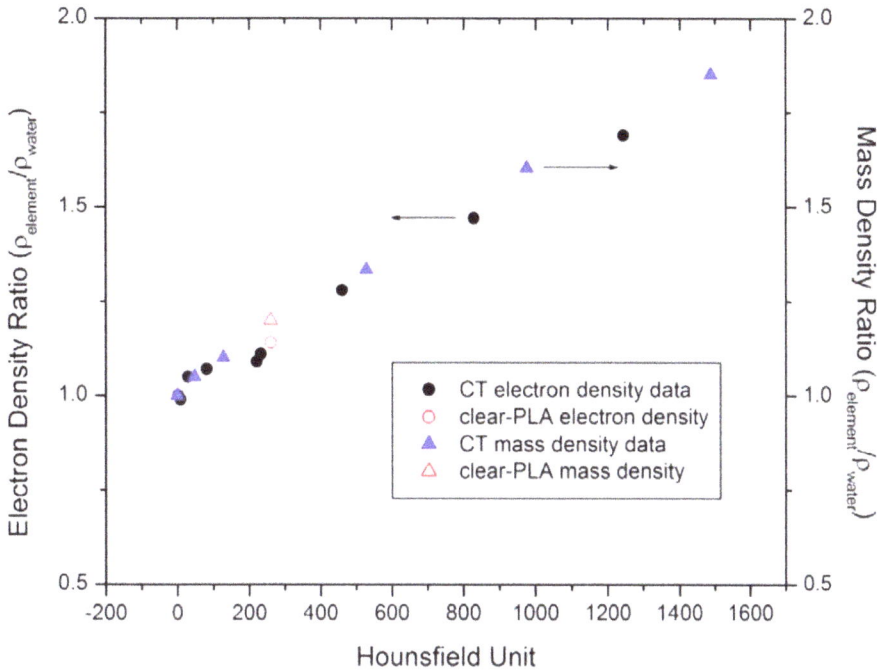

FIGURE 4.6   Electron density and mass density relative to water as a function of CT Hounsfield Units. In this example, the values for printed PLA (hollow symbols) fall close to the measured CT curve used in treatment planning (solid symbols). Figure sourced with permission from [13].

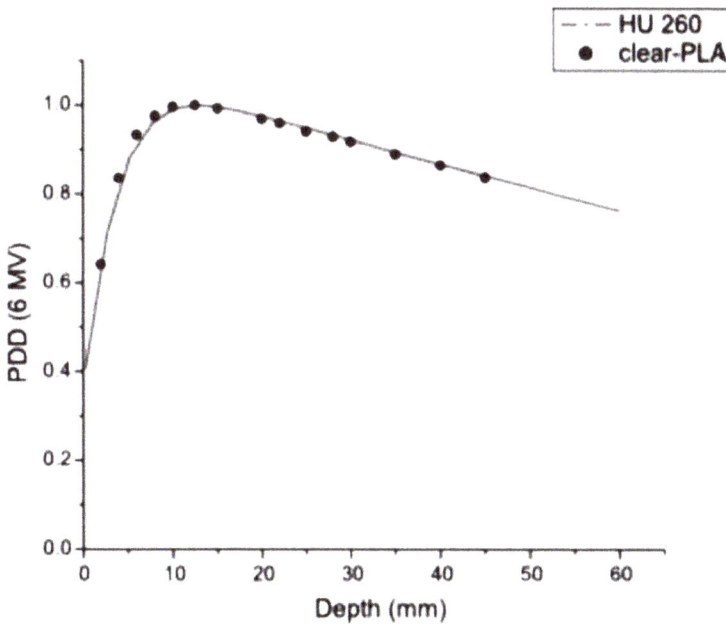

FIGURE 4.7   PDD curves for a 4×4 cm^2 6-MV photon beam, comparing measurements for printed clear PLA with treatment planning calculations when the material HU value is set to 260, producing agreement to within approximately 0.5%. Figure sourced with permission from [13].

It is important to note that the intended use of the material will determine the magnitude of dosimetric effect of any inaccuracy of density assigned to the device in the treatment planning system. For example, if the printed material will be used to create bolus limited to 0.5-mm thickness, a given inaccuracy or uncertainty in density will cause a small dosimetric effect, potentially within allowable treatment planning uncertainties. However, if the material is going to be used to create a large phantom for end-to-end testing, for example, the dosimetric effect may be significant.

Uniformity of Density of Printed Devices

Figure 4.5 also demonstrates variability observed for four different printed materials [12]. For use in photon beam therapy, the printed device must exhibit an expected density within tolerance, but also sufficient uniformity of density throughout its volume. Variability in the density or uniformity may be observed from sample to sample, or even within a single printed object. This may be caused by changes in printer settings, printer malfunction, inconsistencies in feedstock material, or environmental factors such as humidity. An example of unwanted variability in density is shown in Figure 4.8a where a 5-mm-thick FDM-printed PLA chestwall bolus has been imaged using CT, revealing multiple voids as viewed in an axial slice. In Figure 4.8b the same bolus has been reprinted using a TPU material using MJF, showing a different density but excellent material uniformity. The commissioning process should involve printing representative devices in sufficient quantity to characterize expected variability in this regard, and an assessment of the frequency of outliers.

Quality Assurance

As for any technology that is critical in the treatment of patients, 3D printers, printer media, and printed devices must be subject to scheduled and periodic QA. The rigor of QA should be commensurate with the potential magnitude of errors that may be caused by failure modes, the likelihood of errors occurring, and the probability of detecting those

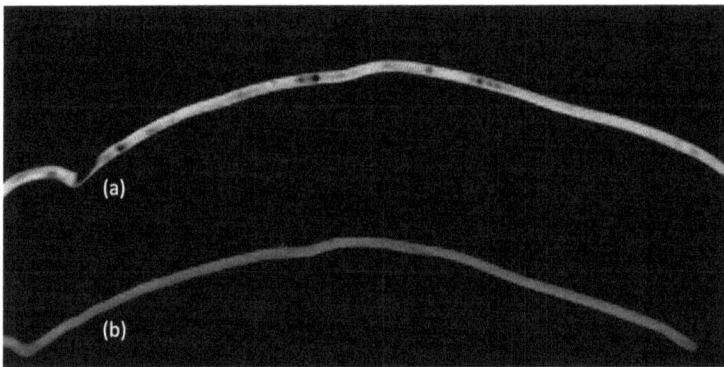

FIGURE 4.8   (a) An example of an axial slice of a 5 mm chestwall bolus printed with PLA using FDM, showing the presence of unwanted material nonuniformity. In (b) the same bolus was reprinted with TPU using MJF, showing excellent material uniformity.

errors. Any observed adverse events or near misses should be recorded and registered in the department's event reporting system. Specific QA guidelines from manufacturers should be followed, but a QA program specific to the equipment and materials used and the devices printed should be developed and implemented. Task group 336 of the American Association of Physicists in Medicine (AAPM) focuses on QA for 3D printing in medical imaging and radiation therapy applications.

A QA program may be established by drawing upon examples already in the radiation oncology department. The program may include machine-specific QA, where the machine in this case is the printer/material combination, as well as patient-specific QA, i.e., testing of individual devices produced. Depending on the stability of the printing, and according to the experience of the clinic, a monthly QA program may be established, e.g., including printing of a standard test object designed to allow evaluation of dimensional accuracy, printed density, scanned HU, and material uniformity. This is analogous to, e.g., monthly QA of a linear accelerator or imaging platform in the clinic. Annually, a complete end-to-end test may be performed using an anthropomorphic phantom to design, print, and deliver a treatment using custom 3D printed bolus.

At the patient level, a QA procedure should be established for every printed device. This may include basic checks for dimensional accuracy (where measurable), measured mass compared to expected mass given the nominal density, and material uniformity, for example. These basic measurements may trigger more in-depth QA if values are detected out of tolerance; for example, CT imaging can be performed to examine for nonuniformities or defects. Alternately, cone beam CT (CBCT) can be performed on first fraction as a QA step examining both the device and correct placement on the patient. A radiation oncology department may elect to apply these QA checks at a high frequency (e.g., for every patient) upon initiation of the 3D printing program and may decrease the frequency with gained experience and regular printer/material QA.

The patient-specific QA steps implemented for 3D printed devices will differ and may be reduced significantly if the 3D printing is outsourced using an OD service. Following fabrication, the 3D printing service may issue a detailed QC certificate-of-analysis showing dimensional accuracy of the fabricated device relative to the design based on high-resolution optical surface imaging, as well as measured mass compared to the expected value, with tolerances applied (e.g., Adaptiiv On Demand, Adaptiiv Medical, Halifax, Canada). This relieves the practitioner of these steps, however the responsibility of accuracy of treatment remains with the clinical team.

CLINICAL CASE STUDIES

Semiflexible Bolus

In 2022, Malone *et al.* published a retrospective study describing their experience with 3D printing in their radiation oncology department and the quality of fit for the first 60 patients treated with patient-specific 3D printed bolus [14]. This study provided an excellent overview of the utility and value of 3D printing over standard sheet and non-custom bolus options. Enrolled patients were categorized into four treatment sites: head and neck

(H&N), pelvis, scalp, and extremities. Based on CBCT imaging at each treated fraction, two observers graded the quality of the bolus fit as poor, acceptable, good, or perfect, according to whether maximal air gaps were larger than 10 mm, 5–10 mm, 1–5 mm, or negligible, respectively. The study evaluated whether fit differed between treatment sites and identified any significant change over the course of treatment. The authors of the study used a relatively inexpensive FDM printer and a common semiflexible TPU filament to print boluses. They used the bolus design tool in their clinical treatment planning system and exported the digital structure to third-party software to convert that design into a 3D printable file. They reported no print failures or issues with the material; however, they did emphasize appropriate bolus design is critical for an accurate fit. The patient's body contour must be accurate in the planning system, including any external immobilization devices. They noted at least one example of a poor fit that was caused by an incorrect body contour. Their overall analysis included 627 distinct fractions. Of these 75.1% of all fractions were rated either good or perfect, 20.6% were acceptable, and 4.3% were rated poor. However, the distribution of grades was not consistent across treatment sites. When considering only pelvis treatments, 20% of fractions were rated poor. Also, H&N and scalp fractions were perfect 22% and 30% of the time, respectively, while pelvis fractions achieved the highest grade only 3% of the time. When they considered changes to fit scores over the treatment course duration, there was no significant trend, but they did note that pelvis cases showed higher variability of fit. The study concluded that using 3D printed bolus not only improved the overall fit, but also replaced labor intensive and imprecise processes of placing manual bolus. Although it was indicated that the total time required may be longer for 3D printing compared to manual methods, the printing itself only happens once and with minimal staff interaction. Treatment staff preferred 3D printed bolus over conventional techniques, reporting simple and fast setup in to placing bolus on patients for each fraction.

Silicone Bolus Fabricated Using a 3D Printed Mold

Instead of 3D printing a bolus directly, it is possible to instead 3D print a mold, then pour silicone to form the bolus. The main advantage is provision of a soft, flexible bolus that is highly conformal to the surface and comfortable for the patient. An additional advantage of the mold approach is completion of 3D printing in a fraction of the time compared to a directly printed bolus given that the mold can be printed at a lower infill, or material density. A skin-safe silicone may be very soft and flexible, e.g., with Shore hardness of 0–30, compared to a Shore hardness of A-88 for a directly printed (yet slightly flexible) TPU bolus. Boluses with softness/flexibility rivaling that of silicone are technically difficult to print directly, requiring much more time, or more sophisticated printing technology. A study by Pollmann et al. [15] describes a workflow to create mold-based silicone boluses, as well as an analysis of the occurrence of air gaps for treatment of 25 H&N patients. Figure 4.9 shows the design and fabrication of a mold-based silicone bolus. Compared to a directly printed bolus, for a mold bolus design there is an additional step to convert the bolus object into a negative, and to create the design for a mold, shown in Figure 4.9b. This can be automated by commercial applications (3DBolus, Adaptiiv

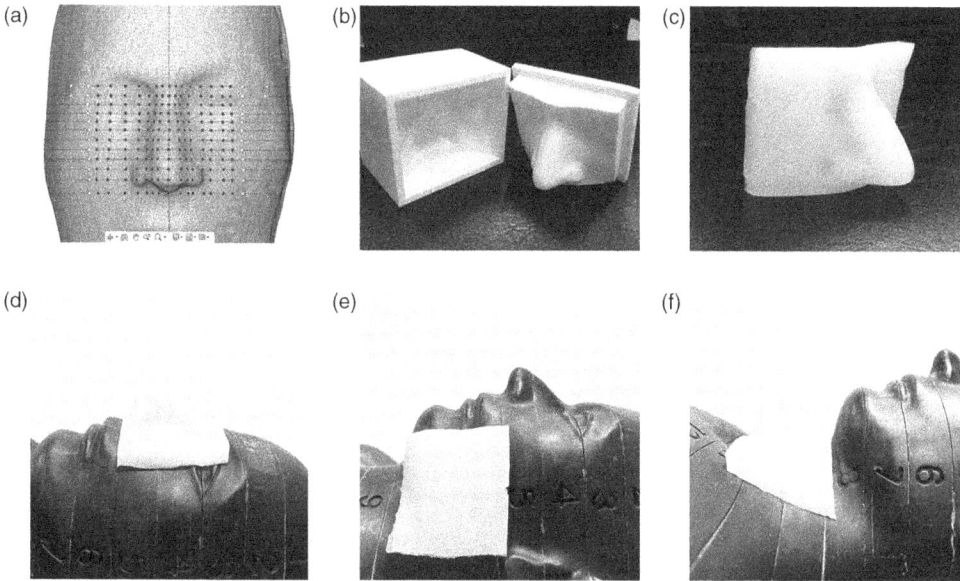

FIGURE 4.9 The process of producing silicone rubber bolus from a mold starting with (a) a model of the bolus area, (b) creation of the 3D printed bolus shell, and (c) the completed silicone rubber bolus. The bottom row shows a silicone bolus on a phantom's nose (d), cheek (e), and neck (f). Figure sourced with permission from [16].

Medical, Halifax, Canada). The bolus mold can be printed with low infill using inexpensive and rapidly printable rigid plastic, allowing for fast fabrication. Once the mold has been printed, a skin-safe silicone mixture is injected and allowed to cure. The curing time is highly variable depending on exactly what mixture is used. Times reported in these studies range from 30 minutes [15] to 24 hours [16]. QA may differ for mold boluses as the material uniformity of the final part is dependent on the pouring and curing of silicone, not variations in printing.

Pollmann *et al.* used this mold procedure to produce 5-mm thick bolus for 25 patients, then performed air gap assessment and *in vivo* dosimetry using radiochromic film to compare to generic sheet bolus. They found that the surface dose accuracy was improved by 2.45% with custom bolus relative to standard bolus (p = 0.038). Air gaps were reduced significantly from 7.9 mm on average to 3.5 mm with custom bolus (p = 0.001). The authors indicated that the immobilization mask was the limiting factor in some cases, interfering with the custom bolus contact with the skin, and that in the future they intend to fabricate the bolus before making the mask to avoid that issue.

Total Scalp Bolus

Scalp bolus was one of the four anatomical categories in the study by Malone *et al.* [14] and found to be an appropriate treatment site for custom 3D printed bolus. A study by Baltz *et al.* [7] reported on an innovative workflow for creating patient-specific 3D printed total scalp that leverages several aspects 3D printing technology to improve treatment and the patient experience. In this workflow, the authors explain that since the scalp is a rigid anatomy, previous imaging can be sourced to design the bolus prior to the

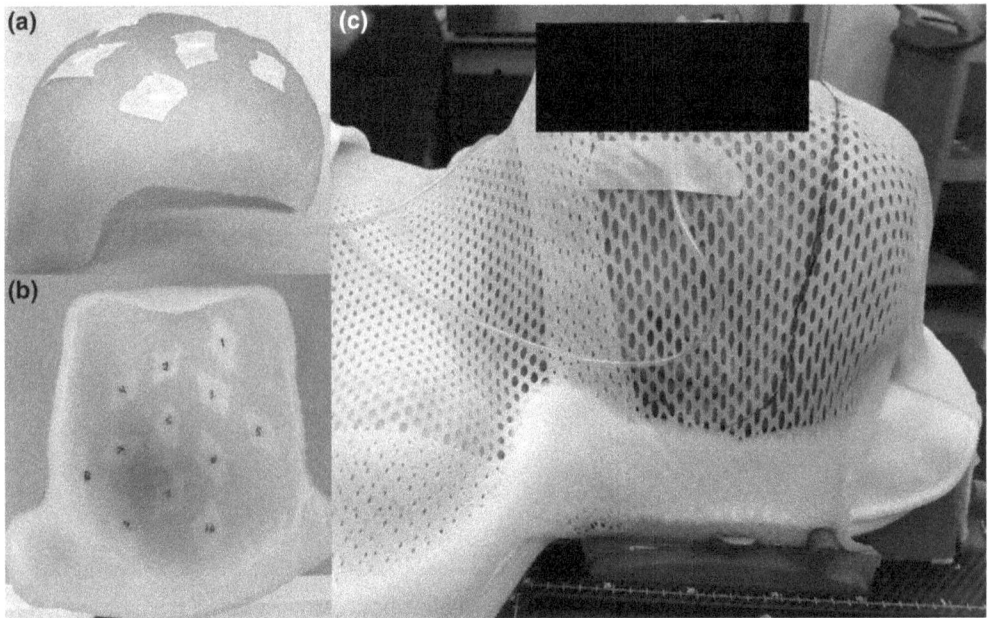

FIGURE 4.10   Patient-specific 3D printed total scalp bolus (a), with in vivo dosimetry locations marked (b), shown fitted on the patient during CT simulation (c). Note that the workflow of printing the custom bolus designed from previous imaging allows the bolus to be placed under the immobilization mask at the time of simulation. Figure sourced with permission from [7].

patient simulation for treatment planning. In this way the bolus can be fit to the patient during simulation, allowing for it to be placed under the immobilization mask as seen in Figure 4.10. In the clinical case described, they used a previous diagnostic CT data set to design the scalp bolus. This reduced the time for simulation to only 20 minutes, compared to the previous workflow that involved fitting several pieces of bolus in a swimming cap, and which took an hour to complete.

Another innovative aspect of this work was the generation of a script executed in the planning system that automatically designs the total scalp bolus and exports it a file for 3D printing. This allowed generation of the 3D printable model in approximately 10 minutes. This automation is complimentary to 3D printing technology and highlights an advantage of digitizing of a previously analog process. The automated approach enforces consistency of design, reduces errors, and expedites the design step. Unlike most cases presented in this chapter that use FDM printers, this study employed a material jetting printer and a material called Agilus-60 to produce the bolus. The authors found that the material to be soft, flexible, and radiologically tissue equivalent. A dosimetric analysis was performed by placing *in vivo* thermoluminescent dosimeters (TLDs) on an anthropomorphic head phantom and on the skin of a treated patient. The average dose error was 2.4% for the phantom study and 5.3% for the patient over three fractions. All measurements were within 10 cGy of the prescribed dose. Air gaps were reduced from 1 to 1.5 cm observed with non-customized bolus to a maximum of 7 mm on the patient with the 3D printed bolus. Overall, their semi-automated workflow to design and fabricate patient specific bolus was superior to their previous standard of care in fit, dose accuracy, and time requirements.

Patient-Specific Phantoms for Photon Therapy

Creation of patient-specific phantoms was among the first 3D printing applications to be developed in radiation oncology. While many commercial phantoms exist for a variety of purposes, 3D printing is a viable method for creating phantoms modeled after real patient anatomy. This allows medical physicists to perform measurements on realistic anatomical geometries. Chapter 10 of this book focuses on 3D printing of phantoms for a broad range of applications. Two examples in photon beam therapy are provided below.

Craft *et al.* [17] published a study describing the fabrication of a phantom based on the CT simulation of a post-mastectomy patient undergoing treatment for breast cancer. Their phantom was designed to be used for end-to-end testing of various delivery techniques for PMRT. The phantom was designed by truncating all anatomy inferior to the navel or superior to the base of the neck. The remaining volume was then sliced in sagittal planes and pockets for dosimeters were incorporated throughout the chest wall, heart, and contralateral breast. The phantom was printed using an inexpensive material extrusion printer and PLA. With application of a correction factor, PLA was found to be useable as a tissue substitute. With the generalizable design, the phantom could be used to deliver and compare a variety of experimental delivery techniques. The study reports that registered images of the assembled phantom and the original patient showed excellent agreement.

Another study describing the use of custom 3D printed phantoms was published by Yoon *et al.* [18]. This study was designed to evaluate the dosimetric accuracy of respiratory-gated volumetric modulated arc therapy (VMAT) for lung stereotactic body radiation therapy (SBRT) treatment. The 3D printed phantoms were not the main focus of the study but essential components in recreating the simulation conditions of the geometry of an actual patient's tumor. To validate dosimetric accuracy, six heterogenous lung phantoms were 3D printed. As seen in Figure 4.11, these phantoms did not include the full patient anatomy, only the tumor and immediately proximal tissue. The phantoms were designed to incorporate radiochromic film and to be received by a commercial respiratory motion platform, allowing motion of the printed tumor to emulate actual respiratory motion. This arrangement allowed the authors to compare the accuracy of the delivered treatment with and without motion, with homogenous or heterogenous phantoms, and using different dose calculation algorithms. While the focus was respiratory-gated VMAT delivery, this study shows the utility of 3D printing in developing custom phantoms for a range of clinical applications.

Immobilization

The use of immobilization is common in radiation therapy to limit inter- and intra-fraction motion for patients. For patients treated for cranial or H&N indications, immobilization is achieved using thermoplastic masks that are manually molded to the patient's head during the simulation imaging session. 3D printing of immobilization is an emerging

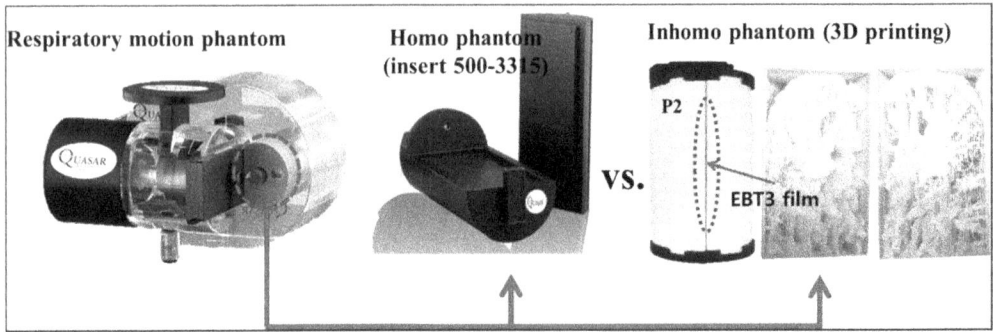

FIGURE 4.11   A demonstration of using a custom 3D printed anatomical lung phantom used in conjunction with existing commercial phantom equipment. The phantom based on patient anatomy was printed to reflect the size and shape of an insert into a commercial respiratory motion phantom. Figure sourced with permission from [18].

technology that may provide benefits to the accuracy of treatment and workflow. A paper by Mattke *et al.* [19] outlines some of these advantages and their experience treating six patients with 3D printed H&N immobilization masks. Source data for immobilizer design can arise from pre-treatment diagnostic MRI, leveraging diagnostic CT data, or via optical surface imaging, allowing the immobilizer to be fabricated prior to simulation. This eliminates the manual fabrication that requires time and effort by the patient and multiple therapists. Importantly, digital design and manufacture will eliminate human error associated with these steps. In concept, customization will become possible, for example, a cut-out for bolus, or openings for patients with claustrophobia. In fact, the authors of the study state that reducing stress and fear for patients was a motivator for 3D printed mask development [19]. While multiple 3D printing technologies may fabricate immobilizers, MJF is capable of printing these devices with high dimensional accuracy and reliability, and can leverage materials with low build-up characteristics to minimize unwanted skin dose [20]. Further detail on immobilization is provided in Chapter 8.

Oral Stents

Oral radiation stents are devices used to position a patient to reduce the incidence and severity of radiation induced oral mucositis that often occurs during radiotherapy of the H&N. A study by Zaid *et al.* [21] describes a workflow to create patient-specific oral stents using a combination of 3D scanning and 3D printing techniques.

Traditionally, fabrication of custom stents is both time consuming and laborious. First, a stone model of the patient's dental impressions is created, a wax model is constructed by hand from that model, which is then used to form a final stent out of resin. While this process could be streamlined by using CT imaging to reconstruct the jaws and teeth, this is prone to artifacts proximal to dental work. The technique developed in the study by Zaid uses an optical 3D scanner to create a digital model of the patient's jaw anatomy by scanning the stone model of the dental impressions. As shown in Figure 4.12, a digital negative is added to the model to create a stent model, which is then 3D printed. This

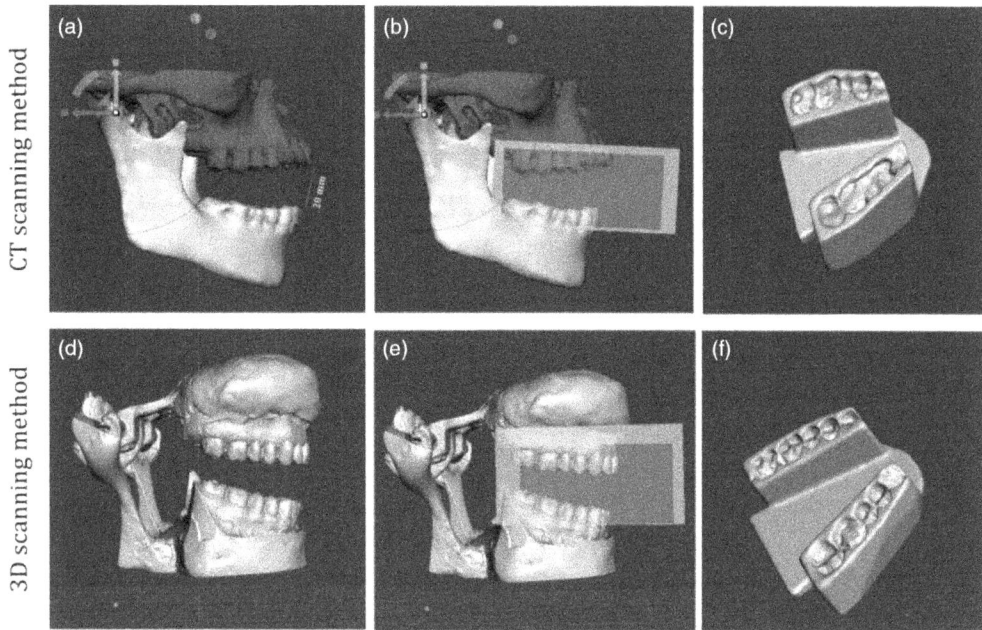

FIGURE 4.12 CT scanning-based (a and b) vs. 3D scanning-based (d and e) processes for designing the final oral stents. The completed stent from CT data is shown in (c) and from 3D scanning shown in (f). Note the much higher detail available from 3D scanning relative to CT. Figure sourced with permission from [21].

study created and tested the fit of stents for three patients using both 3D scanning and CT data as the source for the jaw model. Stents were printed using a vat photopolymerization printer and a dental compatible resin.

The fit of stents created using 3D scanning as the source data was superior to stents based on CT data. Additionally, the optical 3D scanning workflow was faster and less prone to user error because it did not depend on accurate manual segmentation of the jaw bones and teeth, nor was it susceptible to imaging artifacts. This study demonstrates that 3D printing can be used to create novel tools for radiation oncology and that the source data used for the production of those devices is an important consideration.

Veterinary

Most clinicians employing 3D printing to improve patient care in photon radiotherapy are focused on human patients, but the customization afforded by 3D printing also provides solutions for veterinary care. A paper by Martin *et al.* [22] examined one veterinary clinic's experience and the clinical efficacy of using 3D printed bolus compared to standard sheet bolus. All custom boluses were printed with a material extrusion printer and TPU filament. QA was performed on each bolus through visual inspection and using CT to verify that HU values were within 100 HU of expected. By performing CBCT imaging during the treatment course and subsequent dose recalculation, this study quantified differences in fit of bolus and assessed dosimetric effect of air gaps. The study sample included of five dogs and four cats. Patients were treated with both commercial sheet bolus and custom 3D printed bolus in different fractions, with CBCT imaging. Findings demonstrated that for treatments of tumor volumes within the head, 3D printed bolus decreased both air gaps and the dosimetric uncertainty of radiation delivery. The maximum air gaps for head treatments were significantly different between the standard and custom boluses. For sheet bolus, 25% of CBCT slices exhibited a 5 mm gap or larger, and this was reduced to 7% using 3D printed bolus. Overall, the median sheet bolus air gap was 3.6 mm, and for 3D printed bolus it was 2.3 mm. Significant improvements were reported for the cranium, but differences seen for extracranial anatomy were not conclusive. In summary, this study demonstrates the utility of 3D printed bolus over standard sheet bolus, especially in the case of complex patient setup.

REFERENCES

[1] Lobo D, Banerjee S, Srinivas C, et al. Influence of air gap under bolus in the dosimetry of a clinical 6 MV photon beam. *J Medical Phys*. 2020;45:175–181.

[2] Butson MJ, Cheung T, Yu P, et al. Effects on skin dose from unwanted air gaps under bolus in photon beam radiotherapy. *Radiat Meas*. 2000;32:201–204.

[3] Khan Y, Villarreal-Barajas JE, Udowicz M, et al. Clinical and dosimetric implications of air gaps between bolus and skin surface during radiation therapy. *J Cancer Ther*. 2013;4:1251–1255.

[4] Anderson PR, Hanlon AL, Fowble BL, et al. Low complication rates are achievable after postmastectomy breast reconstruction and radiation therapy. *Int J Radiat Oncol Biol Phys*. 2004;59:1080–1087.

[5] Wang KM, Rickards AJ, Bingham T, et al. Technical note: Evaluation of a silicone-based custom bolus for radiation therapy of a superficial pelvic tumor. *J Appl Clin Med Phys*. 2022;23:e13538.

[6] Robar JL, Moran K, Allan J, et al. Intrapatient study comparing 3D printed bolus versus standard vinyl gel sheet bolus for postmastectomy chest wall radiation therapy. *Pract Radiat Oncol*. 2018;8:221–229.

[7] Baltz GC, Chi PM, Wong P, et al. Development and validation of a 3D-printed bolus cap for total scalp irradiation. *J Appl Clin Med Phys*. 2019;20:89–96.

[8] Huq MS, Fraass BA, Dunscombe PB, et al. The report of task group 100 of the AAPM: Application of risk analysis methods to radiation therapy quality management: TG 100 report. *Med Phys*. 2016;43:4209–4262.

[9] Rooney MK, Rosenberg DM, Braunstein S, et al. Three-dimensional printing in radiation oncology: A systematic review of the literature. *J Appl Clin Med Phys*. 2020;21:15–26.

[10] Dipasquale G, Poirier A, Sprunger Y, et al. Improving 3D-printing of megavoltage X-rays radiotherapy bolus with surface-scanner. *Radiat Oncol Lond Engl*. 2018;13:203.

[11] LeCompte MC, Chung SA, McKee MM, et al. Simple and rapid creation of customized 3-dimensional printed bolus using iPhone X True depth camera. *Pract Radiat Oncol*. 2019;9:e417–e421.

[12] Craft DF, Kry SF, Balter P, et al. Material matters: Analysis of density uncertainty in 3D printing and its consequences for radiation oncology. *Med Phys*. 2018;45:1614–1621.

[13] Burleson S, Baker J, Hsia AT, et al. Use of 3D printers to create a patient-specific 3D bolus for external beam therapy. *J Appl Clin Med Phys*. 2015;16:166–178.

[14] Malone C, Gill E, Lott T, et al. Evaluation of the quality of fit of flexible bolus material created using 3D printing technology. *J Appl Clin Med Phys*. 2022;23:e13490.

[15] Pollmann S, Toussaint A, Flentje M, et al. Dosimetric evaluation of commercially available flat vs. self-produced 3D-conformal silicone boluses for the head and neck region. *Frontiers Oncol*. 2022;12:881439.

[16] Chatchumnan N, Kingkaew S, Aumnate C, et al. Development and dosimetric verification of 3D customized bolus in head and neck radiotherapy. *J Radiat Res*. 2022;63:428–434.

[17] Craft DF, Howell RM. Preparation and fabrication of a full-scale, sagittal-sliced, 3D-printed, patient-specific radiotherapy phantom. *J Appl Clin Med Phys*. 2017;18:285–292.

[18] Yoon K, Jeong C, Kim S, et al. Dosimetric evaluation of respiratory gated volumetric modulated arc therapy for lung stereotactic body radiation therapy using 3D printing technology. *Plos One*. 2018;13:e0208685.

[19] Mattke M, Rath D, Häfner MF, et al. Individual 3D-printed fixation masks for radiotherapy: First clinical experiences. *Int J Comput Ass Rad*. 2021;16:1043–1049.

[20] Robar JL, Kammerzell B, Hulick K, et al. Novel multi jet fusion 3D-printed patient immobilization for radiation therapy. *J Appl Clin Med Phys*. 2022;23:e13773.

[21] Zaid M, Bajaj N, Burrows H, et al. Creating customized oral stents for head and neck radiotherapy using 3D scanning and printing. *Radiat Oncol Lond Engl*. 2019;14:148.

[22] Martin TW, Boss M-K, LaRue SM, et al. 3D-printed bolus improves dose distribution for veterinary patients treated with photon beam radiation therapy. *Can Vet J La Revue Veterinaire Can*. 2020;61:638–644.

CHAPTER 5

3D Printing for Electron Therapy

Tiffany Phillips

INTRODUCTION

Three-dimensional (3D) printing applications have been growing in radiation oncology and have become useful in a variety of techniques. Electron therapy is one treatment approach where 3D printing has a potential to make a positive impact patient outcome. As for photon beam therapy, the use of 3D printing for electron therapy will offer the advantages of digitization and automation of manual processes with resultant personalization patient devices [1–3]. However, by also taking advantage of the unique interaction of megavoltage electrons in 3D printable media, additional opportunities are introduced. These new options include sculpting of patients' dose distributions to improve target coverage [4], protective shielding devices to improve sparing of normal tissues, [5–9] and electron field shaping devices [10, 11]. These innovations give rise to new and efficient processes in the clinic leading to improvements in personalized radiotherapy.

BOLUS DESIGN FOR ELECTRON THERAPY

Electron therapy offers the clinical advantage of sparing normal tissues at the distal aspect of the target due to a rapid fall-off of the depth dose. Since it is usually applied in treating superficial volumes, delivering sufficient surface dose is important, and like photon radiotherapy, historically this has been achieved using water equivalent compensators or bolus, such as wax. Electron bolus also reduces dose to healthy tissue beyond the target volume by controlling the depth of dose fall-off, i.e., the practical range of the electron beam. This section describes an innovative technology that extends the functionality of traditional bolus concept that has been enabled by 3D printing. This technology, termed modulated electron bolus (MEB), includes the basic functions of bolus, and through intelligent design of the bolus topology, allows improved conformity of the prescribed radiation dose to the target volume.

 DOI: 10.1201/9781003288404-5

The design and production of MEB is more sophisticated compared to simple uniform thickness bolus used frequently in megavoltage photon radiotherapy. Because of the continuous loss of energy of electrons at a rate of approximately 2 MeV per cm in water-equivalent materials, the thickness of a bolus can be designed to alter the mean energy of electrons impinging on the skin. Moreover, by varying this thickness of a bolus over the area of incidence of an electron beam, the bolus can be designed to modulate the mean energy spatially. At the surface of the skin immediately below the bolus, regions of the electron beam that have traversed lower bolus thicknesses will contain electrons with a larger mean depth range in tissue. Thus, MEB is a patient device that not only fits the patient surface accurately and achieves sufficient surface dose, but also introduces the capacity to precisely shape dose distributions at the deep aspect of a target. This allows improved target coverage, and improved normal tissue sparing at the distal aspect (Figure 5.1).

This general concept is called modulated electron radiation therapy (MERT), an approach that is not new. Even prior to integration of 3D printing, MERT has been explored using several different methods. These include modulation of multiple electron energies and beam weights, and are classified as segmented-field electron conformal therapy (ECT) and intensity-modulated electron therapy (IMET) [12–14]. ECT uses multiple electron fields of various energies and beam weights. IMET employs an inverse planning technique, similar to that used with photons for IMRT, to optimize electron beamlets that are shaped using multileaf collimators. While these implementations of MERT may improve planning target volume (PTV) coverage and normal tissue sparing, they are complex and difficult to implement clinically. The use of custom 3D printed electron bolus therefore shows great promise and is practical to implement.

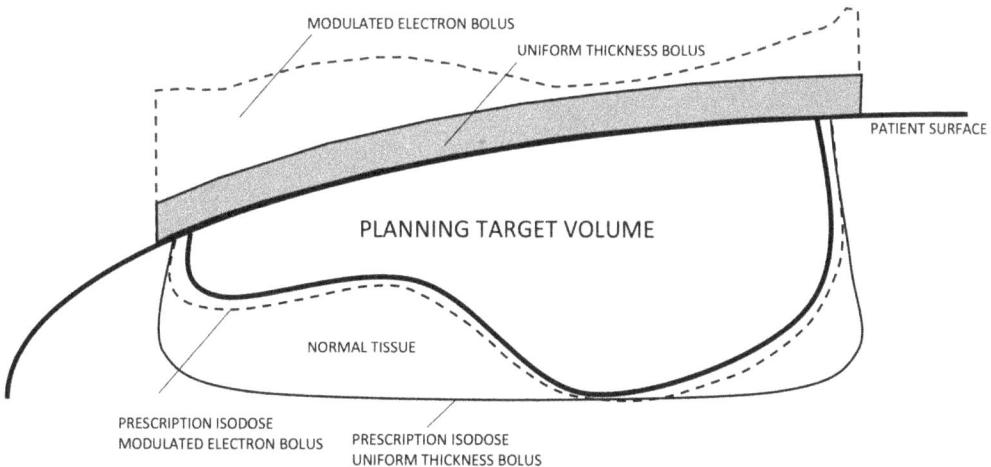

FIGURE 5.1   Compared to a uniform thickness bolus used in electron radiotherapy, a modulated electron bolus (MEB) is designed and 3D printed to allow improved conformity of the prescription isodose surface to the distal aspect of the planning target volume.

Modulated electron beam therapy is achieved using 3D printed bolus customized to the patient surface and accounting for the target shape and electron range. As a result, the isodose surface can be shaped around the target in three dimensions. Initial studies designing custom bolus for electron therapy simply considered the depth along a fan line, from the bolus surface to the distal edge of a target, and set the bolus thickness such that the therapeutic isodose lines covered the target at depth. This approach limited the design with a 2D assumption that the radiation source was in the same plane as the bolus and ignored the heterogeneity of tissue densities. Designing the bolus based on a constant physical depth thus created inaccuracies in the areas of internal air cavities and dense bone, where radiological depth would better approximate the appropriate bolus thickness. Additionally, electrons scatter continuously in bolus media and tissue, the effects of which were not considered. Algorithms developed by Low et al. to allow design of electron bolus with modulated thickness used a pencil beam calculation approach [15]. While not optimal, these addressed some of the original deficiencies by introducing bolus operators into the calculation and performing a 3D dose calculation. The operators modify the original bolus shape to adjust the dose distribution based on physical or effective depths. Operators can also modify bolus margins to ensure adequate coverage near the edges of the target volume. The resultant bolus structure can be included in the patient computed tomography (CT) image set and included in a 3D calculation. The study of Low et al. predated access to 3D printing, thus bolus fabrication was limited to a milling machine. Examples showed improved dose conformality for several cases. However, this approach used a pencil beam 3D calculation, which is known to be limited in coping with regions of heterogeneity.

More recently, Su et al. [4] presented algorithms with the specific intention of 3D printing MEB. These leveraged a commercial electron Monte Carlo (eMC) calculation already commissioned within a radiotherapy department's treatment planning system (Eclipse, Varian Medical Systems, Figure 5.2). Compared to the pencil beam approach, using iterative eMC improves the accuracy of dose distribution by accounting for tissue heterogeneity and contour irregularities. This method enables delivery of conformal dose distributions using an in-house algorithm and 3D printing a bolus of modulated thickness of polylactic acid (PLA). A ray line tracing method provides an initial approximation of bolus thickness, and then is improved upon with each iteration by applying five regional modulation operators. These operators reduce hotspots and increase target coverage. This design algorithm does not require a dose calculation, therefore does not need detailed commissioning separate to the planning system and is easily incorporated into a planning workflow. The output describing the geometry of the final MERT bolus is a standard STL file format that can be used with commercially available 3D printers. This bolus may be printed either at the point-of-care or through an on-demand service. Through clinical examples, investigators demonstrated that the MEB design algorithm can efficiently address variable target shapes, location, and proximity to critical structures [4]. The fabricated MEB substantially reduces the volume of normal tissue irradiated as compared to conventional electron therapy with uniform bolus (Figure 5.3).

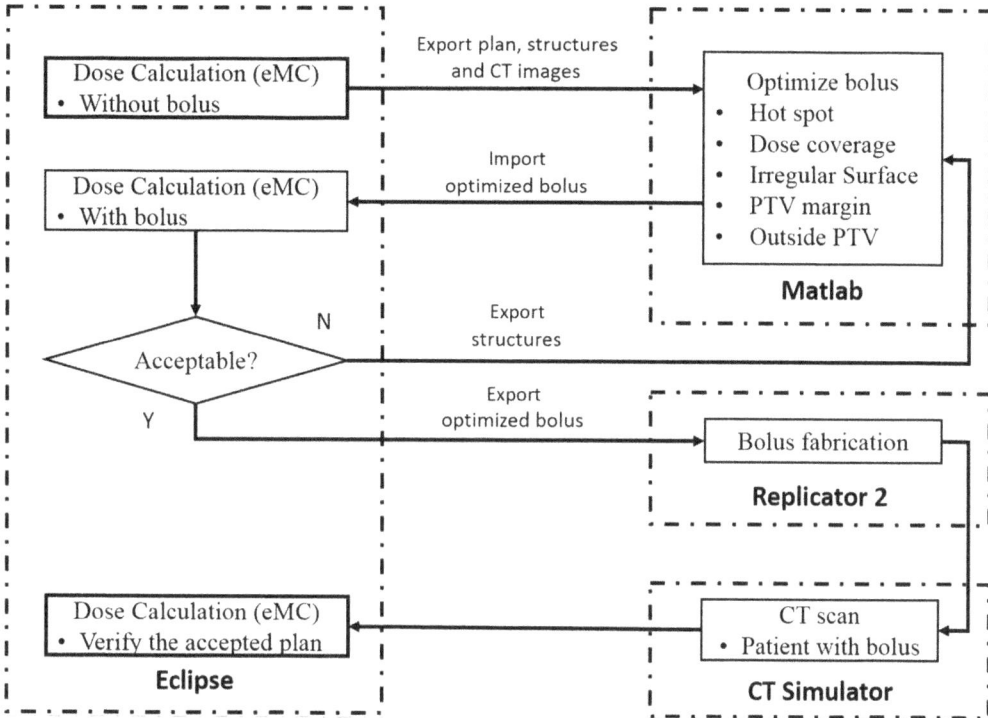

FIGURE 5.2 The approach by Su *et al.* interfaces a commissioned electron Monte Carlo (eMC) dose calculation algorithm within the planning system (Eclipse, Varian Medical) with an iterative modulated electron bolus design algorithm (in MATLAB®). The bolus design is imported into the planning system for final dose calculation and sent to the 3D printer (Replicator 2) for fabrication. Figure sourced with permission from [4].

FABRICATION AND CHARACTERIZATION

Evolution from Milling to 3D Printing

Traditionally, custom electron bolus has been fabricated using a milling machine. This subtractive process begins with a large block of material, for example, paraffin wax, and requires machining a specific design pattern. Aside from wasting material, the milled pattern may be limited in resolution by the end mill size and stepping pattern. Although milled, the resultant bolus may retain the bulky outer block geometry, as illustrated in Figure 5.4 [16]. 3D printing provides the advantages of creating the custom bolus layer by layer with extremely fine resolution, including only the material that is needed for the device, producing devices that would be impossible to create through subtractive milling (e.g., with complex internal structure), and access to a broad selection of printable materials applicable to radiotherapy.

Radiologic Properties of 3D Printed Electron Bolus

The geometrical accuracy of a 3D printing process can be evaluated by printing test objects and comparing fabricated dimensions to those of the design. However, the radiological

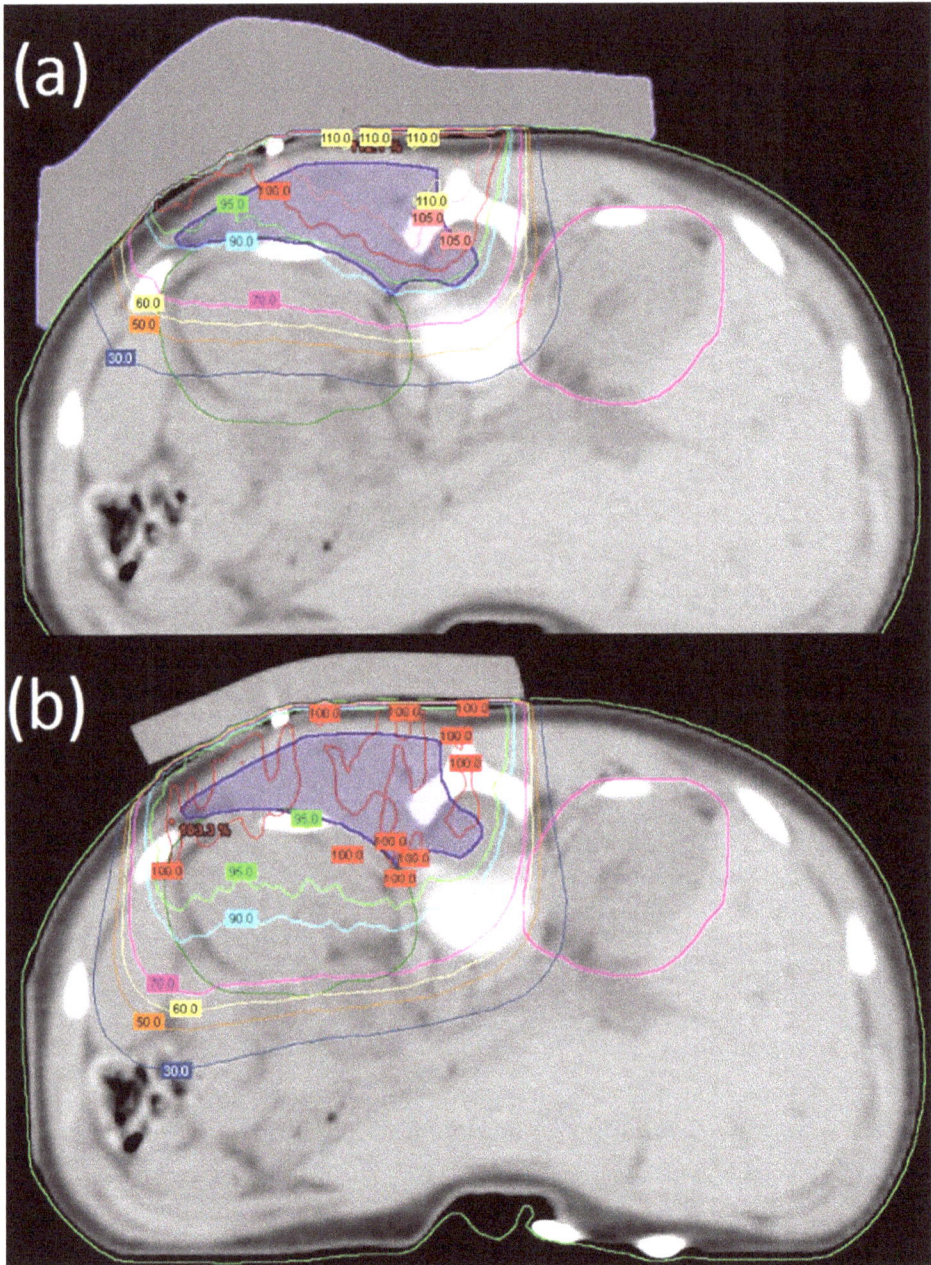

FIGURE 5.3 Treatment plans for a prone patient with rhabdomyosarcoma, showing sparing of the left kidney with MEB (a) compared to bolus of uniform 1-cm thickness (b). Figure sourced with permission from [4].

properties of printed devices must be known, and may be required in the design algorithms discussed above, to ensure dosimetric accuracy. Typical thermoplastics used in fused deposition modeling (FDM) for electron therapy devices include acrylonitrile butadiene styrene (ABS), PLA, and thermoplastic polyurethane (TPU). Other technologies will give access to different materials, for example Multi Jet Fusion (MJF) allows printing with

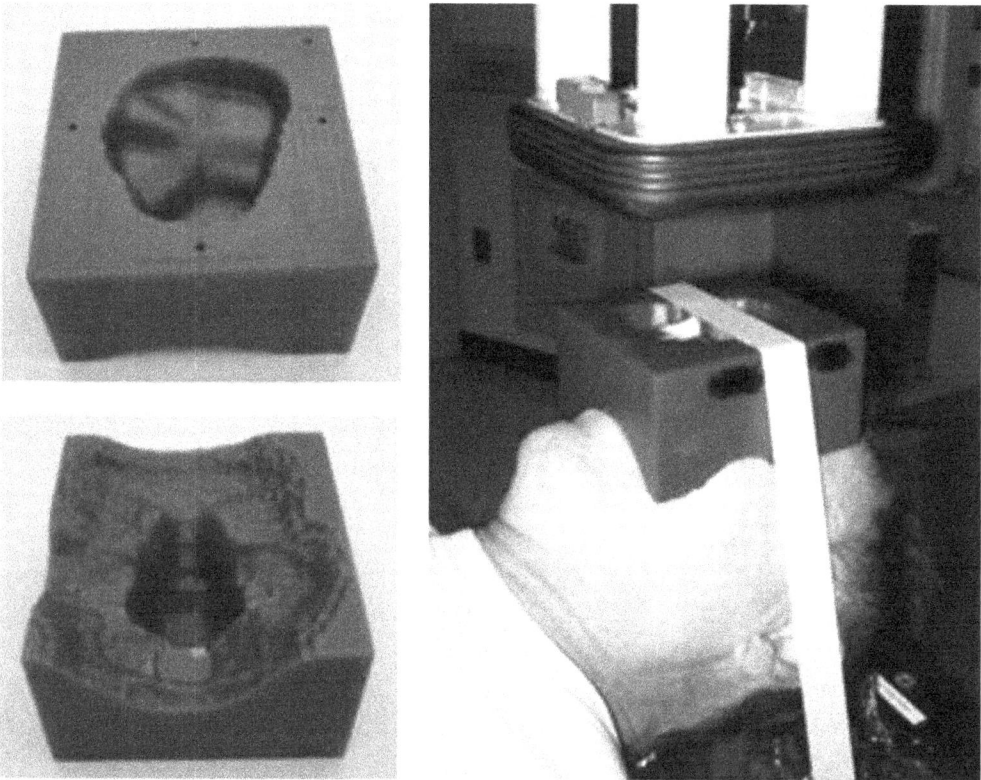

FIGURE 5.4   An electron compensator milled from paraffin wax. Figure sourced with permission from [16].

TPU or polyamide 12 (PA12) polymer. The radiologic parameters relevant to megavoltage electrons are collisional and radiative stopping powers, with collisional stopping power most important for transport in lower atomic number media. However, the characteristic that may be directly measured by the practitioner in the clinic is Hounsfield Unit (HU) determined using CT imaging. This may be related to electron density and relative electron density, which are proportional to collisional stopping power. Several publications are available that address the radiologic properties of 3D printing materials with specific examples of methodology to characterize using computed CT [17–19]. After ensuring that the correct HU, density, or electron density is specified for the device in the treatment plan, validation of the calculated dose is essential. Practical methods for this verification are well described in the literature [4, 17, 18].

Variables Affecting Radiologic Properties
The densities (and thus measured HU) of 3D printed devices are influenced by several factors. For example, if FDM is used, physical properties vary with individual print jobs, different printers, different filaments from various manufacturers, and even different batches of filament stock from the same manufacturer. Different filaments that are nominally the same may exhibit variability in HU, and characterization not only of different

materials, but also individual devices may be necessary [17]. Measured HU values of devices can vary between print jobs, but with careful control of the printing process they may be relatively stable over the course of several weeks [17]. It has been shown that it is important to specify the actual radiologic properties of the material in the treatment planning system, i.e., in terms of density, electron density, or HU [18]. Of concern, Craft *et al.* [17] showed that some materials may not lie on a standard CT curve with respect to the HU/density correspondence. This can lead to dose calculation inaccuracy, and thus it may be necessary to manually specify the HU or density of the device in the planning process. Whether radiologic properties need to be specified on a per-device basis will depend on the variability observed. If material properties show little variability and good material uniformity, a fixed specification of radiologic parameters will suffice in the planning system. However, if a high degree of variability is expected among devices, Craft *et al.* suggest that the physical density of each 3D printed device be determined and accurately assigned in the treatment planning system [17].

For FDM printing, multiple configurable parameters can be set to control the behavior of the printing, including layer height, printing speed, rates of extrusion of the printing material, and 'infill factor'. The infill factor refers to the percentage of a volume that is occupied by the printing medium (and not air). Several studies have shown that different infill factors can be used to mimic various tissues [20–23]. Specific to electron radiotherapy, PLA is shown to be accurately modeled in the treatment planning system when using depth and fluence scaling factors. This was demonstrated across multiple energies for both commercially available treatment planning systems and Monte Carlo approaches [24]. Similarly, tissue equivalence of plastics used for electron dosimetry was studied using the EGSnrc Monte Carlo [25]. Van der Walt *et al.* [26] analyzed dosimetric characteristics of PLA, such as beam profiles and percent depth dose curves for photon and electron energies to determine tissue equivalence and assess the appropriateness of PLA for radiotherapy applications. This study also examined the use of various infills of PLA for tissue equivalence, but for electron specific investigations, 100% infill was used. Percent depth dose curves (PDDs) and profiles were measured for a variety of electron energies. Measured data were compared to the treatment planning eMC calculations and were found to be within acceptable tolerance. Electron beam quality factors of R50 and R80 (the depth of 50% and 80% dose) were also found to be within acceptable tolerance when using PLA 100% infill in 3D printed blocks. Consistent with Craft *et al.* [17] this study showed that varying from 100% infill can induce dose calculation errors if the density to HU relationship is not confirmed. However, using a 100% infill with PLA for 3D printed bolus for electron therapy was shown to be accurately modeled in the treatment planning system and is an acceptable option for eMC calculations.

The variability of radiological properties of devices for electron radiotherapy can be minimized by commissioning the 3D printing process with a defined set of printing parameters. Even while keeping those parameters fixed, however, some variability will exist, and the commissioning process should include a sufficient sample of printed devices to estimate that variability, to establish a baseline. The possibility for variability motivates a QA program overseeing the 3D printing process as well as the devices that it produces. This program should include periodic QC checks on the printer and material, e.g., involving printing measurable test objects where key characteristics, including dimensional accuracy and density, can be checked periodically. The program should also include an aspect of patient-specific QC tests, e.g., measurements on the actual devices for patients. These can include CT imaging the device in advance of treatment to verify HU and material uniformity, as well as CBCT imaging on first fraction to check both material uniformity and correct positioning and fit when applied to the surface of the patient.

3D PRINTING OF ELECTRON APERTURES AND SHIELDING

While MEB represents an innovation improving the accuracy of treatment and optimization of dose distributions, other developments employing 3D printing in electron therapy have focused on devices for electron field shaping [11] and custom shielding devices [6–8, 27].

Electron Apertures

Due to the scatter of electrons in air below the secondary collimation of the linear accelerator, external beam electron therapy requires an applicator with an aperture located proximal (e.g., 5–15 cm) to the patient surface for final field definition. Custom designed apertures for electron radiotherapy can be cumbersome to produce. While the production of these apertures can be done using low melting point alloys such as Cerrobend (containing lead and cadmium) this process is labor-intensive and requires the handling of toxic materials. Skinner *et al.* presented a novel technique of using customized 3D printed plastic shells filled with tungsten ball bearings [11]. Tungsten was chosen for its ease of use and high atomic number. The 3D printed plastic inserts were filled with 2-mm tungsten ball bearings creating a thickness of 12 mm, compared to typical Cerrobend apertures of 15-mm thickness (Figure 5.5). Dose profiles were measured for 5.5-cm circular apertures, as well as representative field shapes for treatment, defined by either Cerrobend or the tungsten-filled, 3D printed shells. These measured profiles were compared to calculated profiles from the planning system, showing excellent agreement up to and including an energy of 16 MeV. Compared to Cerrobend apertures, the dose under the shielding was slightly higher for 16 MeV, thus it may be desirable to increase the thickness for higher energy electron beams. This was the first report showing the potential of implementing a 3D printing approach for electron field shaping devices, offering the advantage of avoiding toxic materials in the clinic and eliminating the manual and labor-intensive procedure of hand cutting and pouring Cerrobend electron apertures. As an alternative approach, high-density materials can be used to print apertures directly using various materials. For example, copper-containing PLA has been investigated for radiotherapy applications [28] where the printing medium is 70% copper by weight. Bronze-containing FDM filament has been used in electron shielding applications [6]. As discussed in Chapter 2, more sophisticated 3D printing technologies can produce metallic parts through powder bed fusion, laser sintering, binder jetting, or metal jet fusion.

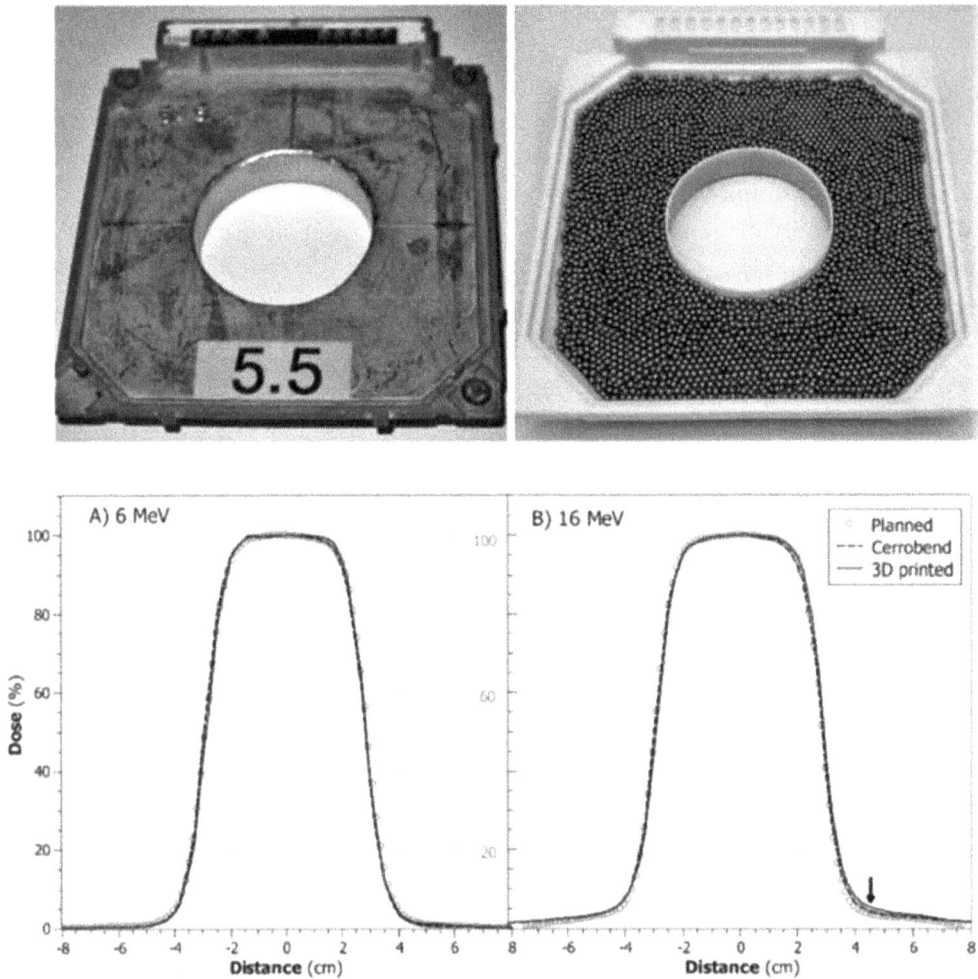

FIGURE 5.5 A traditional alloy metal electron aperture (top left) compared to a 3D printed and tungsten bead-filled aperture (top right) from Skinner *et al*. Measured dose profiles (bottom row) confirm the similarity of dosimetry for 6-MeV and 16-MeV electron beams. Figure sourced with permission from [11].

Skin Surface Shielding for Electron Radiotherapy

Lead shields placed on the surface of the patient are used in superficial photon radiotherapy as well as electron therapy to limit radiation dose to adjacent normal tissues and organs. For electron therapy, these are used in conjunction with Cerrobend electron apertures and provide precise shielding by reducing field size or sharpening field penumbra. Lead shields are typically designed to reduce the underlying dose by at least 95% of the unshielded beam. Prior to the development of 3D printing, on-skin lead shields were fabricated by hand. While clinically adequate, this process is time consuming and labor-intensive. Often these shields are created by making a plaster mold of the patient's face and manually hammering lead onto the plastic face mold. This manual process is prone to nonuniform shielding thickness and uncertainties in the fit of the lead to the patient surface contour. 3D printing of patient-specific shielding devices will improve this process. Initial studies have focused on reducing the labor-intensive workflow by 3D printing the patient's face and using this to form the lead shielding into shape [5], avoiding the need to cast a plaster mold directly on the patient. While eliminating the discomfort for the patient and reducing the time required to create the custom lead shield, the process remained manually cumbersome. This motivated direct printing of shielding that provides sufficient attenuation for electron beams.

Craft *et al.* presented a technique in which patient-specific custom shields can be printed from high-density bronze-based filaments [6]. This case study was the first to present the clinical viability of 3D printed bronze (3DPB) shields as compared to conventionally used handmade lead shields. The percent transmission of the electron beam 3DPB shields is comparable to lead, with 10 and 15 mm of 3DPB sufficient to shield 6 MeV and 9 MeV electron beams, respectively. The report indicates that 3DPB is clinically viable for replacement of manual fabrication of on-skin lead shielding. This technique improves patient comfort and workflow efficiency, while removing the use of toxic lead in the clinic. As the adoption of 3D printing expands in radiation therapy, these initial developments warrant further exploration of high density printing materials.

Scalp Shielding in Total Skin Electron Beam Therapy

Another innovative application unlocked by 3D printing is scalp shielding used during total skin electron beam therapy (TSEBT) [8]. Widespread skin involvement of mycosis fungoides can be treated effectively with TSEBT [29, 30] and low-dose palliative treatment has become the standard of care, offering low toxicity. Of note, the main toxicity observed is alopecia. Temporary and permanent alopecia is expected with doses of 12 and 20 Gy, respectively. Since multiple courses of radiation therapy may be needed, alopecia is a concern for many patients. Historically, lead helmets have been used to shield regions of the scalp in patients receiving more than one course of treatment. These are heavy and uncomfortable for the patient, may present challenges when trying to treat near the hairline, and expose the staff and patient to toxic lead. Examples of these include a helmet made of

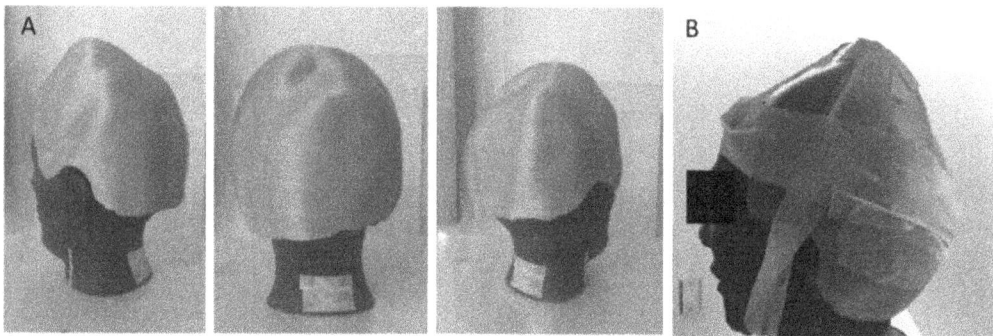

FIGURE 5.6 Patient-personalized 3D printed helmet designed based on 3D optical imaging and printed using FDM, from Rahimy *et al.* Figure sourced with permission from [8].

thermoplastic mask with Superflab bolus [31] and a lead-lined motorcycle half-helmet [32]. 3D printing is advantageous in this application because it can accommodate complex geometries without compromising dose coverage near the hairline, and eliminates the use of toxic lead material. Rahimy *et al.* [8] demonstrated a customized helmet based on 3D optical image data of the scalp, with printing using PLA (see Figure 5.6). The authors also point out that the actual dose received by the scalp can be adjusted based on the designed thickness of the device.

REFERENCES

[1] Park K, Park S, Jeon M-J, et al. Clinical application of 3D-printed-step-bolus in post-total-mastectomy electron conformal therapy. *Oncotarget*. 2016;8:25660–25668.

[2] McCallum S, Maresse S, Fearns P. Evaluating 3D-printed bolus compared to conventional bolus types used in external beam radiation therapy. *Curr Med Imaging*. 2020;17:820–831.

[3] Łukowiak M, Jezierska K, Boehlke M, et al. Utilization of a 3D printer to fabricate boluses used for electron therapy of skin lesions of the eye canthi. *J Appl Clin Med Phys*. 2016;18:76–81.

[4] Su S, Moran K, Robar JL. Design and production of 3D printed bolus for electron radiation therapy. *J Appl Clin Med Phys*. 2014;15:194–211.

[5] Briggs M, Clements H, Wynne N, et al. 3D printed facial laser scans for the production of localised radiotherapy treatment masks – A case study. *J Vis Commun Med*. 2016;39:99–104.

[6] Craft DF, Lentz J, Armstrong M, et al. Three-dimensionally printed on-skin radiation shields using high-density filament. *Pract Radiat Oncol*. 2020;10:e543–e550.

[7] Kwon O, Jin H, Son J, et al. Dose calculation of 3D printing lead shield covered by biocompatible silicone for electron beam therapy. *Phys Eng Sci Med*. 2021;44:1061–1069.

[8] Rahimy E, Skinner L, Kim YH, et al. Technical report: 3D-printed patient-specific scalp shield for hair preservation in total skin electron beam therapy. *Tech Innov Patient Support Radiat Oncol*. 2021;18:12–15.

[9] Sharma SC, Johnson MW. Surface dose perturbation due to air gap between patient and bolus for electron beams. *Med Phys*. 1993;20:377–378.

[10] Miloichikova I, Krasnykh A, Danilova I, et al. Formation of electron beam fields with 3D printed filters. *Aip Conf Proc*. 2016;1772:060018.

[11] Skinner L, Fahimian BP, Yu AS. Tungsten filled 3D printed field shaping devices for electron beam radiation therapy. *PLos One*. 2019;14:e0217757.

[12] Connell T, Alexander A, Papaconstadopoulos P, et al. Delivery validation of an automated modulated electron radiotherapy plan: Validation of an automated modulated electron radiotherapy plan. *Med Phys*. 2014;41:061715.

[13] Klein EE, Vicic M, Ma C-M, et al. Validation of calculations for electrons modulated with conventional photon multi leaf collimators. *Phys Med Biol*. 2008;53:1183–1208.

[14] Al-Yahya K, Verhaegen F, Seuntjens J. Design and dosimetry of a few leaf electron collimator for energy modulated electron therapy. *Med Phys*. 2007;34:4782–4791.

[15] Low DA, Starkschall G, Bujnowski SW, et al. Electron bolus design for radiotherapy treatment planning: Bolus design algorithms: Electron bolus design for radiotherapy treatment planning. *Med Phys*. 1992;19:115–124.

[16] Zeidan OA, Chauhan BD, Estabrook WW, et al. Image-guided bolus electron conformal therapy – a case study. *J Appl Clin Med Phys*. 2011;12:68–75.

[17] Craft DF, Kry SF, Balter P, et al. Material matters: Analysis of density uncertainty in 3D printing and its consequences for radiation oncology. *Med Phys*. 2018;45:1614–1621.

[18] Burleson S, Baker J, Hsia AT, et al. Use of 3D printers to create a patient-specific 3D bolus for external beam therapy. *J Appl Clin Med Phys*. 2015;16:166–178.

[19] Kozee M, Weygand J, Andreozzi JM, et al. Methodology for computed tomography characterization of commercially available 3D printing materials for use in radiology/radiation oncology. *J Appl Clin Med Phys*. 2023;e13999.

[20] Dancewicz OL, Sylvander SR, Markwell TS, et al. Radiological properties of 3D printed materials in kilovoltage and megavoltage photon beams. *Phys Medica*. 2017;38:111–118.

[21] Kairn T, Crowe SB, Markwell T. World congress on medical physics and biomedical engineering, June 7–12, 2015, Toronto, Canada. *Ifmbe Proc*. 2015;728–731.

[22] Madamesila J, McGeachy P, Barajas JEV, et al. Characterizing 3D printing in the fabrication of variable density phantoms for quality assurance of radiotherapy. *Phys Medica*. 2016;32:242–247.

[23] Ricotti R, Ciardo D, Pansini F, et al. Dosimetric characterization of 3D printed bolus at different infill percentage for external photon beam radiotherapy. *Phys Medica*. 2017;39:25–32.

[24] Diamantopoulos S, Kantemiris I, Patatoukas G, et al. Theoretical and experimental determination of scaling factors in electron dosimetry for 3D-printed polylactic acid. *Med Phys*. 2018;45:1708–1714.

[25] Oprea M, Mihailescu D, Borcia C. Monte Carlo evaluation of water equivalency of some plastic materials for realistic electron IORT beams. *J Phys Conf Ser*. 2012;398:012040.

[26] Walt MV der, Crabtree T, Albantow C. PLA as a suitable 3D printing thermoplastic for use in external beam radiotherapy. *Australas Phys Eng S*. 2019;42:1165–1176.

[27] Sharma A, Sasaki D, Rickey DW, et al. Low-cost optical scanner and 3-dimensional printing technology to create lead shielding for radiation therapy of facial skin cancer: First clinical case series. *Adv Radiat Oncol*. 2018;3:288–296.

[28] Ehler ED, Sterling DA. 3D printed copper-plastic composite material for use as a radiotherapy bolus. *Phys Medica*. 2020;76:202–206.

[29] Hoppe RT. Mycosis fungoides: Radiation therapy. *Dermatol Ther*. 2003;16:347–354.

[30] Prince HM, Whittaker S, Hoppe RT. How I treat mycosis fungoides and Sézary syndrome. *Blood*. 2009;114:4337–4353.

[31] Patel CG, Ding G, Kirschner A. Scalp-sparing total skin electron therapy in mycosis fungoides: Case report featuring a technique without lead. *Pract Radiat Oncol*. 2017;7:400–402.

[32] Williams NL, Keller J, Kremmel E, et al. Scalp-sparing total skin electron therapy in mycosis fungoides: Case report highlighting technique and outcome. *Pract Radiat Oncol*. 2016;6:439–441.

CHAPTER 6

3D Printing for Proton Therapy

Clay Lindsay and Cornelia Hoehr

INTRODUCTION

When applied to radiotherapy, the primary difference between photons and charged particles is range. Coulomb interactions between the medium and charged particles result in consistent energy loss, and hence dose deposition, with depth. The lateral and depth profiles of deposited dose depend on the mass of the charged particle, atomic number, and electron density of the medium. Due to their mass, protons (and heavier charged particles) offer a dosimetric advantage over electrons. They are less prone to multiple-coulomb scattering—yielding a more consistent dose profile with depth, and a sharper depth-dose distribution known as a Bragg peak (BP). Preparing a proton beam (most commonly from a cyclotron) for therapy requires energy switching or beam degradation. The energy spectrum of the beam must be modified such that the resulting dose distribution covers the target in depth. The quality of the resulting dose distribution is extremely sensitive to the method and accuracy of beam modulation.

In passive-scatter systems, range is selected through use of field-specific blocks of material in the beam. They may be placed directly on the patient (bolus), or upstream with the collimators (range compensators). Variation in depth is achieved through use of accelerator energy stepping, static scatter-based ridge filters, or modulator wheels. To keep downstream scatter to a minimum, degrading components have classically been plastics or wax. Lateral penumbrae are defined by field-specific high-Z collimators or by a multileaf collimation system. Active-scanning systems don't necessarily require any field-specific upstream modulation. However, applications such as high dose-rate radiotherapy require fast energy switching, which could see benefit from field-specific compensators like in passive systems.

Classically, beam degrading components and collimators have been fabricated using subtractive methods, i.e., milling. Even with modern robotic systems, expertise is still required in the fabrication process. 3D printing offers a more accurate, cost effective, and

 DOI: 10.1201/9781003288404-6

user-friendly mode of fabrication for patient-specific collimators, range compensators, and modulators. This chapter is focused on the application of 3D printing in proton therapy (PT). Physics concepts, component design, and considerations when selecting printing method and material are covered. It is beyond the scope of this chapter to cover the machine-specific causes and solutions of print defects. Instead, we focus on awareness of common defects and their effect on proton dose distributions. Applications to range compensation, energy modulation, collimation, and printed phantoms are reviewed. While not a focus, many of the principles discussed here will also apply to heavy-ion therapies.

BASIC PHYSICS CONCEPTS

We begin with a brief definition of physics concepts in PT. The goal is to cover basics that are important when employing 3D printing—both in print method and material choice.

Proton interactions with matter can be attributed to two sources—Coulomb and nuclear. The rate of energy loss as a proton traverses a medium is:

$$\frac{dE}{dx} = -\rho\left(\frac{S}{\rho}\right) = -\rho\left(\frac{S_{el}}{\rho} + \frac{S_N}{\rho}\right) \tag{6.1}$$

Where ρ is the material density, $\frac{S_{el}}{\rho}$ and $\frac{S_N}{\rho}$ are defined as the electronic and nuclear mass stopping powers. The electronic mass stopping power can be derived from the Bethe-Bloch formula and expressed in the form [1]:

$$\left(\frac{S_{el}}{\rho}\right) = 0.3072 \frac{Z}{A}\frac{1}{\beta^2}\left(\ln\frac{W_m}{I} - \beta^2\right)\frac{MeV}{g/cm^2} \tag{6.2}$$

Where Z is the atomic number, A the atomic mass, $\beta = v/c$, i.e., the particle velocity over the speed of light, I is the mean excitation energy, $W_m = \left(\frac{2m_e c^2\beta^2}{1-\beta^2}\right)$, and m_e is the mass of the electron. Nuclear stopping power does not have a well-modeled closed form. The total mass stopping power is scaled by density, such that it can be tabulated for a variety of materials and proton energies. This quantity increases as proton energy decreases, yielding a spike in energy loss near the end of the track, giving rise to the BP.

Coulomb Interactions

Coulomb interactions scatter incoming protons by an angle depending on impact parameter, medium atomic number, and proton energy. Protons traversing a medium will undergo many such scattering events. This process is known as multiple Coulomb scattering (MCS). Protons of equal energy will have approximately equal *total* path length in a medium. However, the axial depth traversed will be a statistical distribution (roughly Gaussian) due to MCS deflection. This variation in individual proton range is known as *range straggling.*

An idealized mono-energetic proton beam that experiences no range straggling would deposit dose as a sharp peak according to equation (6.2). For a realistic therapeutic beam, the BP has a width associated with the beam energy spread and magnitude of range straggling in the medium. Ideally in a therapeutic beam, energy spread and scatter are minimized to produce the sharpest distal dose falloff possible. Composition and geometric precision of beam degrading components are key to ensuring a high-quality axial dose distribution. These principles also apply to collimators for ensuring sharp lateral beam penumbra. When 3D printing components for PT, attention must be paid to the geometric characteristics of the print. This applies in the sense of quality assurance, but also in the design process.

Nuclear Interactions

As in equation (6.1), nuclear interactions contribute to patient dose via stopping power. In addition, nuclear interactions in beamline components yield secondary neutrons that are difficult to shield. Care must be taken to understand how the placement, geometry, and composition of beamline components will affect secondary dose to the patient. The most effective means of reducing secondary dose are to increase the distance between patient and proton stopping, and beamline shielding including high thermal neutron capture cross sections (e.g., borated polyethylene).

Nuclear interactions may also activate components in or near the beamline. Activation half-lives may be substantial; thus, the material composition of printed components is important from a radiation safety perspective. This is of particular importance if a component is reused often or is placed close to the patient. For any 3D printed component, extraneous materials used in the printing or post-processing (e.g., supports and washes) should also be examined. Any material that could remain on the surface and become activated could be a hazard.

3D PRINTED COMPONENT DESIGN

More so than for photon radiotherapy, PT dose distributions are extremely sensitive to components in the field. 3D printing offers unique benefits in component production and comes with many degrees of freedom, including machine parameters, materials, and print types. In the design process, it is important to consider characteristics of the print method (and machine) such as print direction, infill, layer thickness, and lateral print resolution. How these are addressed will depend on the goal of the component itself. We will discuss potential complications arising from these parameters (and how to avoid them) in the coming sections. First, we describe a basic design strategy in component production. We consider beam degraders in this strategy, but the concepts apply in the same way to collimators (essentially degraders with sufficient thickness to stop the beam).

The purpose of a beam degrader is to pull back proton range in the target. The desired pullback may be a function of axial position (e.g., by using range compensators) or the same value for the whole area of the field (e.g., by using modulator wheels). Degrader design involves calculating the thickness of material required to yield the desired pullback.

Materials may be available in a variety of densities and their stopping powers may be unknown. The concept of *water-equivalent thickness* is used to overcome these issues. For a given thickness T of a material, the *water-equivalent thickness* (T_w) is defined as [2]:

$$T_w = T \frac{\rho}{\rho_w} \frac{\bar{S}}{\bar{S}_w} \tag{6.3}$$

Where ρ is the material density, ρ_w is the density of water, $\bar{S}$ is the material's mean stopping power, and $\bar{S}_w$ is the mean stopping power of water. Water-equivalent thicknesses are tabulated for a range of therapeutic energies and for common materials used in PT [2]. 3D printed degraders may be designed for a target pullback in water by scaling the degrader thickness as in equation (6.3). If print consistency was uniform, stopping power known, and geometric tolerances measured, then standard methods for component design could be employed.

Unfortunately, it is not sufficient for clinical use to assume a uniform print density or rely on approximate stopping powers. The highest quality printers may still produce defects if they malfunction. Even functioning correctly, the density of printed component may be nonuniform, or worse, unpredictable. Additionally, defects may be present on the surface of the print. How these defects and inhomogeneities are distributed, how they depend on print configuration, and their frequency of occurrence will depend on the individual printer used. Geometric defects must be studied and, ideally, accounted for in the fabrication and design process.

Because of the continuous evolution of technology in 3D printing, best practices for specific 3D printers are not addressed here. Instead, the goal is to discuss issues to be aware of when printing components for clinical use. These issues will apply generically to any 3D printing method.

GEOMETRIC CONSIDERATIONS

Geometric accuracy and precision are key in PT. The sharp distal falloff of the BP can only be exploited effectively if there is a high degree of geometric certainty in the components degrading the beam. Geometric effects can be categorized as internal (regularity and density of bulk material) and external (edge and surface defects). Here we discuss four main concepts: geometric accuracy, internal homogeneity, edge defects, and print grid alignment.

Geometric Accuracy

The accuracy of the print is critical for applications to PT. As in equation (6.3), any size mismatch between the print and the intended design leads to a direct effect on the proton range pullback. In absence of outright errors in printing, the resolution of the printer will determine the magnitude of this effect. Print resolution may be specified by manufacturer as two values: resolution in the print direction and resolution in the lateral direction. In order to give the highest pullback accuracy, the printed part should be oriented such that the finer resolution is oriented along the beam direction. This is assuming normal incidence and consistent internal structure.

The magnitude of geometric inaccuracy is determined by the difference between the requested surface/structure position and the possible positions defined by the machine resolution. Depending on the geometry of the print and machine algorithm, a printed surface position may be rounded up or down by, *at most,* the specified resolution. This is best conceptualized in the print direction. A fused deposition modeling (FDM) printer, for example, prints a discrete number of layers. Surfaces defined by print direction must be printed in increments of the slice thickness. Thus, for a 0.2-mm slice thickness machine, a surface requested at 0.17 mm may be rounded to 0.16 mm or 0.18 mm depending on algorithm. This is assuming an integral 0.2-mm slice surface is also requested and a universal offset cannot be introduced. The print algorithm will determine the details of geometric accuracy. Details of the print algorithm may not be explicitly known.

With further development, printer resolutions will likely improve to a point where the resolution becomes irrelevant in this context. Even with modern printers, a 100-μm pullback error seems insignificant. Indeed, it is insignificant and can be accounted for by slightly increasing distal safety margins. However, this effect has wider implications in the context of beam energy modulation. Modulation schemes may be much more sensitive to uncertainties as they rely on a weighted sum of pullbacks.

Figure 6.1 (left) shows an exaggerated cross section of a printed component. With the print direction oriented upwards, the horizontal and vertical walls are restricted to minimum increments of the print direction and lateral resolutions respectively. These increments are not necessarily the same. Figure 6.1 (right) shows a depth-dose curve for modulated BP from an idealized print and for one with 100-μm surface position rounding. The choice of rounding up or down was randomly assigned, leading to up to 3% dose variation in the target region. Here 100 μm represents a 0.3–2% variation in the modulator thickness. This effect on the modulated dose may lead to a greater discrepancy than predicted with just the difference in proton pullback alone.

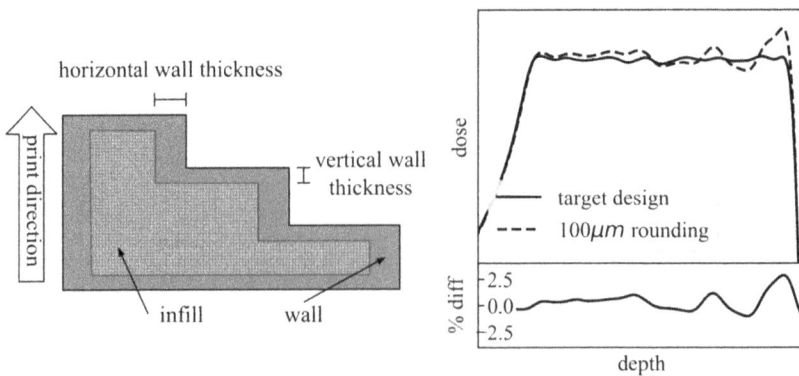

FIGURE 6.1   Diagram of cross section of 3D printed component showing infill and wall definitions (left) and simulated spread out Bragg peaks for an ideal modulator and for one with surfaces rounded to 100 μm (right).

Internal Homogeneity

The homogeneity of the bulk medium is not necessarily consistent between printers, materials or individual machines. Designing components via scaling thickness by the water-equivalent ratio assumes perfect homogeneity. Even set to 100% infill, significant inhomogeneities may occur [3, 4]. The primary effect of inhomogeneities on the resulting dose distribution is known as *BP degradation* [5–9]. Traversing an inhomogeneous medium affects the distribution of MCS, resulting in a widening of the BP. This effect can be caused by structures that are finer than CT scanner or dose calculation resolutions— making them invisible and unable to be modeled in a treatment planning system (TPS). The magnitude of this effect depends on the size and quantity of the heterogeneities [8].

Figure 6.2 shows a degrader containing randomly spaced 50-μm air defects. A schematic of the beam configuration is depicted on the left; the BP resulting from various infill settings is shown on the right. Here the degrader density is scaled such that the same *physical length* of material, and *water-equivalent thickness*, is traversed in all cases. The beam traversing a solid block of PMMA is shown as a solid line, random air defects of 10% and 20% are shown in dotted lines. The effect of increasing the volume of air defects widens the BP and extends the range. On CT, such sub-millimeter defects appear as an average reduction in Hounsfield Units (HU). Assuming a uniform density, as CT would indicate, leads to the discrepancy between solid and dotted lines in Figure 6.2.

Systematic inhomogeneities may also be present in a print. As an example, most FDM printers allow specification of *infill factor*, defined as the percentage of printed volume occupied by the printed medium (and not air) as well as a pattern for this infill (e.g., grid, cross-hatch, or other). The most obvious example of a systematic inhomogeneity is due to infill. If infill is not set to 100%, systematic inhomogeneities are part of the print design. The applicability of the water-equivalent ratio scaling method will depend on the consistency and repeatability of this pattern. Even when set to 100% infill [3,4, 10, 11] there may still be variation in print density across a print. This could occur due to '100% infill' not being truly solid, systematic misprints (layer cracking, warping, wobble), or wall-infill boundaries (see Figure 6.1).

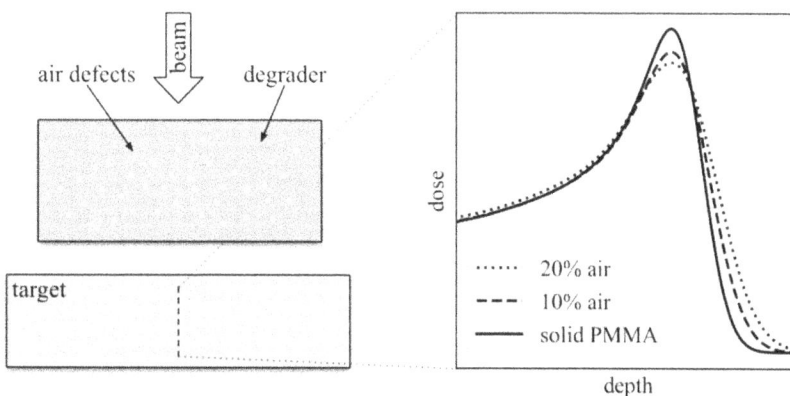

FIGURE 6.2 Diagram of beam configuration impinging on degrader with randomly dispersed air pockets (left) and Bragg peak distributions for solid, 10%, and 20% air infill (right).

Edge Effects

By nature of a printing process, edges of a print maybe be susceptible to print defects. Edge effects may occur in the form of bulging, warping, layer cracking, filament stringing, rounded corners, layer offsets, or other. They may be exasperated by course voxelization, excess support material, print errors, or poor calibration. The net effect of any of these defects is an excess or lack of desired beam-degrading material in the print. Holes will result in an extended proton range; bulges will result in reduced pullback. Such defects may occur on the external surfaces of a printed part, but also internally at infill–wall borders.

Figure 6.3 shows an example of an edge defect for a collimator. The defect protrudes into the beam. The resulting axial dose distribution is then approximated by the sum of two BP's—one at full pullback and one at pullback less the added degrader material. This appears as a 'bump' in the axial dose distribution and a dip in the lateral profile associated with the defect position.

The occurrence of these defects may be sporadic or systematic dependent on geometry. However, the more corners and hard edges, the more likely edge defects may occur. Designing a part to reduce the sharpness of corners and edges may significantly reduce defect frequency. In the context of PT, it is important to perform quality assurance (QA) on the external surfaces of any printed part for edge defects.

Grid/Layer Alignment

At least for FDM printing, infill of a part necessitates a grid infill pattern. Even set to 100% infill, systematic density fluctuations, based on this pattern, can occur. The alignment of the pattern with the proton beam may result in unexpected range changes. The magnitude, probability, and distribution of this effect on the dose distribution will depend on the angle of incidence between the beam and part. Even with the print direction angled at normal incidence with the beam axis, beam divergence and steering may cause variable

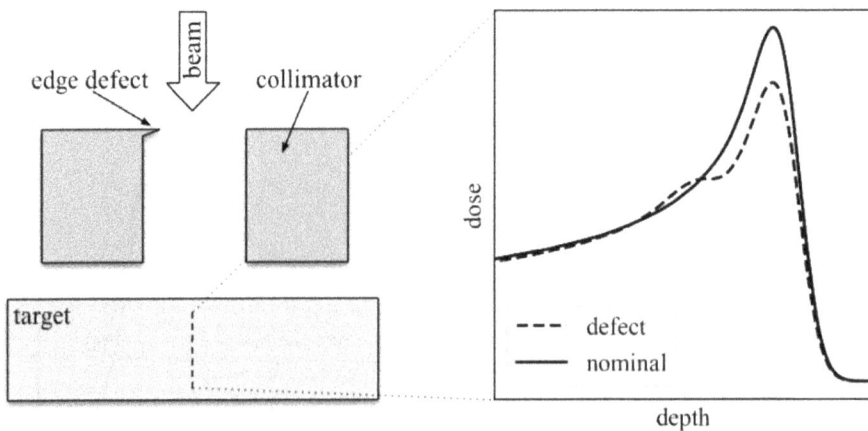

FIGURE 6.3   Diagram of beam configuration showing a collimator with edge defect protruding into beam (left) and resulting Bragg peak distribution showing influence of additional pullback form defect (right).

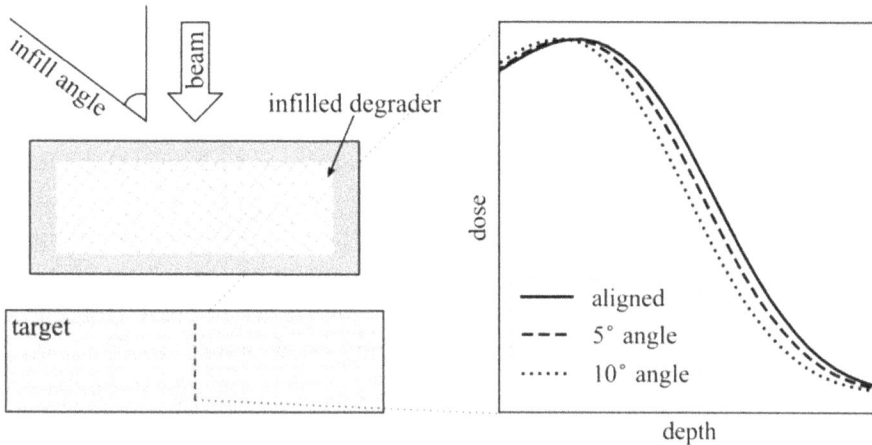

FIGURE 6.4 Diagram of beam configuration showing degrader with patterned infill, where infill is a grid alternating 100% and 90% density voxels (left) and effect of grid angle variation on resulting Bragg peak (right).

incident angle across the beam profile. This is most evident in the case of compensators (passive scatter systems) that are positioned far downstream. Parts placed downstream of an active steering system may also be susceptible to this effect.

Figure 6.4 (left) depicts a cross-section of an infilled degrader. The print is infilled to include a 5% density fluctuation in a grid pattern. Figure 6.4 (right) shows the BP for 0-, 5-, and 10-degree incident beam angles. The magnitude of this effect will increase with decreasing infill setting and increasing beam angle. The result is a variable thickness across the part that is not evident from external measurements or on CT. Care should be taken in part placement and design to minimize this effect.

PRINT MATERIAL CONSIDERATIONS

Materials used in PT are selected according to their desired effect, for example low-Z materials are used for degraders (to reduce scatter) and high-Z materials are used for collimators and scatterers. Outside of this constraint, material choice for printed components involves three main considerations—stopping power, activation profile, and radiation hardness.

Stopping Power

As discussed in the previous section, the overall water-equivalence of a part will depend strongly on the print geometry. From equation (6.3), if stopping power and density are known, the water-equivalence may be calculated. Unfortunately, at the time of writing, there have been few thorough studies performed to determine the stopping power of printed materials independent of their density. This is likely due to the fact that bulk part densities vary widely between printed geometries [3, 4, 12]. Simple parts, such as disks or cubes, can yield a range of density measurements due to variation in external dimensions or internal inhomogeneities. Most often, water-equivalence is measured empirically for a printed bulk part. The resulting water-equivalence may vary widely. If knowledge of a part's density were available, the stopping power for the solid print material could be used to calculate water-equivalence. Ideally, in measuring material stopping power, sizes, shapes, and print orientations would be used. Practically speaking, it may only be possible to perform a limited study and use water-equivalence as a surrogate for a full calculation of stopping power.

It is also possible to use standard CT-based methods to determine stopping power. Variations in density and uncertainties in HU to stopping power conversions limit the accuracy of such an approach. Dual energy CT can greatly improve stopping power measurements [13]. Accuracy is variable depending on structure size, print direction, and material composition. For consistently printed 2×2 cm^2 test objects, dual energy CT predicted proton range pullback within 0.05 and 1 mm over a 2-cm thickness [11].

Table 6.1 shows published stopping power ratios (SPR = S/S_{water}) for a selection of commercial materials. This can be used as an estimate of water-equivalence for a given material, but individual measurements on a variety of prints should be performed for clinical implementation.

Activation

As proton interaction with energies up to 230 MeV leads to activation of the intercepted material, printed materials will be radioactive after irradiation. In the typical plastic materials used for beam shaping, these activation products are from the reactions, e.g., O-16(p,pn)O-15, O-16(p,α)N-13, O-16(p,3(pn))C-11, C-12(p,pn)C-11, O-18(p,n)F-18, or C-12(p,x)Be-7. The half-life of these isotopes are 2 minutes, 10 minutes, 20 minutes, 2 hours, and 53 days, respectively. The largest cross sections are for production of C-11 and O-15, resulting in beam shaping devices that need to be stored for only a short amount of time for the activity to decay to manageable levels.

TABLE 6.1   Published Stopping Power Ratios (SPR) for Commercial Materials Along with Proton Beam Energy and Print Method

	Material	Printer	Print Method	Energy (MeV)	SPR
[3]	ABSPlus	uPrint SE plus	FDM	74	1.22
	ABS	--	FDM	62	
[14]	Accura Bluestone	ProX	SLA	115	1.58
[15]	Acrylic Plastic	Projet HD 3000 plus	Jetted	190	1.16
[13, 16]	PLA	Makerbot Replicator II,	FDM	140	1.1
		Ultimaker 2 Ext.		120	1.18
[16]	PA2200	EOS 3D	SLS	140	0.98
[11]	PolyAmide-12	--	SLS	62	1.01
[11]	PA-Alumide	--	SLS	62	1.16
[11]	PA-Glass Fiber	--	SLS	62	1.22
[11]	TangoPlus	--	Jetted	62	1.12
[11]	TPU	--	SLS	62	1.11
[11]	TuskXC2700T	--	SLA	62	1.14
[3, 11]	VerowhitePlus	Objet 30	Jetted	74	1.15
		--		62	1.17

On the other hand, printing materials with additives, especially metals or ceramics, can lead to long-term activation that necessitates evaluation of activation before reusing the printed part close to the patient. Minimizing dose to the patient as well as to personnel is essential, and appropriate storage needs to be arranged. Also notable is that the support structure of some printing techniques will need to be removed from the printed object. This can sometimes lead to a powdery residue on the surface. When irradiated, this powder can be activated as well and poses a radiation hazard to the personnel handling the device, and care should be taken to remove all loose dust or powder from the object before irradiation.

3D PRINTING APPLICATIONS IN CLINICAL PROTON THERAPY

We now turn to a discussion of applications for 3D printing in clinical PT. Three major applications are discussed: range compensation, energy modulation, and phantoms. Below we give a brief description of each application, the status-quo methods for device fabrication, important considerations when applying 3D printing, published works demonstrating 3D printing for the task, and future developments as the technology improves. Again, we focus on applications to PT, but many concepts are applicable to heavy-ion therapies as well.

Range Compensation

In PT, range compensation refers to the practice of adding a static beam-degrading component to the beam to shift the proton range in the target. This may be a constant pullback for the whole beam or variable across the beam profile. Range compensation is used to account for target inhomogeneities and to compensate for target depth variation (both in surface and distal position), and when proton energy selection may be insufficient or unavailable. Geometric accuracy, internal homogeneity, edge effects, and print-pattern alignment all may influence compensator quality. Compensator positioning is of particular importance. Special attention should be paid to beam angle incidence on the compensator and the effects of infill pattern on water-equivalence. There are two typical positions for range compensators in PT, snout-mounted and on-skin bolus.

Snout-mounted compensators are used widely in passive scatter systems for 2D range shaping. The design process is described by equation (6.3), scaling the compensator thickness by its water-equivalent ratio to yield the desired pullback determined by raytracing to the target. Historically, compensators have been milled from hard wax or plastic (PMMA, Lucite) and mounted on the snout of the treatment head close to the patient. Part resolution has been constrained by the size of the end mill (2–5 mm) and the quality of high-gradient sections depends on the end mill shape [17, 18]. 3D printing alleviates these issues, offering sub-millimeter precision without the tool shape or dimension affecting steep gradient structures. Jet-printed compensators have been shown to have improved geometric accuracy and good agreement with TPS-calculated dose [15]. 2D compensators printed with FDM printers have also been demonstrated to reduce cost and required infrastructure [16].

Snout-mounted compensators have also found application in active scanning systems. For applications that require fast energy switching, static compensators can provide range variation for a single pencil beam. A proposed single-energy pencil beam design employs a dynamic range shifter and static 3D printed field-specific compensators affixed to the snout [19]. This approach allows rapid pencil beam delivery as no energy switching is required. The potential downside is more of the beam must be degraded close to the patient, increasing secondary dose. Pencil beam spot-size requirements must also be considered as they are sensitive to material choice in degraders [20].

Range compensation in the form of bolus is also used in both passive and active PT systems. In cases where skin sparing is not desired or when lateral dose shaping is critical, such as superficial treatment of the head and neck, bolus may be used in place of a snout-mounted design. Reduction of the air gap between compensator and patient significantly aids in controlling pencil beam lateral penumbra [21]. As described in previous sections, air pockets in printed components have a direct impact on proton range. Preliminary studies have shown that replacing a snout-mounted range shifter with patient-specific printed bolus may significantly improve intensity modulated PT plan quality [22]. Simulation and measurements have shown that secondary dose proximal to the target patient is reduced when using on-skin printed bolus for range compensation [12].

The literature is more extensive for 3D printing of bolus in photon and electron therapies. Similar principles apply, however, in that printing parameters have a significant impact on dosimetry [23] and design/fit of bolus may be significantly improved by voxel smoothing or use of a surface scanner [24].

Energy Modulation

The BP dose distribution, to which PT owes its advantages, is not therapeutically useful. The peak is too narrow to uniformly cover any realistic target for treatment. In order to widen the dose distribution in the axial direction, several BPs at different depths are superimposed for a given field. They are weighted to produce a uniform dose distribution over the target region. These BPs may be produced in one of three ways: variable beam degradation over time (modulator wheels), spatial degradation exploiting scatter (ridge filters), or by applying multiple proton beam energies (energy switching). For active scatter systems, energy switching upstream may be a possibility. However, for many passive systems, only one energy is supplied for a given field. Thus, beam degraders must be used for modulation. 3D printing offers several advantages over the standard fabrication techniques for modulators.

Modulator Wheels

For systems that can only apply one energy per field, depth modulation can be achieved by varying the range pullback in time. A modulator wheel is a beam degrader that rotates through a range of thicknesses during treatment. This is simple and effective method for varying pullback in time so long as rotation is fast enough to avoid interplay with beam dynamics. Wheels are commonly implemented as a stepped design and milled from solid pieces of plastic (PMMA, Lucite) [23]. The step height determines the proton range pullback and the step's fractional share of the wheel is its weighting in time. For a passive scatter system, wheels sizes will be constrained by the required maximum field size. It is common for a PT program to house a library of modulator wheels—each associated with a set width of uniform axial dose and optimized for a range of energies.

3D printing has been employed in modulator fabrication to rapidly produce energy and patient-specific modulators, develop optimization methods, test new geometries, and for use as a test case for printed components [3]. Figure 6.5 (left) and (center) show classic modulator wheel designs using FDM and jetted printing techniques. Optimization was done via interpolation on Monte Carlo and the wheel design used water-equivalent scaling. The FDM wheel, made with ABS plastic, has significant surface defects and internal inhomogeneities. The jetted wheel has a much-improved print resolution with more pronounced rounding of sharp edges. Figure 6.6 shows the spread-out Bragg peaks (SOBPs) for the design target, the FDM, and jetted wheels. The jetted wheel's improved homogeneity yielded a much-improved match to the design target. The sharpness of the FDM SOBP was significantly reduced—indicating prominent inhomogeneities in the thinnest step of the FDM print. The high-resolution (20-μm print by 100-μm lateral) PolyJet printer also introduced the option to optimize smooth wheel designs. Standard CNC milling techniques are constrained by drill bit size and shape. Shown in Figure 6.5 (right), the stepless wheel was designed using cubic spline interpolation on Monte Carlo dose distributions. This design avoids sharp-corner defects and exploits more degrees of freedom to improve dose uniformity and distal falloff [25]. This is an example of design-for-fabrication—a design process tailored to the fabrication process that exploits the advantages and avoids disadvantages.

Recent interest in biological studies for high dose-rate therapies, e.g., FLASH therapy, has motivated the design of new platforms for delivery [26]. Printed modulator wheels have been shown to offer rapid prototyping, improved accuracy, and dose rates sufficient for this task [27]. However, spinning modulator wheels are always susceptible to interplay effects. Resonance between beam pulses and a spinning wheel can produce a significantly different dose distributions compared to those planned. Static modulators (ridge filters), potentially in combination with magnetic steering, may help avoid these issues with interplay.

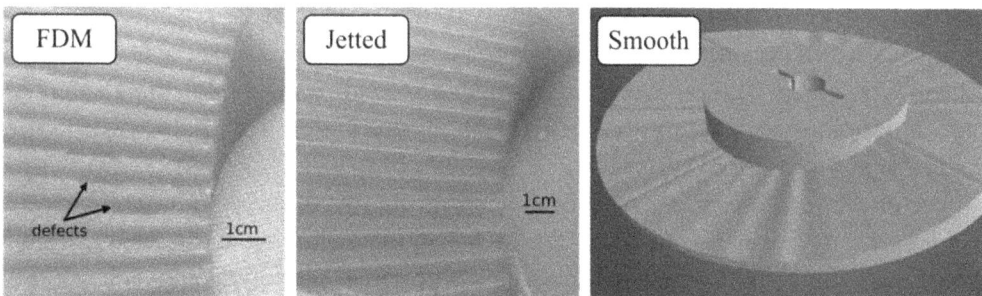

FIGURE 6.5   Photo of FDM printed modulator wheel (left), photo of jet-printed modulator wheel (center), and rendering of stepless modulator wheel design (right). Figure sourced with permission from [25].

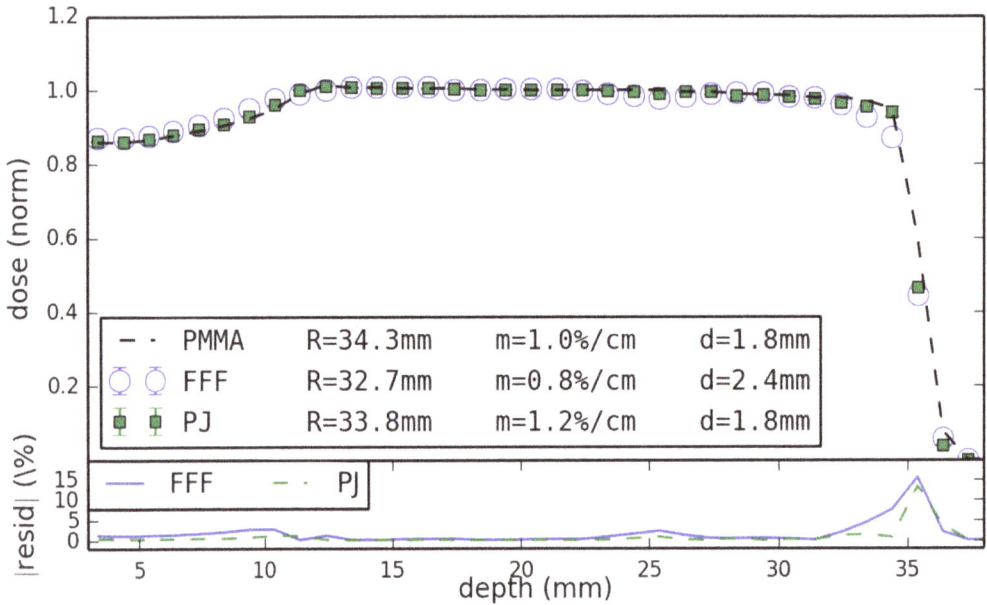

FIGURE 6.6   74 MeV spread out Bragg peaks from modulator wheels fabricated with an FDM (FFF) printer, a jetted (PJ) printer, and milled from solid PMMA. The target modulation width was 23 mm and target range was 34 mm in water. Figure sourced with permission from [3].

Static Modulators

Instead of a varying degrader geometry in time, static modulators rely on scatter through a static component to vary proton range. Depicted in Figure 6.7, static modulators are most often composed of an array of ridges or pyramid-shaped pins. Protons crossing the modulator will traverse a variety of degrading thicknesses. These thicknesses correspond to separate BPs to be applied to a target. Uniform fluence of proton energies across the beam area is achieved through scatter in the component itself. In passive systems, a library of static modulators provides a range of modulation widths for treatment.

Active delivery systems use energy stepping to vary dose with depth. Small spot size and slow energy switching determine the speed of delivery. Combining such a system with a static modulator allows for spreading out of the spot size, requiring fewer (or potentially only one) energy for treatment. Rapid delivery is important to avoid organ-beam timing interplay. It is also necessary for delivery of high dose-rate therapies such as FLASH where the entire treatment must be delivered in under a second. Static modulators that enable these applications must be patient-specific. The complex and high gradient geometries are ideal indications for 3D printing [28].

Recently, several designs have been demonstrated that successfully combine 3D printed static modulators with active scanning systems. Figure 6.7 shows a static modulator design and printed prototype fabricated with jetted photopolymers [29, 30]. The design is optimized for a single beam energy (150 MeV) and includes one 'pin' for each spot in the scanning profile. The total current applied for each spot is then optimized to apply uniform dose to a CT-contoured lung target in a water box. Spot kernels were

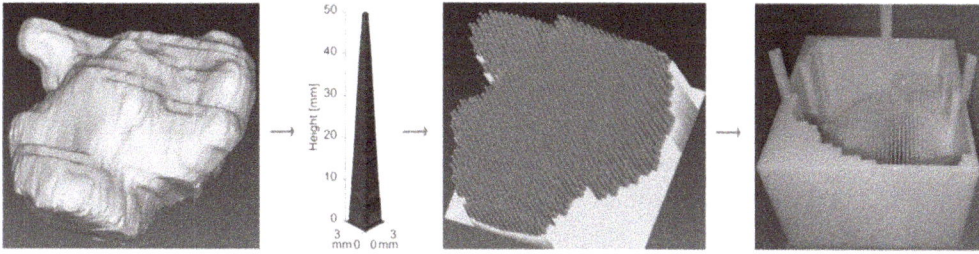

FIGURE 6.7 3D render of target volume (left), render of single pin and entire modulator (middle), and photo of prototype 3D printed modulator with bars for positioning and alignment (right). Figure sourced with permission from [29].

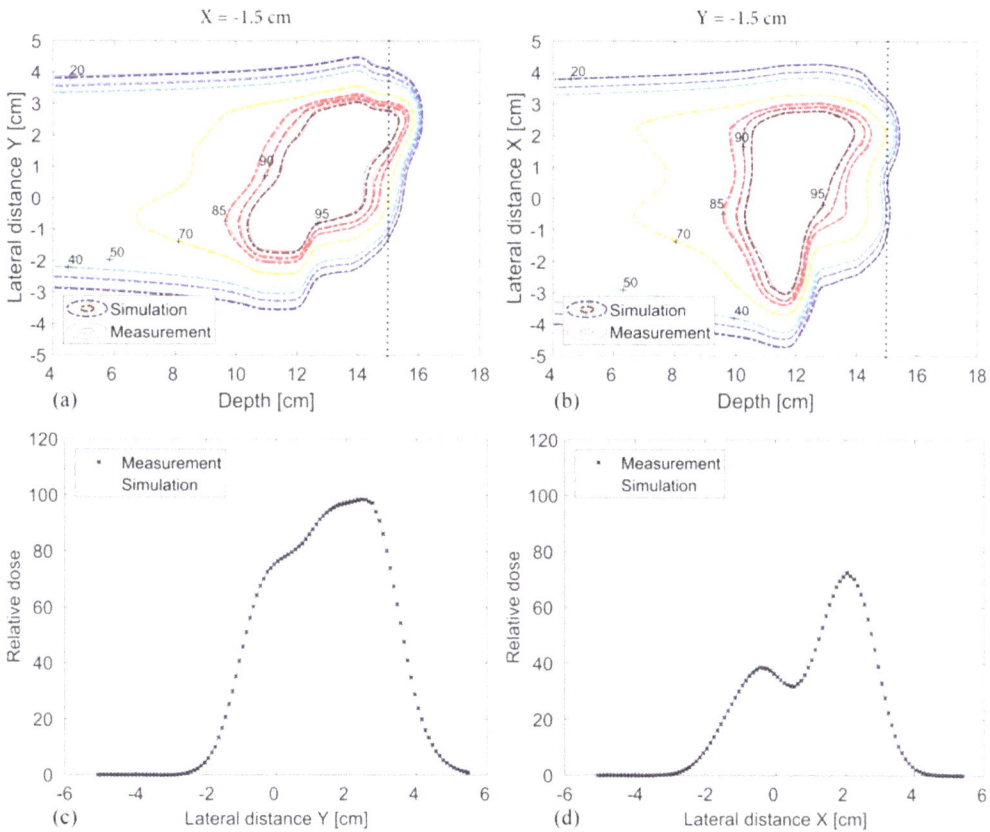

FIGURE 6.8 Isodose lines (upper) and relative dose profiles (lower) for measured and simulated dose to water for scanned 150-MeV proton beam modulated with prototype 3D printed polymer modulator. Figure sourced with permission from [29].

calculated using Monte Carlo [28] and a static pullback compensator was co-optimized in the process. The resulting measured isodoses and profiles in water are shown in Figure 6.8. Dose agreement was excellent, with 99% passing 2%/2mm gamma for 2D slices and the 3D volume. This model was much improved over the previous version [30] that utilized pins half the size, resulting in significantly increased manufacturing artefacts. The same group repeated the study with an aluminum modulator and found comparable results. This prototype and similar designs [31–33] show that 3D printed modulators can enable single-energy scanned treatments that can be delivered at the time scale of seconds.

With these successes, undoubtedly 3D printing will become a key tool in energy modulation for both research and clinical work.

PHANTOMS FOR DOSIMETRY

PT presents unique challenges compared to radiotherapy with photons, including the sensitivity of proton range to heterogeneities, depth of target, and uncertainties of stopping power calculation. Accurate range validation is required to exploit the benefits of the BP falloff. In addition, the dynamics of proton delivery may be vulnerable to organ motion, making it essential to perform end-to-end dosimetry studies that include motion. The use of 3D printed phantoms allows for the creation of heterogeneous and more realistic geometries that can be used to accurately validate proton dose distributions. Here we discuss published applications specifically used in PT dosimetry. Many more studies exist for photon RT applications that are applicable to PT, but we leave those to Chapters 4 and 5 of this book.

3D printing has been widely used in anthropomorphic phantom studies for PT. These CT-based phantoms are printed with the goal of matching the stopping power calculated from CT Hounsfield density. The current state of 3D printing is somewhat limited in the range of densities and materials that can be printed. Despite this, success has been realized using 3D printed phantoms in proton dosimetry. In a study that fabricated a head phantom [10] for 3D gel dosimetry, the near bone-density printed material had unpredictable density variations. In this end-to-end test, where stopping power must be calculated from CT, it was found that CT-based stopping power was discrepant from water column measured by 8%. In addition, variations in CT measured bone stopping power up to 20% were present owing to unintended printed density variations. Despite this, reported range errors were at the 1-mm level. Other head phantom studies have used a similar approach, with water as a tissue surrogate along with dose comparison to film and TPS [34]. Filling a printed phantom with water was effective in this case, with the phantom agreeing with CT within 3% except in areas of fine geometry (sinuses) or skin. Fully printed head phantoms with inlaid dosimeters have also been studied and shown to provide comparable or better agreement to TPS calculated dose than commercially available phantoms [35].

More commonly, 3D printed inserts to mimic local tissue density have been used [36–38]. This is an inexpensive and effective method to enable dosimetry with more realistic local densities. Of particular importance is the study of lung tissue. As discussed earlier, tissue heterogeneities that are not visible on CT can lead to BP degradation in lung. This is difficult to model in the TPS and not well understood experimentally as the tissue is difficult to mimic. Printed lung tissue surrogates comprised of tessellated [39] or CT-based [7] structures allowed for dose measurements that agreed well with Monte Carlo simulation. Printing at sub-millimeter resolution yielded a much more accurate representation of lung tissue than was available.

These studies demonstrate the potential of 3D printing to improve dose calculation verification, despite the limitations of current technology.

Critical in PT is the need to perform end-to-end testing. Because of the inherent uncertainties in many parts of the process, performing dosimetric measurements in patient-realistic scenarios is required for confidence in clinical margins and practices. 3D printing can assist in this, as above, where realistic densities help simulate patient tissue. Furthermore, 3D printing is a simple way to generate large-scale anthropomorphic geometries. A printed thorax phantom allows for more accurate study of interplay between beam dynamics and lung motion [40]. Many head phantoms using 3D printing have been developed for end-to-end or testing of adaptive therapy techniques [10, 34, 36, 41]. Undoubtedly as 3D printing methods improve, more applications for printed dosimeters will emerge. Multi-material printers, or printers that can print a mix of materials, will offer improved stopping power and electron density matching to tissue in the future.

CONCLUSIONS AND LOOKING FORWARD

Proton and ion therapies present unique challenges in delivery and dosimetry that are addressed by improved fabrication techniques offered by 3D printing. 3D printing and novel applications in PT continue to evolve, with the development of more printable materials, variable density prints, variable composition prints, variable hardness of print, inlaid dosimeters, improved density uniformity, and improved reliability. These advancements will be impactful in providing clinicians and researchers with practical solutions that address real challenges in the field.

REFERENCES

[1]   Paganetti H. Proton Therapy Physics. Second Edition, June 30, CRC Press, 2020; 9–26.

[2]   Zhang R, Newhauser WD. Calculation of water equivalent thickness of materials of arbitrary density, elemental composition and thickness in proton beam irradiation. *Phys Med Biol*. 2009;54:1383–1395.

[3]   Lindsay C, Kumlin J, Jirasek A, et al. 3D printed plastics for beam modulation in proton therapy. *Phys Med Biol*. 2015;60:N231–N240.

[4]   Craft DF, Kry SF, Balter P, et al. Material matters: Analysis of density uncertainty in 3D printing and its consequences for radiation oncology. *Med Phys*. 2018;45:1614–1621.

[5]   Urie M, Goitein M, Holley WR, et al. Degradation of the Bragg peak due to inhomogeneities. *Phys Med Biol*. 1986;31:1–15.

[6]   Titt U, Sell M, Unkelbach J, et al. Degradation of proton depth dose distributions attributable to microstructures in lung-equivalent material. *Méd Phys*. 2015;42:6425–6432.

[7]   Baumann K, Weber U, Fiebich M, et al. 3D-printable lung substitutes for particle therapy on the base of high-resolution CTs for mimicking Bragg peak degradation. *Méd Imaging 2019 Imaging Informatics Healthc Res Appl*. 2019;10954:1095414-1095414–1095417.

[8]   Flatten V, Baumann K-S, Weber U, et al. Quantification of the dependencies of the Bragg peak degradation due to lung tissue in proton therapy on a CT-based lung tumor phantom. *Phys Med Biol*. 2019;64:155005.

[9]   Sawakuchi GO, Titt U, Mirkovic D, et al. Density heterogeneities and the influence of multiple Coulomb and nuclear scatterings on the Bragg peak distal edge of proton therapy beams. *Phys Med Biol*. 2008;53:4605–4619.

[10] Hillbrand M, Landry G, Ebert S, et al. Gel dosimetry for three dimensional proton range measurements in anthropomorphic geometries. *Zeitschrift für Medizinische Physik.* 2019;29:162–172.

[11] Michiels S, D'Hollander A, Lammens N, et al. Towards 3D printed multifunctional immobilization for proton therapy: Initial materials characterization: 3D printed immobilization for proton therapy: Materials characterization. *Med Phys.* 2016;43:5392–5402.

[12] Wochnik A, Swakoń J, Olko P. Water equivalence of various 3D printed materials for proton therapy—Monte Carlo simulation, treatment planning modelling and validation by measurements. *Acta Phys Polonica B.* 2020;51:409.

[13] Polf JC, Mille MM, Mossahebi S, et al. Determination of proton stopping power ratio with dual-energy CT in 3D-printed tissue/air cavity surrogates. *Med Phys.* 2019;46:3245–3253.

[14] Cook H, Lambert J, Thomas R, et al. Development of a heterogeneous phantom to measure range in clinical proton therapy beams. *Phys Medica.* 2022;93:59–68.

[15] Ju SG, Kim MK, Hong C-S, et al. New Technique for Developing a proton range compensator with use of a 3-dimensional printer. *Int J Radiat Oncol Biol Phys.* 2014;88:453–458.

[16] Zou W, Fisher T, Zhang M, et al. Potential of 3D printing technologies for fabrication of electron bolus and proton compensators. *J Appl Clin Med Phys.* 2014;16:4959.

[17] Wagner MS. Automated range compensation for proton therapy. *Méd Phys.* 1982;9:749–752.

[18] Yoon M, Kim J-S, Shin D, et al. Computerized tomography-based quality assurance tool for proton range compensators: Computerized tomography-based QA tool for proton range compensators. *Méd Phys.* 2008;35:3511–3517.

[19] Kang M, Wei S, Choi JI, et al. A universal range shifter and range compensator can enable proton pencil beam scanning single-energy Bragg Peak FLASH-RT treatment using current commercially available proton systems. *Int J Radiat Oncol Biol Phys.* 2022;113:203–213.

[20] Shen J, Liu W, Anand A, et al. Impact of range shifter material on proton pencil beam spot characteristics: Range shifter material for proton pencil beam. *Méd Phys.* 2015;42:1335–1340.

[21] Safai S, Bortfeld T, Engelsman M. Comparison between the lateral penumbra of a collimated double-scattered beam and uncollimated scanning beam in proton radiotherapy. *Phys Med Biol.* 2008;53:1729–1750.

[22] Michiels S, Barragán AM, Souris K, et al. Patient-specific bolus for range shifter air gap reduction in intensity-modulated proton therapy of head-and-neck cancer studied with Monte Carlo based plan optimization. *Radiother Oncol.* 2018;128:161–166.

[23] Biltekin F, Yazici G, Ozyigit G. Characterization of 3D-printed bolus produced at different printing parameters. *Méd Dosim.* 2021;46:157–163.

[24] Dipasquale G, Poirier A, Sprunger Y, et al. Improving 3D-printing of megavoltage X-rays radiotherapy bolus with surface-scanner. *Radiat Oncol Lond Engl.* 2018;13:203.

[25] Lindsay C, Kumlin J, Martinez DM, et al. Design and application of 3D-printed stepless beam modulators in proton therapy. *Phys Med Biol.* 2016;61:N276–N290.

[26] Jolly S, Owen H, Schippers M, et al. Technical challenges for FLASH proton therapy. *Phys Medica.* 2020;78:71–82.

[27] Kourkafas G, Bundesmann J, Fanselow T, et al. FLASH proton irradiation setup with a modulator wheel for a single mouse eye. *Méd Phys.* 2021;48:1839–1845.

[28] Simeonov Y, Weber U, Penchev P, et al. 3D range-modulator for scanned particle therapy: Development, Monte Carlo simulations and experimental evaluation. *Phys Med Biol*. 2017;62:7075–7096.

[29] Simeonov Y, Weber U, Schuy C, et al. Development, Monte Carlo simulations and experimental evaluation of a 3D range-modulator for a complex target in scanned proton therapy. *Biomed Phys Eng Express*. 2022;8:035006.

[30] Simeonov Y, Weber U, Schuy C, et al. Monte Carlo simulations and dose measurements of 2D range-modulators for scanned particle therapy. *Zeitschrift für Medizinische Physik*. 2021;31:203–214.

[31] Holm KM, Weber U, Simeonov Y, et al. 2D range modulator for high-precision water calorimetry in scanned carbon-ion beams. *Phys Med Biol*. 2020;65:215003.

[32] Zhang G, Gao W, Peng H. Design of static and dynamic ridge filters for FLASH-IMPT: A simulation study. *Méd Phys*. 2022;49:5387–5399.

[33] Maradia V, Colizzi I, Meer D, et al. Universal and dynamic ridge filter for pencil beam scanning particle therapy: A novel concept for ultra-fast treatment delivery. *Phys Med Biol*. 2022;67:225005.

[34] Makris DN, Pappas EP, Zoros E, et al. Characterization of a novel 3D printed patient specific phantom for quality assurance in cranial stereotactic radiosurgery applications. *Phys Med Biol*. 2019;64:105009.

[35] Kamomae T, Shimizu H, Nakaya T, et al. Three-dimensional printer-generated patient-specific phantom for artificial in vivo dosimetry in radiotherapy quality assurance. *Phys Medica*. 2017;44:205–211.

[36] Nenoff L, Matter M, Charmillot M, et al. Experimental validation of daily adaptive proton therapy. *Phys Med Biol*. 2021;66:205010.

[37] Gorgisyan J, Lomax AJ, Rosenschold PM af, et al. The dosimetric effect of residual breath-hold motion in pencil beam scanned proton therapy – An experimental study. *Radiother Oncol*. 2019;134:135–142.

[38] Dimitriadis A, Palmer AL, Thomas RAS, et al. Adaptation and validation of a commercial head phantom for cranial radiosurgery dosimetry end-to-end audit. *The Br J Radiol*. 2017;90:20170053.

[39] Koketsu J, Kumada H, Takada K, et al. 3D-printable lung phantom for distal falloff verification of proton Bragg peak. *J Appl Clin Méd Phys*. 2019;20:86–94.

[40] Mayer R, Liacouras P, Thomas A, et al. 3D printer generated thorax phantom with mobile tumor for radiation dosimetry. *Rev Sci Instruments*. 2015;86:074301.

[41] Neppl S, Kurz C, Köpl D, et al. Measurement-based range evaluation for quality assurance of CBCT-based dose calculations in adaptive proton therapy. *Med Phys*. 2021;48:4148–4159.

CHAPTER 7

Applications in Brachytherapy

Amanda Cherpak and Krista Chytyk-Praznik

INTRODUCTION

Although brachytherapy is one of the oldest forms of radiotherapy, it can be argued that, compared to external beam therapy, many of its essential tools have benefited from only incremental advancements over the past decades. This situation has changed dramatically with the incorporation of 3D printing, which now promises to compliment or disrupt multiple brachytherapy technologies by offering true personalization of patient setup and treatment delivery. For example, existing brachytherapy applicators may be personalized to offer improved dosimetry particular to a patient's geometry of target volumes and organs-at-risk (OARs). In other approaches, generic applicators are discarded entirely in favor of *de novo* bespoke 3D printed devices, for example, that introduce new options for improving fit to the patient and for optimizing source trajectories.

This chapter begins with a discussion of 3D printable materials that are applicable to brachytherapy, including both tissue-like and shielding media. Examples of 3D printable tools are described that fulfill unmet needs, ranging from apparatus for precise source calibration, to phantoms allowing realistic training experience. Various clinical applications are described that highlight the broad array of innovations that have been unlocked by 3D printing in surface, breast, and gynecological brachytherapy. Finally, given that 3D printing is a fairly new approach now intersecting brachytherapy practice, practical implications for workflow are discussed.

3D PRINTING MATERIALS FOR BRACHYTHERAPY APPLICATIONS

A wide range of materials are available for 3D printing; however, brachytherapy applications introduce stringent requirements, limiting the potential options. As in most patient applications, materials must be biocompatible, however specific requirements depend on intended use of the device, i.e., whether it makes contact with intact skin or mucosal surfaces, as well as the duration of application. The invasive nature of

DOI: 10.1201/9781003288404-7

inter- and intra-cavitary brachytherapy treatments also requires applicators to be steriliz-able. Manufacturers have supported these needs by introducing several printing materials that adhere to the International Standard ISO-10993, and the United States Pharmacopeia (USP) standards for biocompatibility. Chapter 3 of this book provides a comprehensive discussion of these requirements. Personalized applicators with individualized catheter channels aim to offer minimal perturbation of dose, and therefore should be approxi-mately water equivalent. This allows for compatibility with standard treatment planning systems that utilize TG-43 dose calculation algorithms [1]. Recent work has also explored patient-specific shielding using 3D printed high-Z materials [2, 3]. Materials used in con-junction with brachytherapy sources must be investigated to understand the impact of the material on the radiation dose distribution [4]. Brachytherapy sources emit low-energy (kV) radiation, so the photoelectric effect has a more significant contribution to the total radiation attenuation coefficient compared to megavoltage radiation. The cross section is therefore proportional to the 4–5th power of the atomic number (Z) of the attenuating material and inversely proportional to the third power of the photon energy [5]. The first 3D printed brachytherapy applicators were constructed using material attenuation coefficients for a high dose rate (HDR) Ir-192 brachytherapy source [6, 7]. Initial results demonstrated that this method was promising, however recent studies have furthered material characterization with absolute and relative dose measurements [4].

Tissue-Equivalent Materials

Table 7.1 summarizes properties of various material candidates for brachytherapy applications. Two commonly-used 3D printing materials are polylactic acid (PLA) and acrylonitrile butadiene styrene (ABS). Both materials are inexpensive and available for fused deposition modeling (FDM) printing. PLA may be biocompatible but due to a low softening temperature it cannot be sterilized by steam autoclave [8] so it must be sterilized using other methods such as ethylene oxide, gamma or electron beam irradiation. It can also be cleaned with surface disinfectants; however, some cleaning agents can degrade the material over time [9]. ABS is not certified biocompatible [10]. Similar to PLA, it exhibits significant dimensional deviations after steam sterilization and therefore should be cleaned using the abovementioned alternative methods [8].

The effects of PLA and ABS on the dose distribution from an Ir-192 source were investigated in air using both an ion chamber and radiochromic film [4]. Samples up to 30-mm thick were printed with infill percentage between 95% and 100%, and measurements showed dose deviations from water to be within measurement uncertainty (Figure 7.1). Theoretical calculations show that the attenuation coefficient of PLA is slightly lower than that of water for Ir-192. For ABS, the effective atomic number was higher than that of water, resulting in greater attenuation. Although 100% infill may be specified in 3D printer settings, completely homogeneous density is not achieved in practice, e.g., due to very small but unavoidable gaps between printed layers. In this work it was thus hypothesized that this characteristic may offset the higher attenuation of the material itself.

Another study [13] developed the 'MARM' phantom (Figure 7.2) and a standard procedure to investigate the properties of PLA and ABS with irradiation by a Ir-192

TABLE 7.1   Examples of Commonly Used Materials Suitable for 3D Printing in Brachytherapy

Material	Biocompatible[a]	Sterilizable	Water Equivalence
Acrylonitrile butadiene styrene (ABS)	Not certified	Not suitable for steam autoclave. Alternative method must be used.	Within measurement uncertainty. *Measured dose within 0.94%, 0.5–1.5 cm from source, ion chamber and radiochromic film.* [11]
Polylactic acid (PLA)	Yes	Not suitable for steam autoclave. Alternative method must be used.	Within measurement uncertainty. *Measured dose within 2.3%, 0.5–1.5 cm from source, ion chamber and radiochromic film.* [4]
Polycarbonate-ISO (PC-ISO)	Yes	Yes	Within measurement uncertainty. *Measured dose within 1%, 1–6 cm from channel, Gafchromic film.* [12]
Polyetherimide (PEI)	Yes	Yes	Attenuation similar to water. Quantified using Monte Carlo simulation. [2]
Polyphenylsulfone (PPSF/PPSU)	Not certified	Yes	Attenuation similar to water. Quantified using Monte Carlo simulation. [2]
Polyether ether ketone (PEEK)	Yes	Yes	Attenuation similar to water. Quantified using Monte Carlo simulation. [2]
Polyamide 12 (PA12/NPA)	Yes	Not suitable for steam autoclave. Alternative method must be used.	Attenuation similar to water. Quantified using Monte Carlo simulation. [2]
Dental SG	Yes	Yes	No published results.

Note: [a]Biocompatible: defined by the IUPAC (International Union of Pure and Applied Chemistry) as the capacity to be in contact with a living system without producing an adverse effect. ISO 10993 entails a series of standards for evaluating the biocompatibility of medical devices to manage biological risk (adopted by FDA).

source, with the phantom accommodating both film and ion chamber detectors. Results demonstrated that dose measurements differed by 2.3% (PLA) and 0.94% (ABS) from those measured in water within a clinically relevant range of 0.5–1.5 cm from the source (Figure 7.3). The overall dose uncertainty associated with the measurement setup (electrometer, ion chamber, source positioning) was ±3%. The difference attributed to the PLA and ABS samples was therefore considered to be clinically insignificant. This result satisfies the relevant tolerance for dose uncertainty in brachytherapy accuracy of 5% [14].

PC-ISO is another commercially available 3D printing material. It is a certified biocompatible polycarbonate material that has been used for gynecological applicators [12]. It is not suitable for sterilization by steam autoclave, however, gamma radiation and ethylene oxide are viable alternatives. Radiation attenuation of the material has been evaluated using a custom film dosimetry apparatus (Figure 7.4) that accepts Gafchromic film for

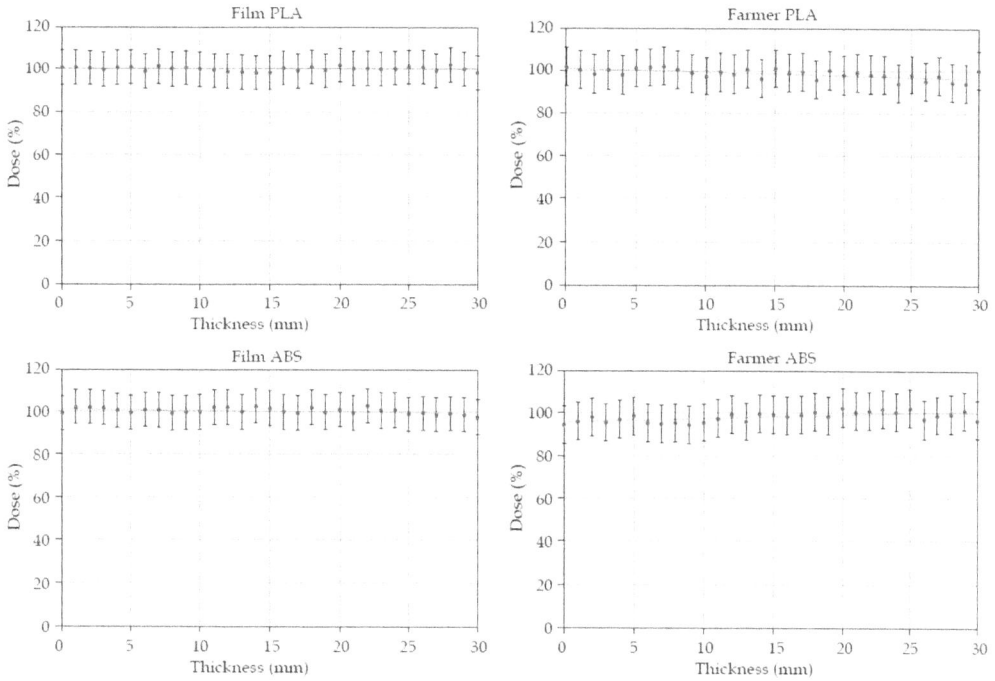

FIGURE 7.1   Average dose and measurement uncertainty as a function of thickness of PLA (top row) and ABS (bottom row) samples. All measured doses are within measurement uncertainty of dose calculated in water. Figure sourced with permission from [4].

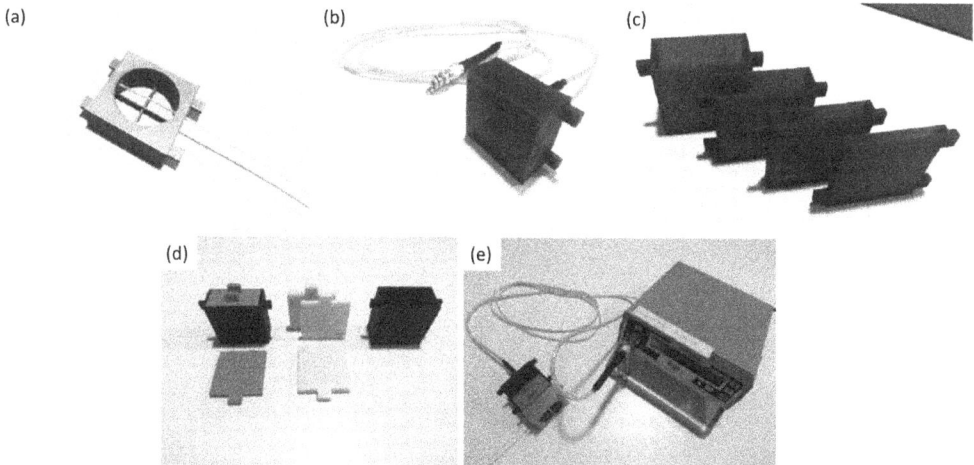

FIGURE 7.2   The MARM phantom showing (a) a catheter in its holder, (b) placement of the ion chamber, (c) a set of boxes of different dimensions, (d) inserts of PLA, ABS and water, and (e) the complete phantom with detector an electrometer. Figure sourced with permission from [13].

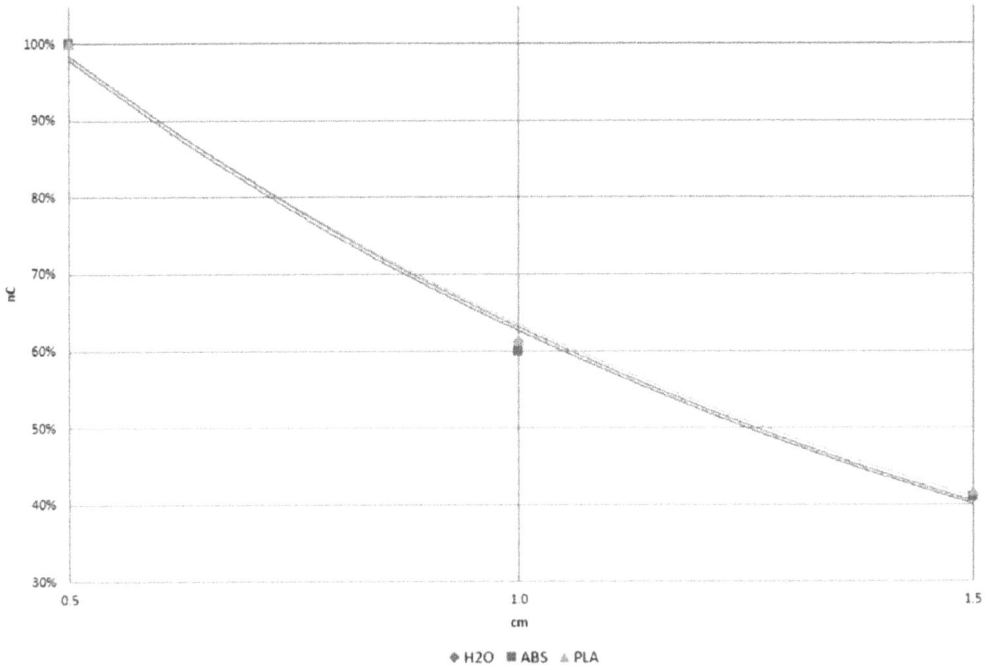

FIGURE 7.3   Measured percentage depth dose for an Ir-192 source in water compared to in ABS and PLA. Figure sourced with permission from [13].

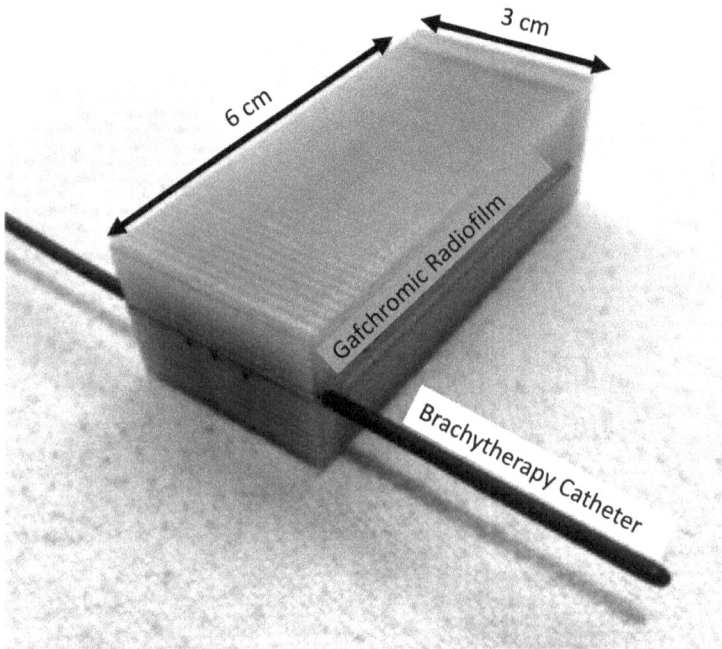

FIGURE 7.4   Test apparatus including a 6-French catheter inserted into a channel in a PC-ISO and containing Gafchromic film. The measurement was repeated with a water-equivalent phantom. Figure sourced with permission from [12].

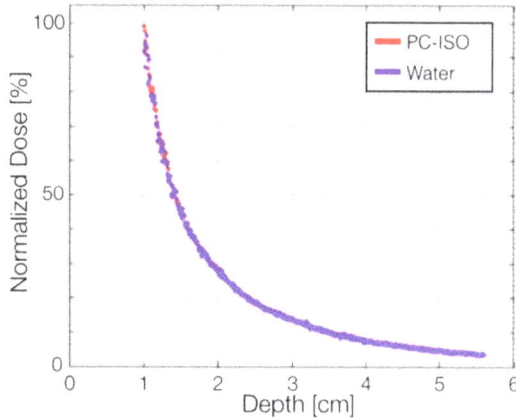

FIGURE 7.5 Percent depth dose measured with Gafchromic film, comparing PC-ISO to water, showing agreement within 1% over a depth from 1 to 6 cm from the source channel. Figure sourced with permission from [12].

measurement of percent depth dose curves. Corresponding measurements acquired in water showed agreement within 1% over distances of 1 to 6 cm from the source channel (Figure 7.5). Variation increased to 4% to 7% for measurements taken in air.

Many material options exist for both FDM and Multi Jet Fusion (MJF) printing, and the list of candidates is expanding continuously. In addition to the well-studied materials mentioned above, other candidates include nylon polyamide (NPA), polymethyl methacrylate (PMMA), polyetherimide (PEI, e.g., ULTEM), polyphenylsulfone (PPSF/PPSU), polyether ether ketone (PEEK), and stereolithography (SLA)-printing resins such as Dental SG (Formlabs, Inc.), and polyamide 12 (PA12) (HP). Semeniuk *et al.* used Monte Carlo simulations to investigate the effects of several of these biocompatible materials on the dose distribution from a generic vaginal vault [2]. The material to be investigated occupied the volume labelled 'test material' in Figure 7.6 and dose from an Ir-192 source was scored from the outside wall of the applicator (radius 1.8 cm) to 10 cm from the source. Nine materials considered in this study resulted in similar, water-like distributions, as shown in Figure 7.7.

High-Z Materials

Intensity modulation of Ir-192 distributions and organ-at-risk sparing can be achieved by incorporating high density and high atomic number materials into specific regions of brachytherapy applicators. Commercially available options include vaginal vault applicators with wedge inserts comprised of shielding materials [15]. Such wedges are limited with respect to size and solid angle (i.e., a quarter-wedge or half-wedge), and options are not patient-specific or fully adaptable to different clinical scenarios. An alternative that has been proposed is to use 3D printing of high-Z filament to build personalized shielding into patient-specific applicators [2, 3].

One material candidate is 3D printable tungsten-loaded plastic (WPLA). This filament (Filamet™, The Virtual Foundry, WI) consists of 95% tungsten powder and 5% plastic

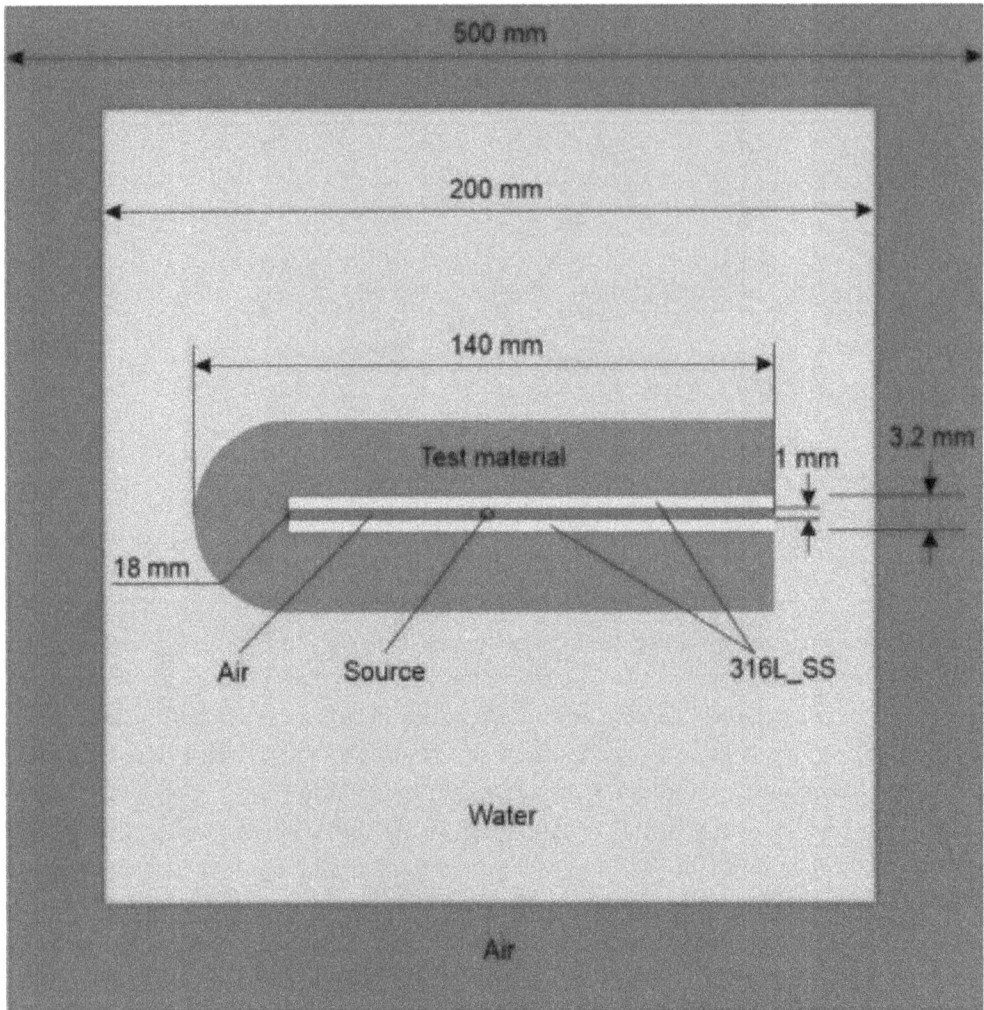

FIGURE 7.6 Geometry of a generic HDR brachytherapy applicator for testing of dosimetry of 3D printable materials using Monte Carlo simulation. Figure sourced with permission from [2].

by weight, giving a bulk density up to 9 g/cc. This mass density gives a half-value layer of approximately 4 mm for an Ir-192 source [3]. One study that investigated the use of WPLA in a vaginal vault applicator design used an outer shell comprised of an ISO 10993 certified biocompatible plastic so that the tungsten material is not in contact with the patient surface. Several versions of a vaginal applicator were simulated with differing configurations of shielding material, as shown in Figure 7.8. Monte Carlo simulations were performed to model the dose from applicators with multiple configurations of shielded material incorporated. The 3D printable tungsten-PLA composite shielding material was simulated with weight fractions of 0.0028 H, 0.025 C, 0.0222 O, and 0.95 W, i.e., 95% tungsten by weight and with a mass density of 9 g/cc. Dose was also calculated using the Acuros BV algorithm (Varian Medical Systems) for comparison. It should be noted that the highest density material that can be simulated in Acuros BV is stainless steel, with a density of 8 g/cc, therefore differences between MC and Acuros can be

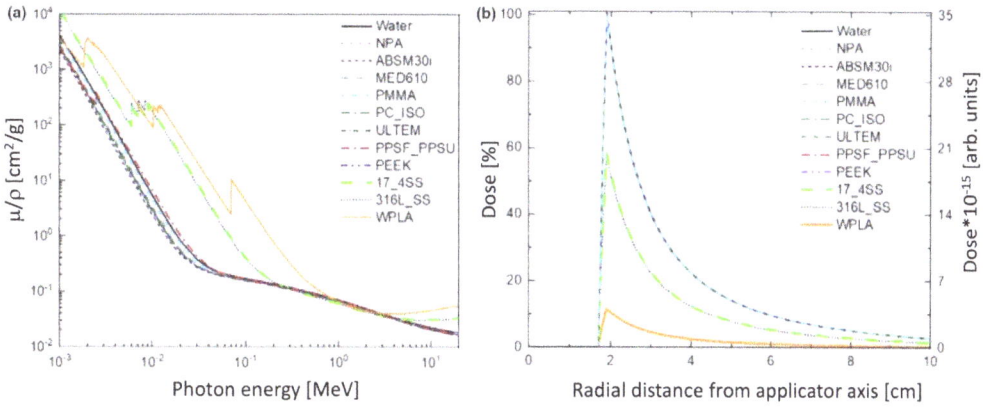

FIGURE 7.7 (a) Mass attenuation coefficients for various printable materials as a function of energy, including candidates that are tissue-like as well as candidates for shielding and (b) dose profiles for the same materials in water, for the generic applicator shown in Figure 7.6. Figure sourced with permission from [2].

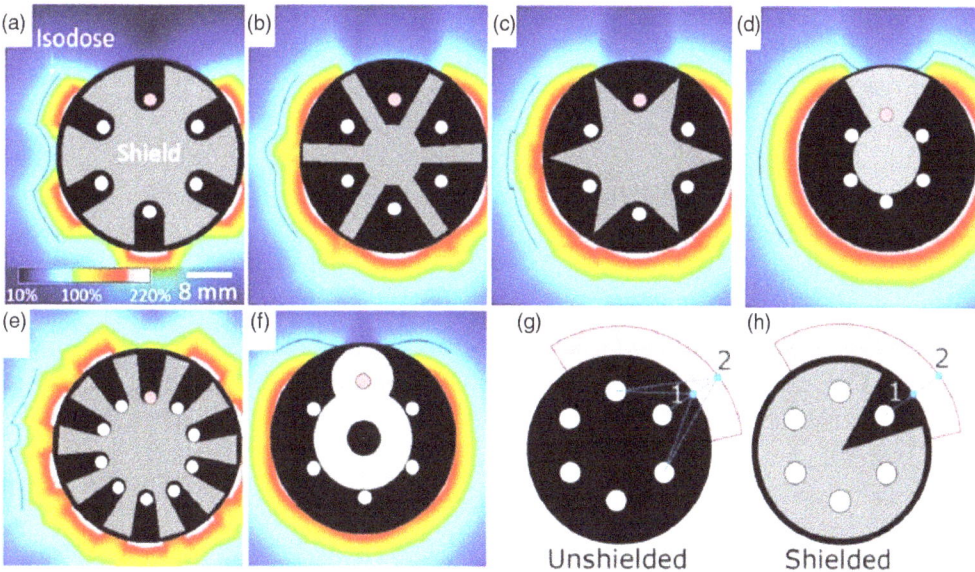

FIGURE 7.8 (a–f) Configurations from Skinner et al., where gray is the tungsten-filled volume, black is filled with water, and white and pink circles show active and inactive channels, respectively. (g and h) The concept that a line of sight to just one source will yield a more rapid dose fall off. Figure sourced with permission from [3].

attributed to differences in attenuation of the modeled shielding materials. Figure 7.9 shows the significant reduction in transmission possible as profiles are taken through differing thicknesses of WPLA [3].

The report by Semeniuk et al. also studied WPLA, as well as two variations of stainless steel (17_4SS, 316L_SS) [2]. The first type, 17_4SS, is a common and exceptionally durable type of steel used in a diverse variety of industries and applications. The prefix 17_4 refers to its composition, i.e., approximately 17% chromium and 4% nickel. The

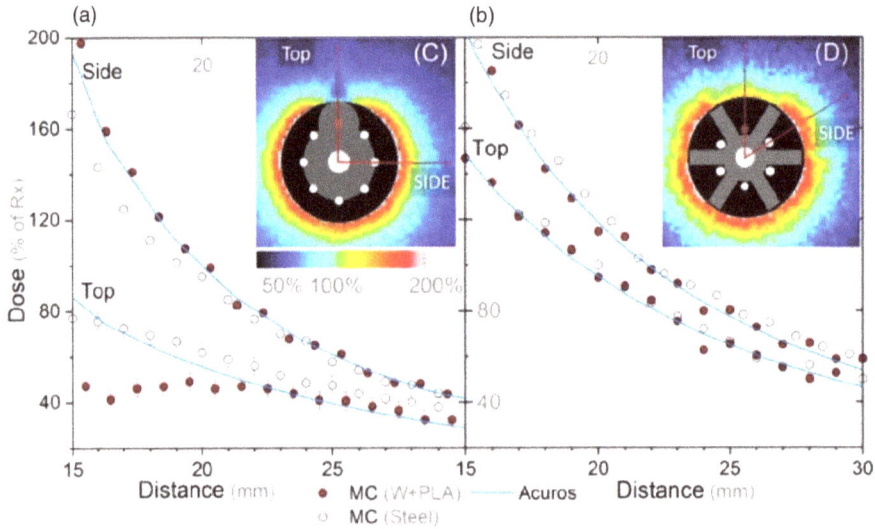

FIGURE 7.9   Dose profiles shown for two shielding configurations from Skinner et al., comparing Monte Carlo to Acuros dose calculation results. Figure sourced with permission from [3].

second type of stainless steel, 316L_SS, is comprised of 16%–18% chromium and 10%–14% nickel. The densities of the stainless steel materials are 7.75 g/cm³ (17_4SS), 8 g/cm³ (316L_SS). Unlike WPLA, both stainless steel types are biocompatible. In the Monte Carlo study, all three materials (WPLA, 17_4SS, and 316L_SS) decreased transmission of an Ir-192 source to varying degrees, as seen in Figure 7.7. Dose profiles from the two stainless steel materials were similar, both shielding the radiation at the applicator surface to approximately 60% of the value for transmission through water alone. When stainless steel was used, transmission dropped to approximately 20% at a distance 13 mm from the applicator surface. The third material, WPLA, offered even greater shielding, with transmission dropping to just above 10% at the applicator surface and to approximately 5% at 13 mm from the surface. It should be noted that, to date, the use of stainless steel in 3D printing brachytherapy applications remains in development.

DEVICES ENABLED BY 3D PRINTING IN BRACHYTHERAPY

Medical specializations have long devised their own equipment to fulfill particular functions. Maxillofacial, neurological, and orthopedic surgery were among the first areas to adopt 3D printing due to specific needs of equipment in those disciplines as well as the desire to reduce long operating room times [16, 17]. Custom implants and prosthetics, anatomical models for surgical planning and surgical guides were the most common devices printed. Brachytherapy is a highly specialized technique, so it is not unexpected that this area of radiation oncology has given rise to dedicated equipment and phantoms for routine use that may not be available commercially. Devices manufactured using 3D printing include those for routine quality assurance and patient-specific training phantoms.

Quality Assurance Equipment

Specification of source strength (also known as Reference Air Kerma Rate, or RAKR) is required for routine quality assurance in hospitals with brachytherapy programs. While many radiotherapy departments use a well-type chamber traceable to a primary standards laboratory for these measurements, not all laboratories will have the capability to produce a brachytherapy standard. The ability to calibrate the source with a Farmer-type ionization chamber in air is beneficial where there is no brachytherapy calibration available, or where a secondary check is desired. The literature contains examples of custom jigs created to fulfill the calibration conditions needed for a cylindrical ion chamber measurement, but these are often affected by setup and positional uncertainties, as well as uncertainty in scatter corrections and attenuation factors. Simpson-Page *et al.* [18] designed and 3D printed a jig for RAKR determination in air (Figure 7.10), with an uncertainty of 3.75%. As reported, this jig is easy to set up, customizable to accommodate any cylindrical ion chamber, and has been tested in several facilities. The 3D printing file for the jig is publicly available for download.

Precise source calibration is essential in brachytherapy, but other sources of error exist, such as those affecting source dwell position, application of correct units, and those related to performance of equipment and software. Major adverse incidents in brachytherapy have been linked to errors in the channel length for applicators, and the relationship that length has with the first dwell position relative to the anatomy. Otani *et al.* proposed a pre-treatment verification that involves a replica transparent applicator that was manufactured with a 3D printer using transparent resin [19]. The model was

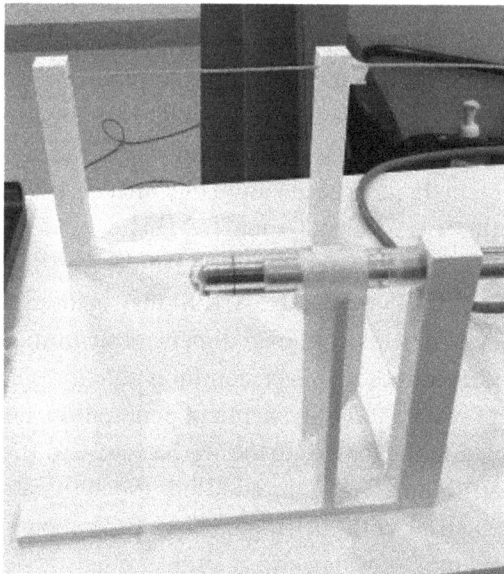

FIGURE 7.10   Printed jig allowing positioning of a PTV 30013 ionization chamber at a set distance from the brachytherapy source for RAKR measurement. Figure sourced with permission from [18].

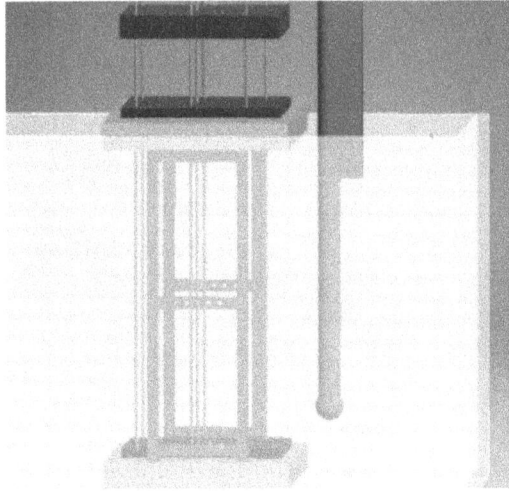

FIGURE 7.11   Phantom allowing positioning of the ultrasound probe to perform distance, resolution and needle template-to-electronic grid alignment in the axial plane. Figure sourced with permission from [22].

designed from CT datasets of the applicator, as well as plans from the vendor (Nucletron, Elekta AB, Stockholm, Sweden). After the replica was validated against the original applicator radiographically, the planned dwell and check cable positions were observed with a digital camera and positioning error was calculated.

Brachytherapy must be supported by a comprehensive quality assurance program addressing possible failure modes, and this should include end-to-end testing. Bassi *et al.* created a full end-to-end test and an HDR audit for the cancer centers in Ireland using a 3D printed phantom that accommodates a planning target volume (PTV) Farmer chamber, Gafchromic EBT3 film, and three thermoluminescent dosimeters (TLDs) [20]. The authors found good agreement and reproducibility among the centers for all dosimetry devices and demonstrated the ease of setup and use of the system.

Some QA tests in brachytherapy occur annually, including testing of the ultrasound system, as specified in the AAPM Task Group 128 [21]. Low dose rate (LDR) seeds and HDR needles for prostate brachytherapy are inserted under transrectal ultrasound (TRUS) guidance. A phantom (e.g., CIRS Model 045, CIRS) may be used to check the resolution and geometric constancy of objects of known dimensions within the treatment planning system as imaged with ultrasound. However, common phantoms do not allow simple and effective assessment of grayscale visibility, depth of penetration, and template alignment. Leong *et al.* [22] created a liquid-based phantom that satisfied the requirements of TG-128 in a single phantom (Figure 7.11). In addition, the authors were able to complete the QA 25 to 45 minutes faster with the single phantom, compared to a standard (CIRS Model 045) phantom and tank of water, and at a substantially lower cost.

Training and Verification Phantoms

The manual insertion of brachytherapy applicators motivates the development of dedicated training and simulation phantoms. Such phantoms allow practice sessions without a patient to evaluate new techniques, to troubleshoot difficult anatomy and to provide valuable experience to trainees.

One of the earliest examples of 3D printing in brachytherapy was presented by Ryu *et al.* [23]. 3D TRUS images from five patients were used as part of a planning study investigating the effect of using oblique versus parallel needle trajectories to treat prostate cancer with LDR brachytherapy, for patients who have pelvic arch interference. A phantom study to test the ability of a 'mechatronic device' in inserting oblique needles via a needle guide used a 3D printed mold to create a 60-cc prostate model from agar (to mimic the speed of sound in tissue) and tungsten powder (for added for CT contrast). The agar prostate was positioned within a phantom container to affix the prostate position, and a machined pelvic arch insert and ultrasound probe were added before the container was fully filled with agar (Figure 7.12). Planned needle and seed positions were compared to CT images of the needle track, showing mean seed displacement within millimeters.

Prostate phantoms have also been developed for education of trainees. Shaaer *et al.* [24] designed a prostate phantom based on a typical patient's TRUS imaging (Figure 7.13). A prostate mold was created via 3D printing and was filled with gelatin, graphite powder, and water to create the prostate. The simulated tissue surrounding the prostate in the cylindrical phantom omitted the graphite. The resulting phantom was generally rated 'good' to 'very good' by radiation oncologists for quality and realism for scanning and insertion.

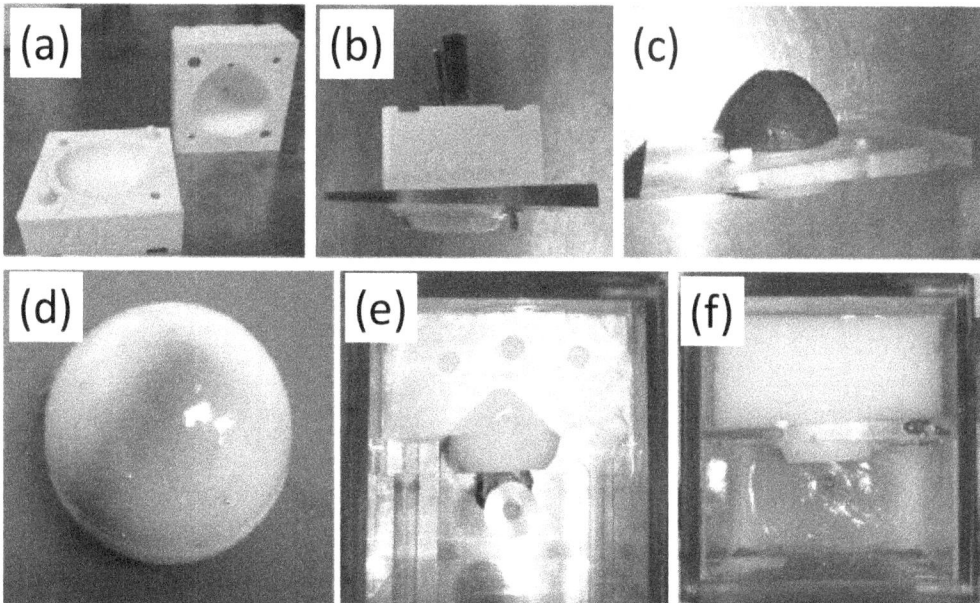

FIGURE 7.12 Fabrication of an agar prostate phantom showing (a) a 3D printed prostate mold, (b) use of a compound plate for pouring, (c) the resultant prostate model, (d) encasement of the prostate in a sphere with fiducials, (e) pouring of the upper half of the phantom, and (f) addition of a simulated pubic arch prior to pouring the lower half of the phantom. Figure sourced with permission from [23].

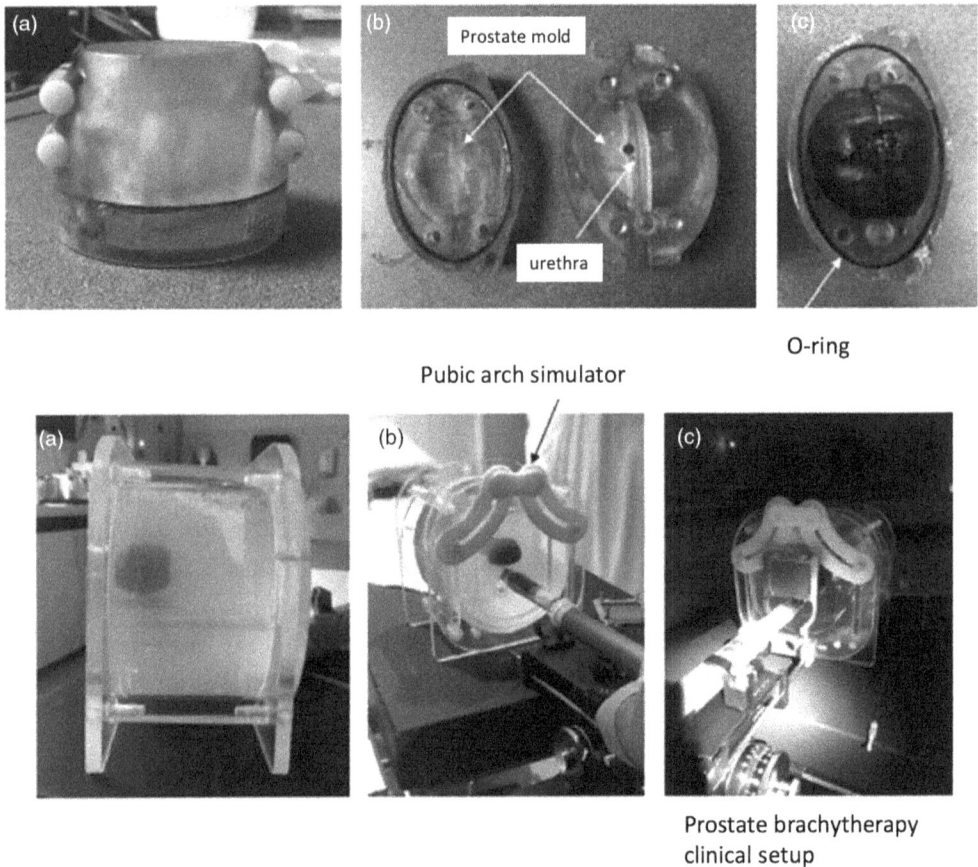

FIGURE 7.13 Fabrication of a 3D printed mold to produce a gelatin/graphite prostate (upper row) and use of the prostate in a cylindrical TRUS phantom (lower row). Figure sourced with permission from [24].

Gynecological phantoms are also of interest, allowing practice of suturing and needle insertions outside of the operating room. Nattagh *et al.* [25] used 3D printing to create a gynecologic phantom consisting mostly of gelatin (Figure 7.14). The vaginal cavity and uterus molds were designed using computer-aided design (CAD) software, with dimensions specified by a radiation oncologist. The gelatin uterus was thinly coated in rubber to better mimic the elasticity of a real uterus. The phantom was reusable, allowing 50 applications of the TRUS probe and 20 suturing sessions. The transparent design was found to be of benefit. Kadoya *et al.* [26] created a female pelvis phantom to evaluate the results of deformable image registration algorithms for CT images with and without a brachytherapy applicator. A bladder and uterus, created from 3D printed molds with silicone and urethane, respectively, were added to a plastic phantom for manipulation.

A reported decline of brachytherapy utilization prompted Campelo *et al.* [27] to create a phantom for use in brachytherapy training (Figure 7.15). The authors aimed to simulate normal and pathological cervical conditions using multi-material PolyJet printing. Patient anatomy for the phantom was modeled using magnetic resonance imaging

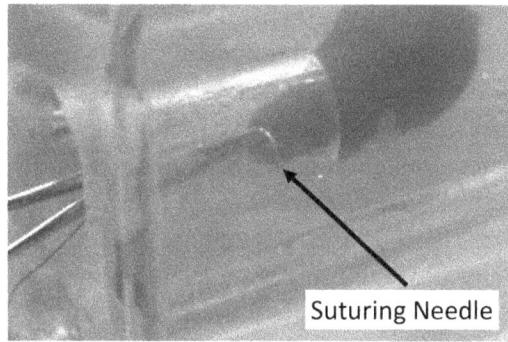

FIGURE 7.14   Gynecological phantom showing practice of suturing at the cervix. Figure sourced with permission from [25].

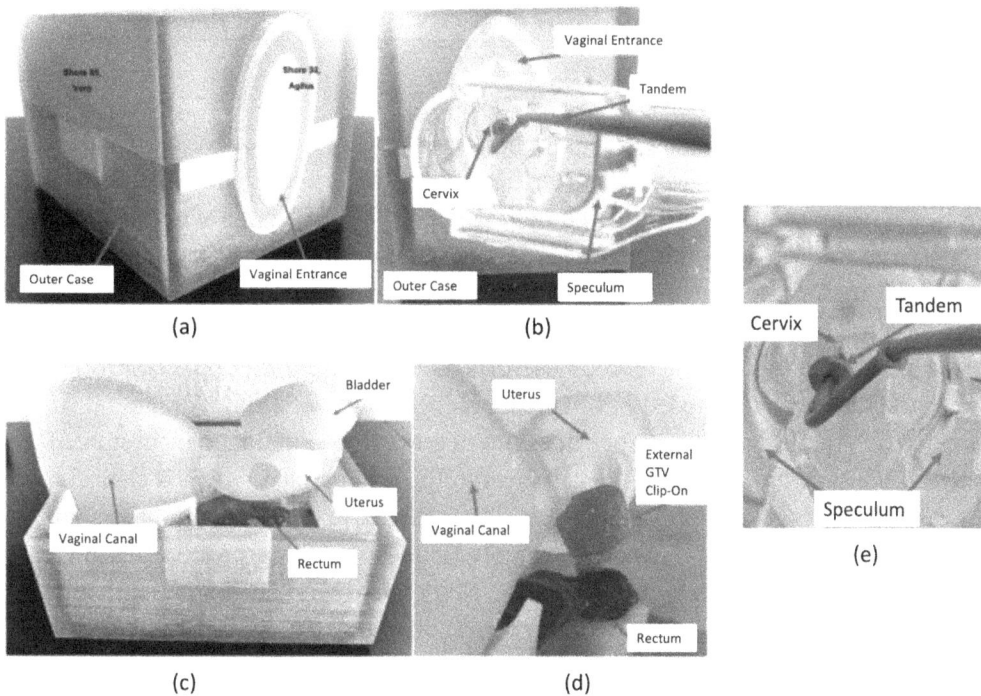

FIGURE 7.15   The gynecological phantom from Campelo et al., showing (a) the closed phantom setup, (b) the speculum entering the vaginal canal, (c) the 3D printed bottom of the case containing the organs of interest, (d) attachment of a GTV on the uterine body, and (e) application of a tandem and speculum during simulated treatment. Figure sourced with permission from [27].

(MRI) and CT data from 50 patients with locally advanced cervical cancer. High risk (HR) clinical target volumes (CTVs) were contoured on T2-weighted MRI images in the treatment planning system. CT data were used to print a vaginal canal, uterus, rectum, and bladder. Three anteverted and one retroverted uterus, along with four different gross tumor volumes (GTVs), derived from the contoured HR-CTVs, were designed. The CAD designs were then printed on a PolyJet printer, with each tissue material printed with a

Young's modulus determined experimentally in previous work. The phantom has yet to undergo an evaluation study by physician residents.

3D printing has also been used for verification of new techniques. Lugez *et al.* [28] created a phantom consisting of a series of prostate templates to hold HDR prostate needles in many catheter configurations. The authors tested electromagnetic (EM) tracking for catheter reconstruction. Silva *et al.* [29] investigated bladder surface dosimetry during gynecological HDR brachytherapy by creating a phantom composed of PMMA, based on patient data. Optically stimulated luminescent dosimeters (OSLDs) and radiochromic film measurements agreed with the planning system to within 10%, leading the researchers to conclude that their phantom design could be used to evaluate *in vivo* dosimetry methods, to validate algorithms, and to further investigate dose points in a patient-realistic phantom.

CLINICAL EXAMPLES OF 3D PRINTING IN BRACHYTHERAPY

Surface Brachytherapy

Superficial tumors, for example, squamous cell carcinoma (SCC) or basal cell carcinoma (BCC), are often treated with electron beams or low energy X-rays. Unfortunately, treatment planning and delivery are complicated with these methods when the treatment area is large, or the patient skin surface is complex. Tumors on irregular surfaces are often candidates for surface brachytherapy, traditionally requiring laborious and manual fabrication of molds. This has involved creation of a plaster of the treatment area to create a wax mold containing catheters, or use of a Freiburg flap-type applicator. There are drawbacks to these customized but manual brachytherapy solutions. A material such as wax may fit a patient's anatomy but does not necessarily maintain a consistent distance between the catheters and from the catheters to the skin surface, which is critical to the delivered dose distribution. Flap applicators are difficult to localize without attaching to an external system (for example, a thermoplastic mesh mask), a process that increases fabrication time. 3D printing introduces the new capacity to match a patient's anatomy precisely, as well as the option of defining personalized catheter trajectories.

An early example of FDM to create a surface brachytherapy applicator was described in 2006 by Schreiber *et al.* [30] who optically scanned a patient and used CAD to design the applicator (Figures 7.16 and 7.17) and the catheter channels. The 2-mm diameter channels were 10 mm apart, 5 mm from the skin surface, with a continuous 25-mm radius of curvature for the entire length of the channels. The study reported that the design and fabrication were more efficient than for a typical workflow, and that the precision of the catheter channel modeling was superior to conventional devices. 3D printers were less accessible at the time of that study, and the applicator was printed off-site at a 'special model center'.

Nearly a decade later, Harris *et al.* [14] investigated the accuracy of a 3D printed applicator using a low-cost, in-house printer. An ABS applicator with in-printed catheter channels was designed in the treatment planning system (Nucletron Oncentra v4.3) and imported

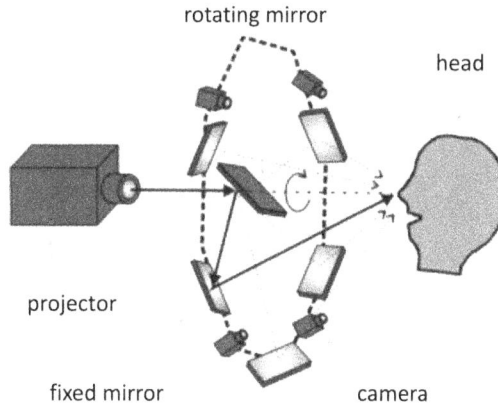

FIGURE 7.16   Schematic depicting optical imaging of the patient for surface brachytherapy applicator design in 2006 by Schreiber et al. Figure sourced with permission from [30].

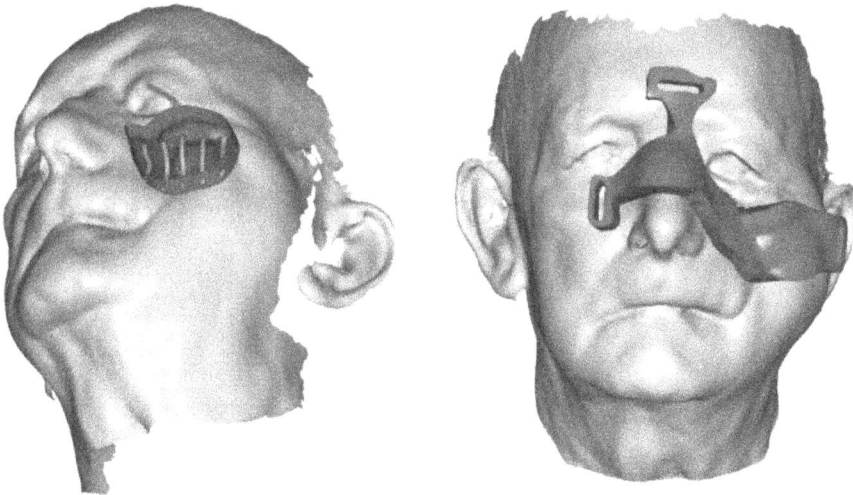

FIGURE 7.17   A view of the catheter trajectories of a surface brachytherapy (left) and the full applicator designed in CAD (right). Figure sourced with permission from [30].

into MATLAB® (Mathworks) for pre-processing before printing. The study examined print accuracy versus orientation of the catheters (vertical or horizontal), reprint accuracy, reproducibility of the catheters in the channels, and accuracy of channels of various radii of curvature (Figure 7.18). Printed applicators showed a dimensional accuracy of within 0.5 mm and 1.0 mm parallel and perpendicular to the build plate, respectively. The catheter channels were 3.5 mm in diameter to allow room for 2-mm catheters to be inserted, but this also allowed inadvertent positioning error of 1 mm. Dosimetric measurements showed that attenuation was about 1% higher through the ABS material from 1 to 3 cm from the source, and within 0.5% at distances 3 to 5 cm away, relative to water.

In 2016, a phantom study examining the use of in-house 3D printed surface applicators was undertaken with examples of comparative treatment plans using 3D printed or

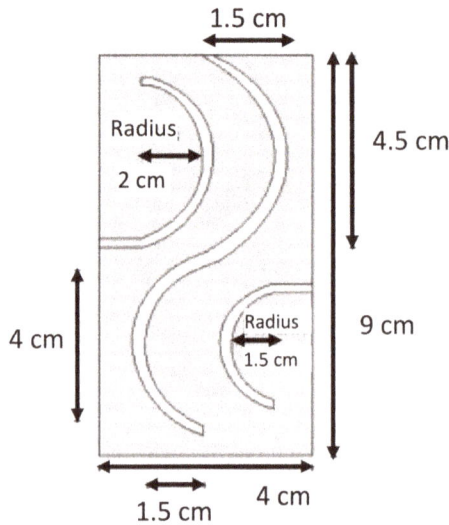

FIGURE 7.18   Cross section of a phantom used to test the accuracy of catheter channels of various radii of curvature. Figure sourced with permission from [14].

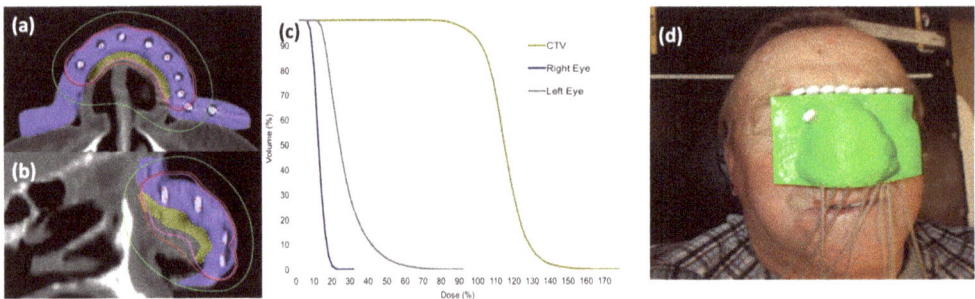

FIGURE 7.19   A treatment plan including a 3D printed surface brachytherapy to treat a lesion on the nose, showing the dose distribution (a and b), dose volume histograms for the CTV and eyes (c) and the physical applicator applied to the patient (d). [31, 32]. Figure sourced with permission from [32].

Freiburg flap applicators [31]. Examples were shown for the ankle and nose, comparing the accuracy of the applicators in fitting to the patient surface, as well as key calculated dosimetric parameters. The 3D printed applicators yielded a smaller volume of air gap between the applicator and the phantom surface, while the calculated dose distributions were comparable or better than the Freiburg flap. An applicator for a BCC patient was printed in preparation for clinical use (Figure 7.19) [31, 32].

Since then, further phantom studies evaluating dose distributions and materials have been carried out [4, 33–35] with several case studies demonstrating treatment at disease sites that would be difficult with manual mold methods, including fingers [36, 37], leg [38], nose [39], and penis [40–42]. Figure 7.20 shows an example of treating an extensive lesion on the shin with a custom FDM-printed surface applicator designed in the Adaptiiv 3DBrachy application (Adaptiiv Medical, Halifax, Canada).

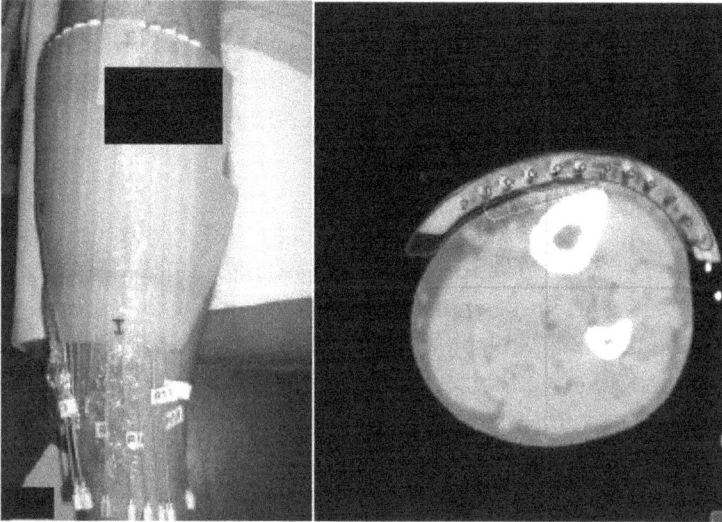

FIGURE 7.20   A 3D printed applicator treating multiple lesions on the shin (left) and an axial slice of the associated treatment plan (right). Figure sourced with permission from [43].

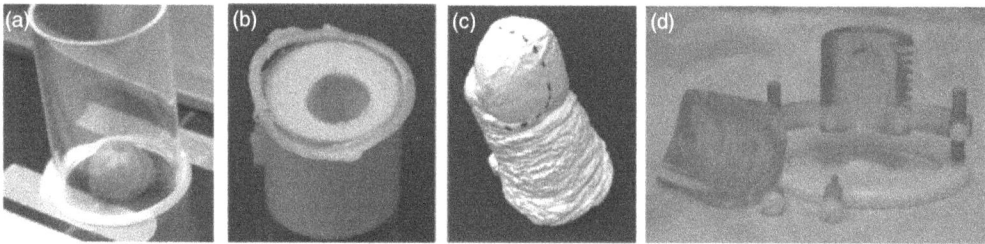

FIGURE 7.21   A negative impression of the penis was formed using dental alginate (a and b) allowing production of a dental stone (c) that was scanned to generate a stereolithography file, allowing definition of catheter trajectories 4 mm from the penile surface. Figure sourced with permission from [41].

Penile brachytherapy, used typically for SCC, can be challenging with regard to immobilization of the anatomy and stabilization of the brachytherapy catheters. D'Alimonte et al. [41] used a dental alginate to create a negative impression of the penis, which was then scanned with a laser-based imager to generate a digital SLA file (Figure 7.21). The applicator was applied to the patient for the planning CT. In another example, Saldi et al. [42] acquired a CT dataset of the patient in the supine position, which was used to delineate the penis and lesion, and to generate a personalized applicator in CAD. The 3D printed applicator was then placed on the patient for the planning CT, with a thermoplastic mask that was applied to the patient to retract the foreskin, expose the glans and hold the penis vertical. In both studies, the urethra was delineated to monitor and limit the dose to the structure.

The benefits of digital design of applicators, compared to typical laborious fabrication with wax and other materials, was demonstrated by Jones et al. [39]. This group created a plan to treat BCC of the nose with customized catheter curvatures, varying distances from the patient surface to take advantage of the inverse-square law fall-off of HDR brachytherapy and incorporating shields for the eyes (Figure 7.22). These features were adjusted manually and were not inherently optimized.

Breast Brachytherapy

Historically, HDR interstitial breast brachytherapy has involved inserting multiple catheters in a desired configuration under ultrasound guidance [44, 45]. One commonly used template, the Kuske applicator, provides a uniformly spaced grid for catheter guidance (Figure 7.23) while at the same time immobilizing the breast [46]. The number and configuration of catheters is limited by the template used for insertion [47] and constrained to a uniformly spaced array.

3D printing has been employed to design personalized templates with the flexibility of defining a patient-specific spacing and configuration of catheters [46, 47]. Personalized templates may also allow for more comfortable patient immobilization [46]. The first

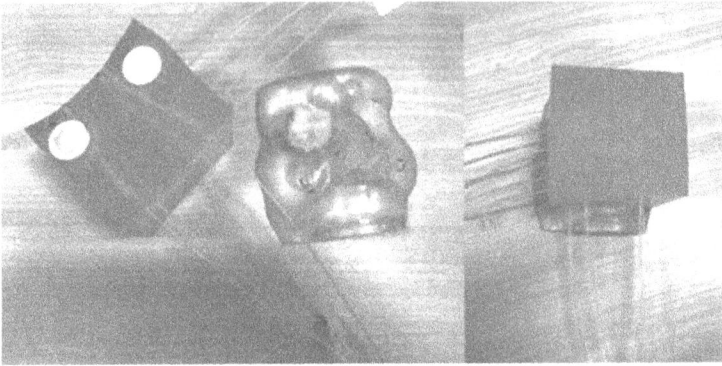

FIGURE 7.22 The 3D printed brachytherapy applicator by Jones et al., including thermoluminescent dosimetry inserts. Figure sourced with permission from [39].

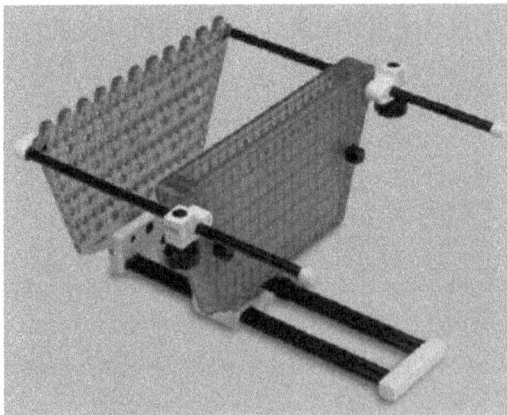

FIGURE 7.23 The Kuske applicator for breast brachytherapy. Figure sourced with permission from [46].

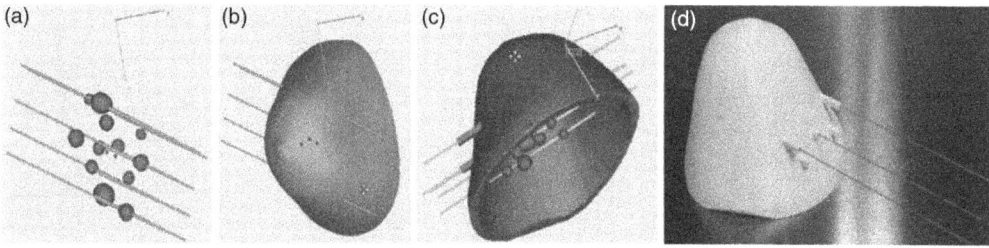

FIGURE 7.24 Planned catheters for a personalized breast template (a), the catheters relative to the breast volume (b), the designed template (c), and the 3D printed template with catheters through the guide holes (d). Figure sourced with permission from [46].

study to apply 3D printed templates to breast brachytherapy used pre-operative CT to localize the tumor site and to create a plan for catheter insertion [46]. A personalized template was designed and printed to both guide catheter insertion and to immobilize the breast tissue during the procedure (Figure 7.24). Workflow and template printing were tested using an agar-based breast phantom and catheter position was verified with post-implant CT. Large variations in agreement between planned and actual catheter positions were noted, ranging from 2 to 10 mm. In one case only one of five needles exited the phantom in the designed exit hole, leaving four needles abutting the side of the template. In the second trial, two of the five needles exited through the designated exit hole. Inaccuracies in catheter position were attributed to positioning of the template post-printing. The technique was refined, adding fiducial markers to the breast tissue to guide template placement and increasing the length of the needle guide in template. These improvements resulted in a marked increase in accuracy of catheter placement, reducing the maximum position error to 8 mm.

Another study investigated the use of personalized breast brachytherapy templates for real-time 3D ultrasound-guided treatments. The templates were printed with a sterilizable bioplastic and applied during insertion into an agarose-based breast phantom [47]. A significant improvement in target coverage was demonstrated when using the personalized 3D printed template compared to the Kuske template. The personalized template also allowed for a reduction in the total number of catheters from an average of 14 to 12. The dose homogeneity index (DHI) of the PTV was reduced with the personalized template, however values were within recommendations from the American Brachytherapy Society. It was found that the DHI was further reduced with experience, suggesting a learning curve [47]. The main limitation of the workflow proposed was the time needed for printing, which took 2 hours using locally available resources. It was proposed that a medical grade, production 3D printer could reduce printing time, providing the tools for a clinical trial protocol [47].

As discussed earlier in this chapter and in Chapter 3, biocompatibility and sterilization are important considerations in brachytherapy treatment. Regardless of the sterilization method used, the process can place a heavy burden on clinical resources in terms of both time and cost. This is especially true for intraoperative brachytherapy, where applicators are placed inside the breast tissue to deliver electronic brachytherapy immediately after

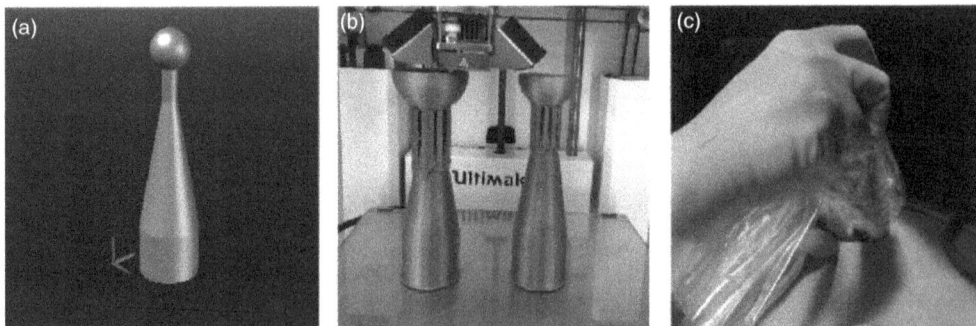

FIGURE 7.25 A CAD file for a 2.5-cm sizing tool for IORT (a), printing of sizing tools using FDM (b) and a sizing tool being used during the procedure (c). Figure sourced with permission from [48].

lumpectomy. The typical workflow for intraoperative electronic breast brachytherapy (IORT) involves testing multiple sterilized applicators to find the appropriate size to fill the surgical void. Applicators are costly and must be replaced after a specified number of sterilizing cycles. A 2016 study developed a 3D printed sizing tool for post-lumpectomy IORT [48]. The tool could be used to quickly determine lumpectomy cavity size and identify the best fitting applicator. This created cost savings by avoiding unnecessary sterilization of applicators that are the wrong size. The tool was printed using a PLA material that is not approved for high temperature sterilization. It was therefore sheathed in a plastic bag similar to covers used for ultrasound probes, as seen in Figure 7.25. The brachytherapy sizing tools were created and printed in five days with cost savings of 30%–50% compared to similar manufacturer-made surgical tools.

Intracavitary Gynecological Brachytherapy

Intracavitary gynecological cylindrical applicators are commercially available in several diameters, typically ranging from 2.5 cm to 4.0 cm in 0.5 cm increments. A patient's vaginal vault may not match the exact diameter of an available cylinder and may exhibit a variable diameter throughout its volume. If an applicator is ill-fitting, there is risk that the applicator is too loose and may move from its initial planning position, or too tight and be painful/uncomfortable for the patient, or there may be air gaps between the target area and the applicator. Any of these scenarios may introduce problems with setup reproducibility and create areas of the patient that could have an excess of dose delivered or areas that are not adequately treated.

Early reports of 3D printing in gynecological brachytherapy described a patient with endometrial cancer who was referred for vaginal cuff brachytherapy [6, 49]. Upon physical examination, the ideal cylinder for vaginal cuff treatment featured a diameter that did not exist in the vendor's product line, in this case, 2.75 cm. An appropriately sized cylinder was prototyped that could accommodate the vendor's standard central vaginal tube (Figure 7.26). The cylinder was printed using PC-ISO thermoplastic, an early commercial material that was shown to be 3D printable, biocompatible, sterilizable, and

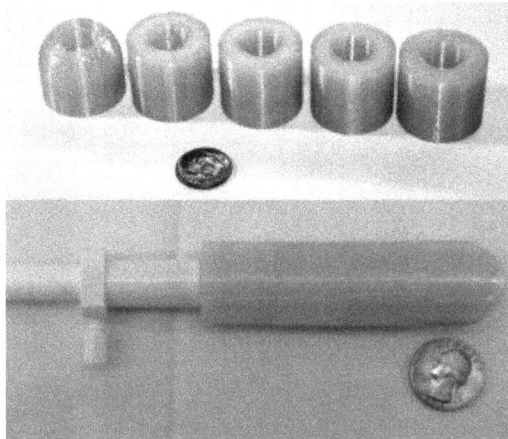

FIGURE 7.26   3D printed segments of the cylinder applicator with a user-defined diameter (top) that may be stacked onto a plastic rod with a central source channel (bottom). Figure sourced with permission from [49].

approved by the FDA [13]. Placement was verified with gold fiducials that were inserted into the patient's vaginal cuff.

Post-hysterectomy vaginal anatomy can be atypical due to the location of the tumor and the surgical methods used, presenting anatomy that is incompatible with a cylindrical applicator. Yan *et al.* [50] compared the dosimetry of plans using 3D printed applicators to those with an in-house multichannel cylinder applicator (including one central and six peripheral catheters for more dose customization) for 48 patients. To design the 3D printed applicator, contrast-soaked gauze was inserted into the vagina of the patient and a CT image was acquired. The packing was contoured to create the shape of the applicator. Peripheral catheters were placed 5 mm from the surface of the applicator, with 10-mm spacing between catheters. The digital model of the applicator was then exported and 3D printed (Figure 7.27). Patients were CT-simulated once again with applicators in place, for treatment planning. Dosimetrically, the 3D printed applicators could deliver a higher dose that was more conformal to target volumes.

While the work of Yan *et al.* was primarily a planning study, Mohammadi *et al.* [51] evaluated their SLA resin printed applicators using EBT3 radiochromic film measurement and Monte Carlo simulation, with comparison to treatment planning system dosimetry. Monte Carlo simulated and measured results were within 2%, showing acceptable agreement.

Most innovations using 3D printing in brachytherapy have focused on HDR brachytherapy with Ir-192. Since electronic brachytherapy sources are of a much lower energy, findings in HDR may not be applicable to electronic brachytherapy where photons are generated using a miniature X-ray tube. Lee *et al.* [52] printed cylindrical applicators with a range of diameters, lengths, and infill percentages, and calculated dose distributions using Monte Carlo simulation to compare to measurement with an electronic brachytherapy source. The authors found that by controlling infill percentages, appropriate dose

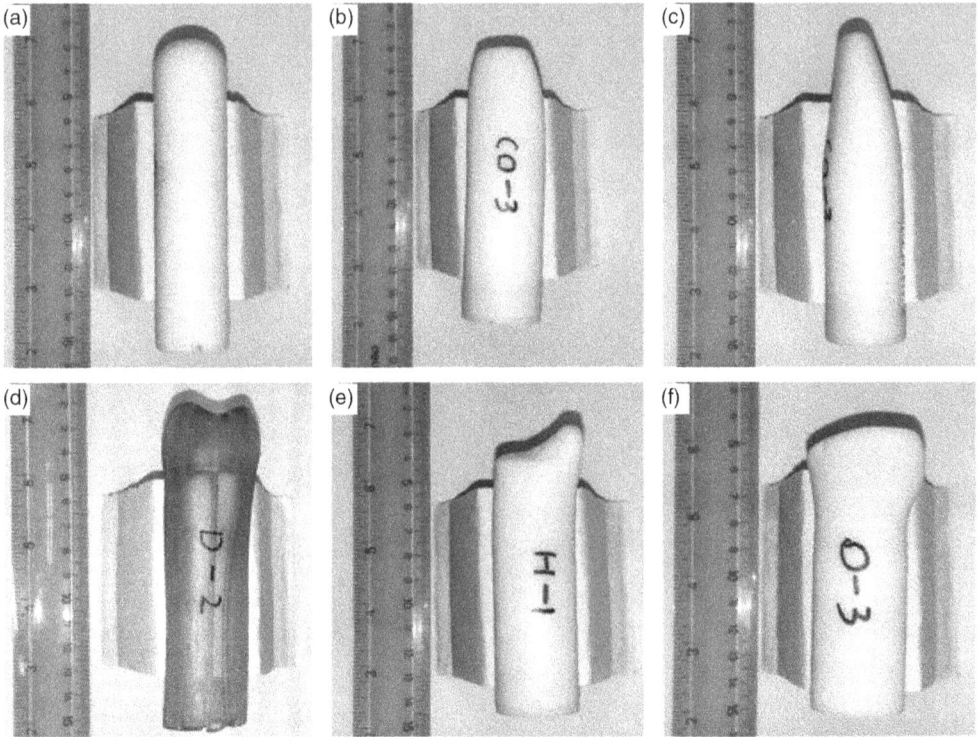

FIGURE 7.27   3D printed gynecological applicators from the study of Yan et al. Figure sourced with permission from [50].

and depth-dose profiles can be produced with the range of applicator sizes, and by optimizing the dwell positions and times, a uniform dose distribution can be achieved.

Most groups using 3D printing in brachytherapy have employed a combination of treatment planning systems and CAD software to create novel applicators. The commercial software 3DBrachy (Adaptiiv Medical, Halifax, Nova Scotia, Canada) includes a brachytherapy module in addition to its 3D printed bolus functionality. Adaptiiv has created the patient-personalized 'Halifax Cylinder' [53] that can be designed using the brachytherapy module. When printed using SLA, the applicator dimensions are accurate to within 0.2 mm, including catheter trajectories developed in the software according to the geometry of the treatment plan. This allows for fast creation of intracavitary applicators in a validated software solution.

Interstitial Gynecological Brachytherapy

More extensive disease (e.g., target thickness greater than 5–10 mm) typically requires interstitial needles. Sethi *et al.* [6] included two interstitial patients in their case studies. One patient presented with recurrent endometrial cancer of the vaginal cuff and was referred for palliative brachytherapy. The printed applicator was 2 cm in diameter, with six peripheral channels spaced 1 cm apart (Figure 7.28). Another patient presented with an extensive vulvar mass to be treated with a printed applicator that was 3.5 cm in diameter with 10 peripheral channels for interstitial insertion and one central tandem channel. Both applicators were fabricated with PC-ISO.

MRI is an invaluable imaging modality when interstitial implants are required. Lindegaard *et al.* demonstrated the use of MRI in designing personalized 3D printed vaginal templates to be used in conjunction with a commercial ring and tandem applicator for locally advanced cervical cancer [7]. A 3D printed ring was designed, identical in dimensions to the ring inserted for the CT and MRI pre-planning imaging. The ring included customized channels for needle trajectories. The needles were then implanted to the depths defined in the pre-plan. In another study where patients' plans were suboptimal with standard ring and tandem applicators, 3D printed applicators were developed using the standard applicators in pre-plans [54]. The authors mimicked the design of the standard applicators and added interstitial needle trajectories to better treat patients' advanced disease (Figure 7.29). A similar concept is the 'Montreal split-ring' (Adaptiiv Medical, Halifax, Nova Scotia, Canada) that is a CT/MR applicator designed from a commercial applicator [53, 55] within the 3DBrachy software application. Early examinations of this device showed that the printed applicators were accurate to within

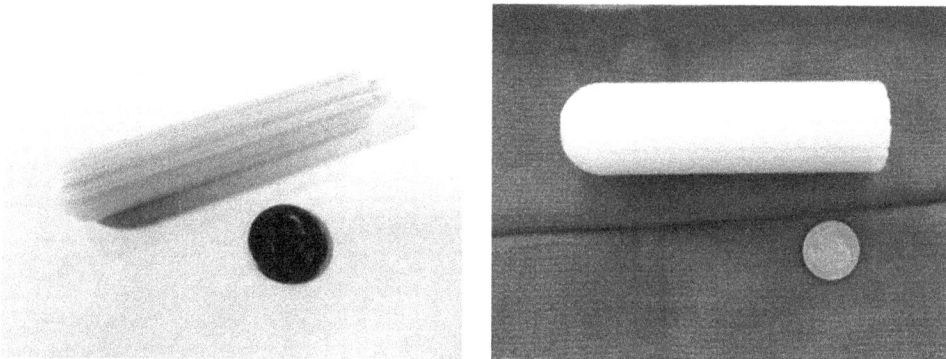

FIGURE 7.28   A 2-cm diameter vaginal cylinder featuring six external channels and one central catheter channel (left) and a 3.5-cm diameter cylinder with ten external channels and one central tandem channel (right). Figure sourced with permission from [6].

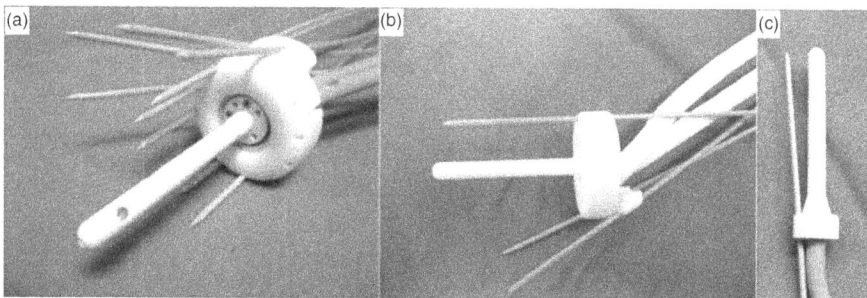

FIGURE 7.29   A 3D printed add-on ring with custom needle guides (a), 3D printed tandem and ring (b) and 3D printed tandem with a single needle at a 15-degree angle (c). Figure sourced with permission from [54].

(a) (b) (c)

Patient #1   Patient #2

Segmentation of axial MR images

Concatenation of segmented contours

Surface mesh modeling

(d)

Patient #1

Patient #2

Personalised needle applicator models
—— Vaginal vault (segmentation)   — ·· — Needle channels
···· Tumor (segmentation)   ——— Applicator reconstruction channel

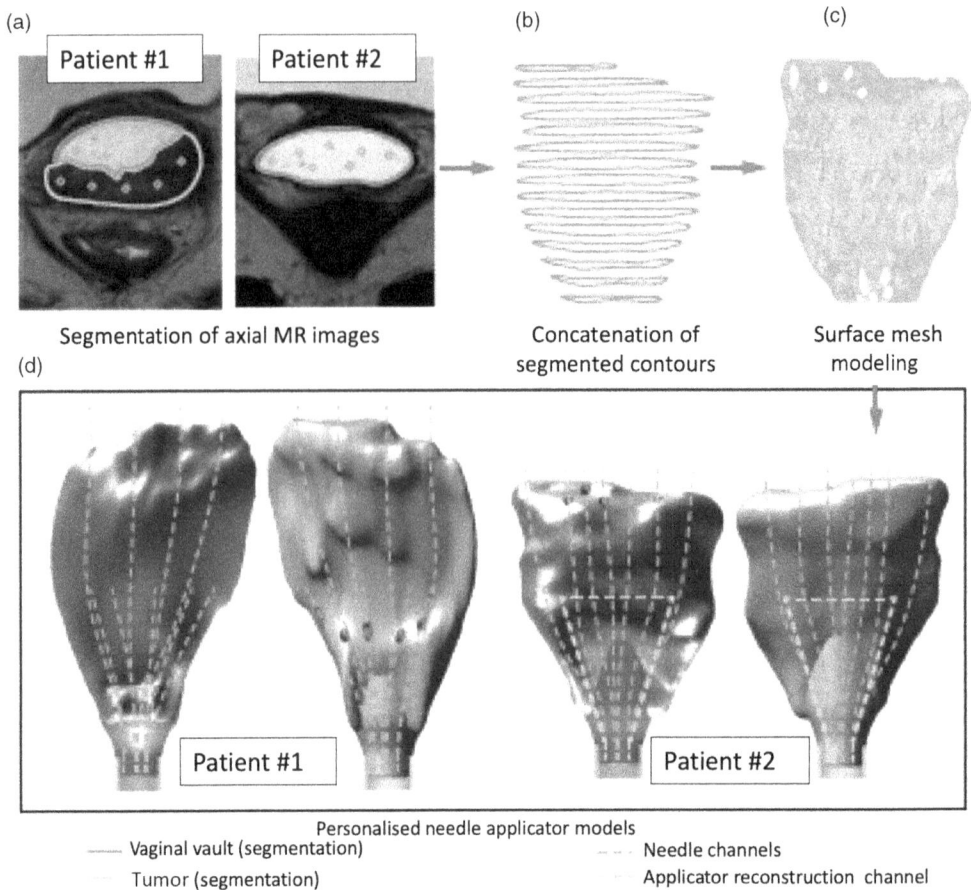

FIGURE 7.30   Illustration of processing steps in creating a personalized vaginal applicator, including (a) segmentation on MRI data, (b) and (c) handling of contour data to produce a surface mesh model, and (d) example applicators for two patients with needle channels. Figure sourced with permission from [57].

0.2 mm. For non-cervical tumors, Sekii *et al.* acquired CT and MR images with cylinders inserted into vaginal cancer patients with advanced disease, and 3D printed cylinders containing interstitial needle paths [56].

Some investigators have created applicators that are not derived from the geometry of commercial applicators but are based entirely on the patient's anatomy. Laan *et al.* [57] used pre-brachytherapy MRI imaging and an aqueous gel injected into the patient's vaginal vault to design entirely personalized applicators (Figure 7.30). Needle trajectories were determined manually during the planning stage, including channels printed within the applicator to accommodate 6F catheters. This study indicated that a minimum radius of curvature of at least 35 mm should be maintained to limit the force of needle insertion.

Intensity Modulated Brachytherapy
Intensity modulated brachytherapy (IMBT) involves the use of applicators capable of producing asymmetric dose distributions by modulating the source fluence at particular

points in the patient. The concept of using a higher density material (such as lead or stainless steel) to shield an OAR has been an option for some time, with shielded ovoids or cylinders available commercially. The options for intensity modulation can be categorized as employing static shielding or dynamic shielding [58]. In static IMBT, the shield that is present in the source or applicator does not move relative to patient tissues. Examples include an I-125 eye plaque with gold shields or a cylinder applicator with a shield in the direction of the rectum. With dynamic IMBT, the shield can be rotated or translated to better adapt the dose delivered to the patient. For example, the applicator may include a rotating tungsten cylinder to reduce dose in a particular direction. In 3D printed applicators, static shielded IMBT is used almost exclusively for gynecological treatment.

A personalized example of IMBT was presented by Semeniuk *et al.* [2] who simulated generic and patient-specific applicators, with the latter featuring high density shielding volumes. Dosimetry from these applicators was evaluated using Monte Carlo modeling. The design of the patient-specific applicator was determined using a novel raytracing algorithm to calculate the thickness and location of the shielding (Figure 7.31). Dose distributions were calculated for sample patient cases using the patient-specific applicators (Figure 7.32). The results showed that although the OARs were adequately shielded with the designs, this might be achieved at the expense of target volume coverage, suggesting refinements to the raytracing and need for optimization. The shielding was 'binary', i.e., it occupied the full volume of the applicator for ray-lines that intersected OARs. In concept, the shielding thickness could also be modulated to achieve a more flexible IMBT delivery.

Biltekin *et al.* [59] designed an IMBT applicator to be used as an alternative to interstitial brachytherapy where the tumor is larger than 1 cm. As seen in Figure 7.33, the applicator includes four interior chambers designed to house source transfer channels for a 5F plastic catheter or, alternatively, shielding materials (aluminum, stainless steel, Cerrobend), while the central channel is used to insert a vendor-provided tandem. Applicator fixation tools were also 3D printed. This work validated the positions of dummy markers in the applicator, and the accuracy of dwell positions, comparing delivered dose distributions to

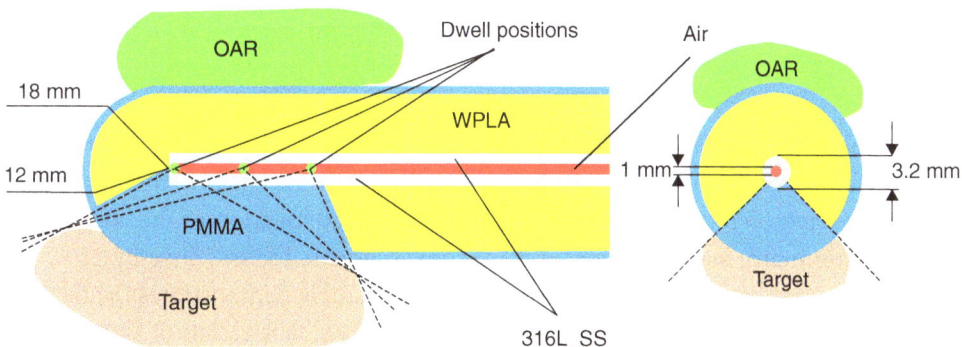

FIGURE 7.31 A modeled cylindrical applicator including 3D printed material (PLA containing tungsten) in all regions other than where ray lines intersect the target volume. Figure sourced with permission from [2].

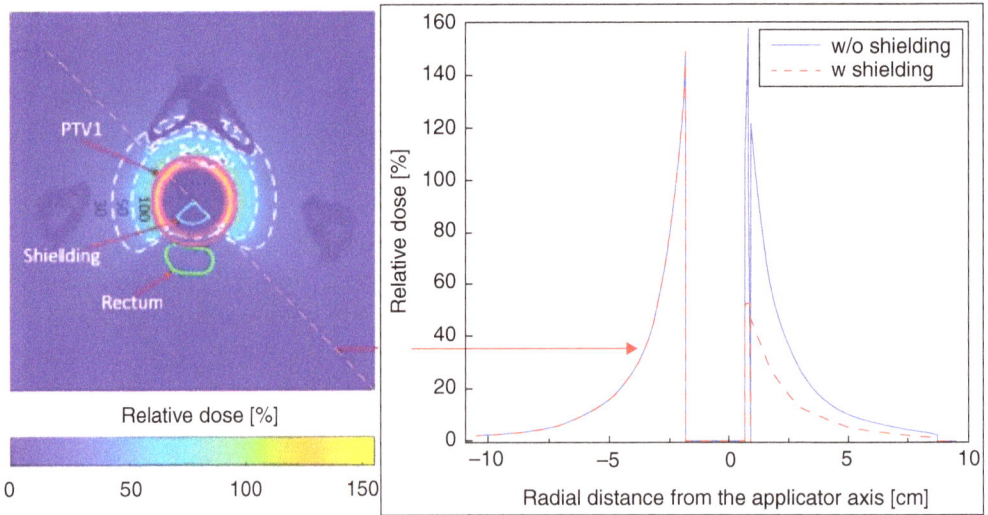

FIGURE 7.32 Dose distribution for an applicator depicted in Figure 7.31 (left) and dose profiles along the dashed yellow line without and with shielding (right) showing the amount by which dose may be reduced with this design. Figure sourced with permission from [2].

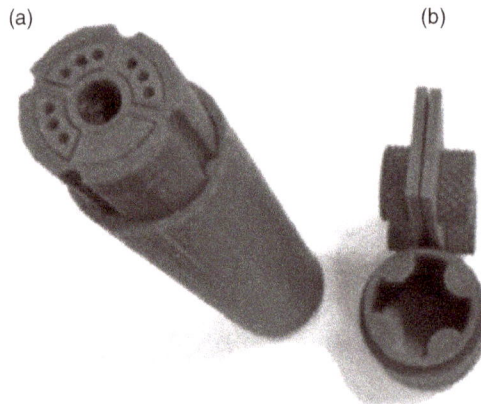

FIGURE 7.33 Prototype of an IMBT applicator showing removable sections in the applicator that may be filled with source channel inserts or with shielding (a) and auxiliary fixation tools (b). Figure sourced with permission from [59].

treatment plans. All positional tests agreed within 1 mm. Gamma analysis showed high pass rates for 1% dose/1 mm criteria, and absolute point dose measurements agreed to within 4% compared to planned values. Examining the attenuation of the compensator materials, aluminum, stainless steel, and Cerrobend attenuated the dose by 15%, 35%, and 75% when compared to PLA (Figure 7.34). This example demonstrates the flexibility of 3D printing in creating innovative prototypes, however fabrication of the applicator itself does not require 3D printing in that it is not entirely patient-personalized.

An IMBT applicator may need to incorporate variable path lengths of shielding material, depending on the location and dimensions of target volumes and OARs relative

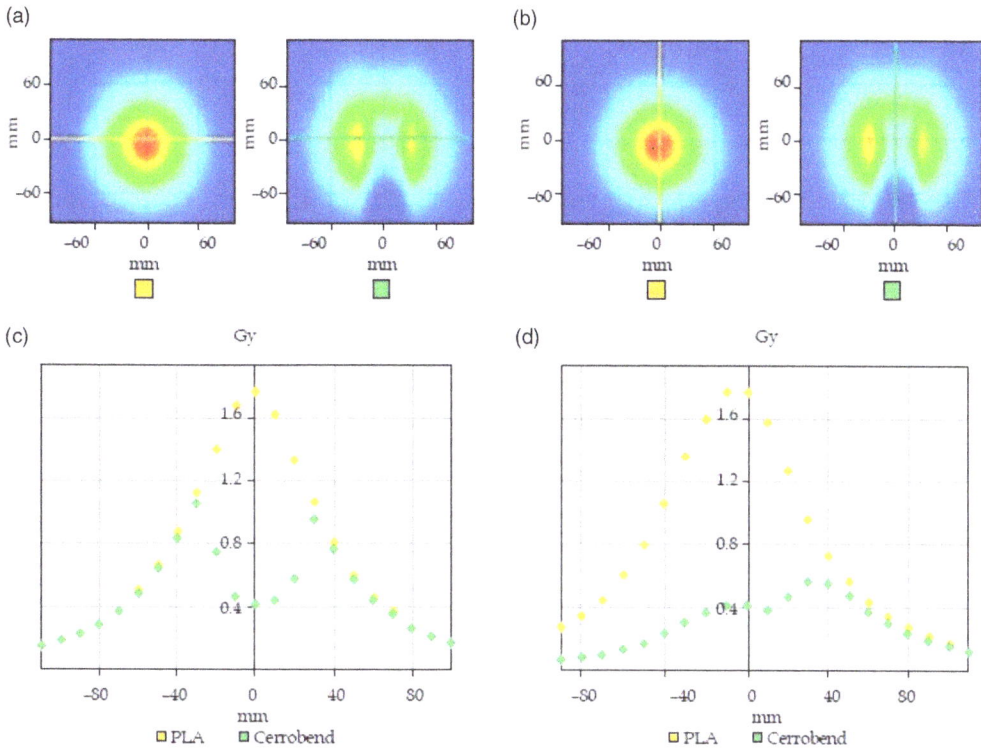

FIGURE 7.34 Measured dose distributions (a and b) for the applicator shown in Figure 7.33 where *x*- and *y*-axis dose profiles are shown in (c) and (d) for applicators containing PLA or Cerrobend shielding. Figure sourced with permission from [59].

to source positions. The challenge is in determining the appropriate, or even optimal, thicknesses of shielding. Skinner *et al.* [3] developed a 2D dose calculation model to quickly optimize shielding using an efficient dose calculation for each source position (Figure 7.35). This was done in two dimensions, taking into account attenuation, inverse square law fall-off and a weighting factor to account for the relative dwell time of each source. The shielding designs were calculated using both Monte Carlo (using TOPAS) and Acuros BV (Varian Medical Systems) to provide quantitative results. The 2D dose calculation algorithm matched the robust calculations qualitatively. The shielding material was printed using a filament that consisted of 95% tungsten powder and 5% plastic. The outer applicator shells were printed with a biocompatible, sterilizable plastic.

Sohn *et al.* [60] presented an inverse optimization model to design a 3D printed gynecological applicator via the gradient descent method. The model generated the optimal thickness and dwell time for each source dwell position. The proposed applicator includes adjustable 5 mm-long shielded segments along the length of the tandem (Figure 7.36). Each segment can provide a different degree of shielding by adjusting the rotation in 60-degree increments. The model was evaluated with 2D phantom and patient cases. The IMBT applicator was printed with tungsten using a 3D metal printer. Dosimetric validation was left to future work.

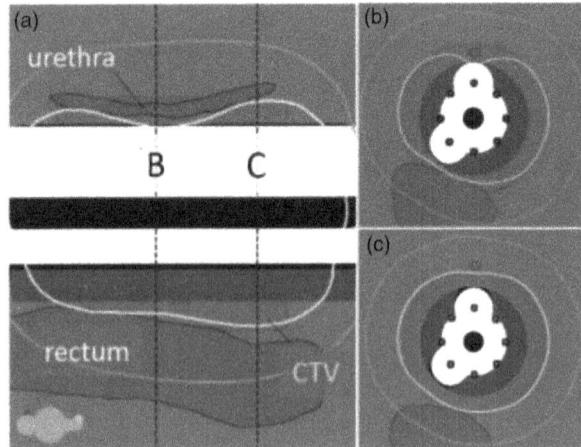

FIGURE 7.35   Example IMBT applicator with shielding shown in white, capable of sparing urethra and rectum while providing sufficient coverage of the clinical target volume. Figure sourced with permission from [3].

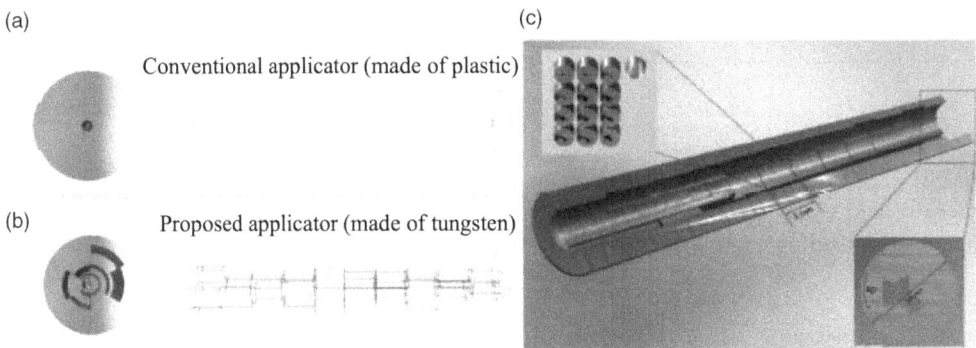

FIGURE 7.36   A conventional cylinder design (a) compared to the novel tungsten IMBT applicator (b and c) designed by Sohn et al. Figure sourced with permission from [60].

CLINICAL WORKFLOWS INCORPORATING 3D PRINTING INTO BRACHYTHERAPY

Incorporating 3D printed tools, applicators, and templates introduces several new steps to the brachytherapy procedure. Relevant patient information such as the outline of the body contour or the shape of an intracavitary volume must be acquired to allow for the design and manufacturing of 3D printed devices. This may require pre-planning imaging, physical impressions [41], photogrammetry [35], or optical scanning methods [30] to acquire surface anatomy. Pre-planning must be completed to optimize catheter positions or trajectories and dose distributions. Depending on available resources, 3D printing may require a few hours to several days, or may be outsourced using an on-demand service, providing biocompatible and sterilizable materials. Once the device is created, quality assurance should be done to verify its integrity and accuracy and sterilization or cleaning need to be completed. Semeniuk *et al.* [2] have described an example workflow

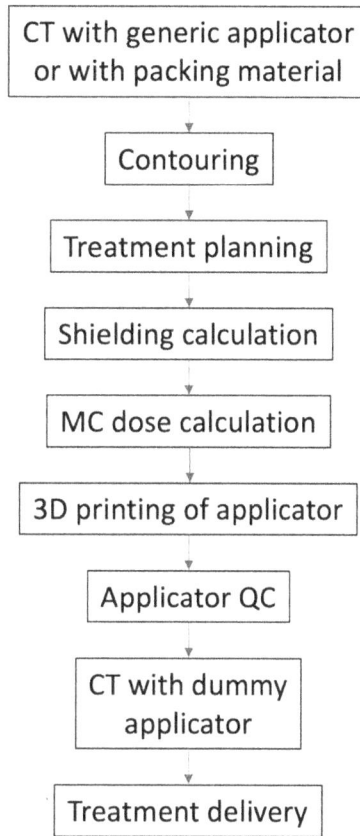

FIGURE 7.37 Example workflow for design and use of a gynecological applicator incorporating shielding. Figure sourced with permission from [3].

for gynecological HDR brachytherapy applicators incorporating shielding, depicted in Figure 7.37.

Whether the device is a template for catheter insertion [46, 47] or an intracavitary applicator with intensity modulation [2], correct positioning on or within the patient is critical to achieve accuracy of treatment delivery. This may require pre-treatment imaging with the device, or a component of the device in place. Skinner *et al.* suggested verifying the placement of a 3D printed vaginal vault with shielding by imaging the patient on the day of treatment with a dummy applicator in place [3]. Once proper positioning is verified, the intended device can be placed inside of the dummy 'shell' applicator in a fixed position.

Although 3D printing may introduce new steps in the workflow, it should be recognized that existing and standard workflows in brachytherapy are already highly variable in terms of steps and time required. Targeted gynecological treatment requires a pre-planning MRI with the intended applicator in place to enable accurate treatment planning. HDR prostate brachytherapy requires an initial TRUS volume study to assess eligibility for the procedure as well as a real-time ultrasound during insertion. In contrast, simple vaginal vault brachytherapy can be done without any image guidance for planning or insertion.

Thus, while the use of 3D printed devices may add additional steps, the additional work required may be comparable to the variability of procedures in existing brachytherapy approaches.

REFERENCES

[1] Rivard MJ, Butler WM, DeWerd LA, et al. Supplement to the 2004 update of the AAPM Task Group No. 43 Report: Supplement to AAPM TG-43 update. *Med Phys.* 2007;34:2187–2205.

[2] Semeniuk O, Cherpak A, Robar J. Design and evaluation of 3D printable patient-specific applicators for gynecologic HDR brachytherapy. *Med Phys.* 2021;48:4053–4063.

[3] Skinner LB, Niedermayr T, Prionas N, et al. Intensity modulated Ir-192 brachytherapy using high-Z 3D printed applicators. *Phys Med Biol.* 2020;65:155018.

[4] Bielda G, Zwierzchowski G, Rostan K, et al. Dosimetric assessment of the impact of low-cost used in stereolithography in high-dose-rate brachytherapy. *J Contemp Brachyther.* 2021;13:188–194.

[5] L'Annunziata MF. Handbook of radioactivity analysis. Elsevier, 2012; https://doi.org/10.1016/C2009-0-64509-8

[6] Sethi R, Cunha A, Mellis K, et al. Clinical applications of custom-made vaginal cylinders constructed using three-dimensional printing technology. *J Contemp Brachyther.* 2016;8:208–214.

[7] Lindegaard JC, Madsen ML, Traberg A, et al. Individualised 3D printed vaginal template for MRI guided brachytherapy in locally advanced cervical cancer. *Radiother Oncol.* 2016;118:173–175.

[8] Dautzenberg P, Volk HA, Huels N, et al. The effect of steam sterilization on different 3D printable materials for surgical use in veterinary medicine. *Bmc Vet Res.* 2021;17:389.

[9] Luchini K, Sloan SNB, Mauro R, et al. Sterilization and sanitizing of 3D-printed personal protective equipment using polypropylene and a single wall design. *3D Print Med.* 2021;7:16.

[10] Cunha JAM, Flynn R, Bélanger C, et al. Brachytherapy future directions. *Semin Radiat Oncol.* 2020;30:94–106.

[11] Harris BD, Nilsson S, Poole CM. A feasibility study for using ABS plastic and a low-cost 3D printer for patient-specific brachytherapy mould design. *Australas Phys Eng S.* 2015;38:399–412.

[12] Cunha JAM, Mellis K, Sethi R, et al. Evaluation of PC-ISO for customized, 3D Printed, gynecologic 192-Ir HDR brachytherapy applicators. *J Appl Clin Med Phys.* 2014;16:5168.

[13] Pera O, Membrive I, Lambisto D, et al. Validation of 3D printing materials for high dose-rate brachytherapy using ionisation chamber and custom phantom. *Phys Med Biol.* 2021;66:18NT04.

[14] Beaulieu L, Tedgren ÅC, Carrier J-F, et al. Report of the task group 186 on model-based dose calculation methods in brachytherapy beyond the TG-43 formalism: Current status and recommendations for clinical implementation: TG-186: Model-based dose calculation techniques in brachytherapy. *Med Phys.* 2012;39:6208–6236.

[15] Sureka CS, Aruna P, Ganesan S, et al. Computation of relative dose distribution and effective transmission around a shielded vaginal cylinder with Ir192 HDR source using MCNP4B: Shielded vaginal cylinder dose distribution using MCNP4B. *Med Phys.* 2006;33:1552–1561.

[16] Rengier F, Mehndiratta A, Tengg-Kobligk H von, et al. 3D printing based on imaging data: Review of medical applications. *Int J Comput Ass Rad*. 2010;5:335–341.

[17] Tack P, Victor J, Gemmel P, et al. 3D-printing techniques in a medical setting: A systematic literature review. *Biomed Eng Online*. 2016;15:115.

[18] Simpson-Page E, Hamlett L, Lew D, et al. 3D printed brachytherapy jig for Reference Air Kerma Rate calibration. *Phys Eng Sci Med*. 2021;44:1141–1150.

[19] Otani Y, Sumida I, Nose T, et al. High-dose rate intracavitary brachytherapy pretreatment dwell position verification using a transparent applicator. *J Appl Clin Med Phys*. 2018;19:428–434.

[20] Bassi S, Berrigan L, Zuchora A, et al. End-to-end dosimetric audit: A novel procedure developed for Irish HDR brachytherapy centres. *Phys Medica*. 2020;80:221–229.

[21] Pfeiffer D, Sutlief S, Feng W, et al. AAPM Task Group 128: Quality assurance tests for prostate brachytherapy ultrasound systems. *Med Phys*. 2008;35:5471–5489.

[22] Leong B, Ostyn M, Oh S, et al. Technical Note: The design, construction, and evaluation of a liquid-based single phantom solution for TG128 brachytherapy ultrasound QA. *Med Phys*. 2019;46:1024–1029.

[23] Ryu B, Bax J, Edirisinge C, et al. Prostate brachytherapy with oblique needles to treat large glands and overcome pubic arch interference. *Int J Radiat Oncol Biology Phys*. 2012;83:1463–1472.

[24] Shaaer A, Alrashidi S, Chung H, et al. Multipurpose ultrasound-based prostate phantom for use in interstitial brachytherapy. *Brachytherapy*. 2021;20:1139–1145.

[25] Nattagh K, Siauw T, Pouliot J, et al. A training phantom for ultrasound-guided needle insertion and suturing. *Brachytherapy*. 2014;13:413–419.

[26] Kadoya N, Miyasaka Y, Nakajima Y, et al. Evaluation of deformable image registration between external beam radiotherapy and HDR brachytherapy for cervical cancer with a 3D-printed deformable pelvis phantom. *Med Phys*. 2017;44:1445–1455.

[27] Campelo S, Subashi E, Meltsner SG, et al. Multi-Material 3D printing in brachytherapy: Prototyping teaching tools for interstitial and intracavitary procedures in cervical cancers. *Brachytherapy*. 2020;19:767–776.

[28] Lugez E, Sadjadi H, Joshi CP, et al. Improved electromagnetic tracking for catheter path reconstruction with application in high-dose-rate brachytherapy. *Int J Comput Ass Rad*. 2017;12:681–689.

[29] Silva RMV, Belinato W, Macedo LE, et al. Anthropomorphic phantom to investigate the bladder dose in gynecological high-dose-rate brachytherapy. *Brachytherapy*. 2015;14:633–641.

[30] Schreiber S, Reitemeier B, Herrmann T, et al. A Process for making cutaneous radiation applicators based on digital data. *Strahlenther Onkol*. 2006;182:349–352.

[31] Clarke S, Yewondwossen M, Robar J. Sci-Thur PM – Brachytherapy 06: 3D printed surface applicators for high dose rate brachytherapy. *Med Phys*. 2016;43:4934–4935.

[32] Zhao Y, Moran K, Yewondwossen M, et al. Clinical applications of 3-dimensional printing in radiation therapy. *Med Dosim*. 2017;42:150–155.

[33] Ricotti R, Vavassori A, Bazani A, et al. 3D-printed applicators for high dose rate brachytherapy: Dosimetric assessment at different infill percentage. *Phys Med*. 2016;32:1698–1706.

[34] Bassi S, Langan B, Malone C. Dosimetry assessment of patient-specific 3D printable materials for HDR surface brachytherapy. *Phys Medica*. 2019;67:166–175.

[35] Bridger CA, Reich PD, Santos AMC, et al. A dosimetric comparison of CT- and photogrammetry- generated 3D printed HDR brachytherapy surface applicators. *Phys Eng Sci Med*. 2022;45:125–134.

[36] Aldridge S, Jones E-L, Tonino A, et al. Skin HDR brachytherapy treatment using a mould made with a 3D printer. *Brachytherapy*. 2016;15:S147–S148.

[37] Taggar A, Barnes E, Martell K, et al. 3D printed individually customized high-dose-rate brachytherapy applicator for treatment of chronic digital Psoriasis. *Brachytherapy*. 2019;18:S22.

[38] S C, G B, B A-PJ. High dose rate 192-Ir-Brachytherapy for Basal Cell Carcinoma of the Skin using a 3D printed surface mold. *Cureus*. 2019;11:e4913.

[39] Jones E-L, Baldion AT, Thomas C, et al. Introduction of novel 3D-printed superficial applicators for high-dose-rate skin brachytherapy. *Brachytherapy*. 2017;16:409–414.

[40] Voros L, Cohen GN, Piechocniski PW, et al. Custom mold technique with 3D printed applicator "Shell" in Penile HDR Brachytherapy. *Brachytherapy*. 2017;16:S49–S50.

[41] D'Alimonte L, Ravi A, Helou J, et al. Optimized penile surface mold brachytherapy using latest stereolithography techniques: A single-institution experience. *Brachytherapy*. 2019;18:348–352.

[42] Saldi S, Zucchetti C, Fulcheri CPL, et al. High-dose-rate brachytherapy with surface applicator in penile cancer. *Brachytherapy*. 2021;20:835–841.

[43] Chytyk-Praznik K, Oliver P, Allan J, et al. Design of custom, 3D-printed surface brachytherapy applicators. *Med Phys*. 2020;47:e-737.

[44] Major T, Fröhlich G, Lövey K, et al. Dosimetric experience with accelerated partial breast irradiation using image-guided interstitial brachytherapy. *Radiother Oncol*. 2009;90:48–55.

[45] Cuttino LW, Todor D, Arthur DW. CT-guided multi-catheter insertion technique for partial breast brachytherapy: Reliable target coverage and dose homogeneity. *Brachytherapy*. 2005;4:10–17.

[46] Pompeu-Robinson A, Kunz M, Falkson CB, et al. Immobilization and catheter guidance for breast brachytherapy. *Int J Comput Ass Rad*. 2012;7:65–72.

[47] Poulin E, Gardi L, Fenster A, et al. Towards real-time 3D ultrasound planning and personalized 3D printing for breast HDR brachytherapy treatment. *Radiother Oncol*. 2015;114:335–338.

[48] Walker JM, Elliott DA, Kubicky CD, et al. Manufacture and evaluation of 3-dimensional printed sizing tools for use during intraoperative breast brachytherapy. *Adv Radiat Oncol*. 2016;1:132–135.

[49] Sethi R, Cunha JAN, Mellis K, et al. 3D printed custom applicator for high-dose-rate intracavitary vaginal cuff brachytherapy. *Brachytherapy*. 2014;13:S93.

[50] Yan J, Qin X, Zhang F, et al. Comparing multichannel cylinder and 3D-printed applicators for vaginal cuff brachytherapy with preliminary exploration of post-hysterectomy vaginal morphology. *J Contemp Brachyther*. 2021;13:641–648.

[51] Mohammadi R, Siavashpour Z, Aghdam SRH, et al. Manufacturing and evaluation of multi-channel cylinder applicator with 3D printing technology. *J Contemp Brachyther*. 2021;13:80–90.

[52] Lee JH, Kim HN, Lim HS, et al. Three-dimensional-printed vaginal applicators for electronic brachytherapy of endometrial cancers. *Med Phys*. 2019;46:448–455.

[53] Basaric B, Morgan L, Engelberts C, et al. PO-0177 A new software for designing patient-specific sleeves for the Montreal split-ring applicator. *Radiother Oncol.* 2021;158:S140–S141.

[54] Logar HBZ, Hudej R, Šegedin B. Development and assessment of 3D-printed individual applicators in gynecological MRI-guided brachytherapy. *J Contemp Brachyther.* 2019;11:128–136.

[55] Kamio Y, Roy M, Morgan L, et al. PO-0192 Prototype testing the 3D-printed Montreal split-ring applicator (GYN) using biocompatible materials. *Radiother Oncol.* 2021;158:S152–S153.

[56] Sekii S, Tsujino K, Kosaka K, et al. Inversely designed, 3D-printed personalized template-guided interstitial brachytherapy for vaginal tumors. *J Contemp Brachyther.* 2018;10:470–477.

[57] Laan RC, Nout RA, Dankelman J, et al. MRI-driven design of customised 3D printed gynaecological brachytherapy applicators with curved needle channels. *3D Print Med.* 2019;5:8.

[58] Callaghan CM, Adams Q, Flynn RT, et al. Systematic review of Intensity-Modulated Brachytherapy (IMBT): Static and dynamic techniques. *Int J Radiat Oncol Biol Phys.* 2019;105:206–221.

[59] Biltekin F, Akyol HF, Gültekin M, et al. 3D printer-based novel intensity-modulated vaginal brachytherapy applicator: Feasibility study. *J Contemp Brachyther.* 2020;12:17–26.

[60] Sohn JJ, Polizzi M, Kang S-W, et al. Intensity modulated High Dose Rate (HDR) Brachytherapy using patient specific 3D metal printed applicators: Proof of concept. *Frontiers Oncol.* 2022;12:829529.

CHAPTER 8

3D Printed Patient Immobilization

James L. Robar

PATIENT IMMOBILIZATION AND PROBLEMS WITH THE STATUS QUO

Radiation therapy relies critically on accurate patient positioning to deliver the required dose to target volumes while minimizing toxicity to surrounding healthy tissues. Inter-fractional error will be present due to the variability of setting up a patient between sessions, and the magnitude of this variability would increase without immobilization. However, image guidance systems incorporated to treatment units (such as cone beam CT) offer means to minimize this source of error. Intra-fractional error, i.e., that caused by patient motion during the treatment itself, on the other hand, certainly necessitates patient immobilization. Most commonly, immobilization is applied to the cranium and head-and-neck (HN), although it may also be used for breast, extremities, and other sites.

Early methods of forming patient immobilization involved creating a positive model of the patient anatomy for vacuum forming a plastic such as Perspex [1]. Over the past decades the standard method has involved heating a thermoplastic (TP) mesh, e.g., to 70°C, using a hot water bath or oven and directly forming over the patient's anatomy. While used widely in the practice of radiation therapy (RT), there are several fundamental problems with this approach, as follows.

1. The fit and quality of the TP shell produced, and thus its performance in patient positioning, will depend on the skill of the human fabricating the device. While it is possible to produce high-quality TP masks manually, this is not guaranteed, and a poorly made device, e.g., showing gapping between the shell and skin surface, can degrade patient positioning accuracy on treatment [2]. Qualitative studies demonstrate that healthcare providers are cognizant of this source of error as one that may compromise patient outcomes [3].

2. Many patients show significant anxiety while wearing a mask, and this anxiety is most prevalent early in the treatment process, including at fabrication time [4].

 DOI: 10.1201/9781003288404-8

Surveys among patients have shown that the immobilizer fabrication is more uncomfortable than the therapy itself, with 75% of patients indicating that they would like to avoid the mask-making process [5]. Sharp *et al.* [6] indicated that the immobilizer fabrication process, combined with the stress of cancer diagnosis, can lead to a state of panic. If this anxiety persists from time of immobilizer fabrication through treatment, it may even lead to treatment interruption [4]. It has been shown that customizing the immobilizer for the patient (by creating openings, etc.) may reduce this anxiety [7], however truly personalizing immobilizers in this regard requires manual prost-processing, i.e., cutting of the mesh by hand.

3. The manual method of immobilizer fabrication is both human and capital resource intensive. Typically, more than one radiation therapist is required to form an immobilizer. The process includes multiple steps, requiring time to heat the TP, time to form, and a period allowing the immobilizer to cool on the patient so that it is not shrinking independently of the anatomy. In total, this may require up to one hour [5]. In addition, many facilities perform this procedure in the CT imaging suite, which ties up this valuable capital resource.

4. Multiple additional operational drawbacks exist, including the need to occupy clinic space with hot water baths or ovens to heat the TP as well as the need to source and stock bulky raw materials.

WHY 3D PRINTING FOR PATIENT IMMOBILIZATION?

These various shortcomings were articulated by the research team of Sanghera in 2002, who provided among the earliest descriptions of additive manufacturing of immobilizers [8]. It is notable that this proposal was made a full decade before the eventual widespread accessibility of 3D printing, which occurred following the expiry of foundational patents. Since that time, the 3D printing of immobilization has garnered significant interest within radiation oncology research and clinical communities. There are several reasons for this, as described below.

1. With a 3D printing approach, the patient would be relieved of the fabrication process. Thus, the first experience of the patient in the RT clinic would not have to be an unpleasant one. The immobilizer design would be based on 3D imaging that has been acquired previously (e.g., MRI data [9]) or imaging that may be acquired rapidly, e.g., via optical surface imaging [10].

2. The dependence of immobilizer quality and performance would no longer be subject to human error during manufacturing. As an end-to-end digital process, both the design and fabrication of immobilizers could be stringently controlled.

3. The mechanical aspects of the immobilizer could be systematically engineered, rather than simply resulting from a largely uncontrolled fabrication process. For example, the immobilizer design could include thicker regions at points known to be more critical for immobilization, e.g., brow, bridge of nose, upper mandible.

4. Some 3D printing techniques allow selection of printing media that may be advantageous from a dosimetric point of view, potentially even reducing toxicity of treatment. This could include, for example, the use of materials that lower dose build-up and thus reduce erythema and desquamation [11]. While the source of skin toxicity in radiotherapy is multifactorial [12], certainly the radiological path length of traditional immobilization has been identified as a cause. This factor is particularly important, e.g., for immobilization of the intact breast where skin toxicity and poor cosmesis is common [12–14].

5. Multiple patient devices required for a treatment course could be integrated into a single design through 3D printing. For example, instead of a manual (and potentially cumbersome) combination of patient bolus with the immobilizer, both devices could be unified in a single design, while ensuring that the bolus is always positioned correctly and in contact with the skin. This would also serve to streamline patient setup at treatment time and potentially introduce efficiencies. Integration of immobilizing components with other devices, e.g., brachytherapy applicators, is also possible.

6. Conversion to a digital process means that design modifications become possible, e.g., openings for eyes, mouth, tracheostomy, etc., that are fully customized to the patient. In addition, some printing technologies, e.g., Multi Jet Fusion (MJF) or powder jet printing, allow for color printing on the top surface, introducing options for patient labels, set-up markers such as cross-hairs, or even patient-friendly customizations such as patterns or images on the surface, e.g., superhero images for pediatric patients.

APPROACHES TO DESIGN AND FABRICATION OF 3D PRINTED IMMOBILIZERS

Various approaches have been followed in producing 3D printed immobilizers in the R&D setting. These efforts have leveraged different imaging modalities to provide input data, a range of software tools for design, as well a number of different printing technologies and media. Below we discuss examples that highlight the range of these methods.

Although the early report by Sanghera [8] was published over two decades ago, this work was prescient in that it identified a dilemma regarding the source image data: if CT is needed as input information to the design process, it would be required in advance; yet the RT planning process normally requires CT acquisition with the patient positioned in the immobilizer. This implies the need for two CT imaging sessions, which would not be acceptable in most practices. Therefore, digital surface photogrammetry (DSP) was used in this work to capture the relevant cranial anatomy. DSP acquisition was extremely fast (~8 ms) and provided the required resolution for the design task. The 'immobilizer' in this study was rudimentary (Figure 8.1), consisting merely of a solid shell of the anterior surface of the face extending to the cranial vertex. It was printed using fused deposition modeling (FDM) and acrylonitrile butadiene styrene (ABS) 400 TP, a process that

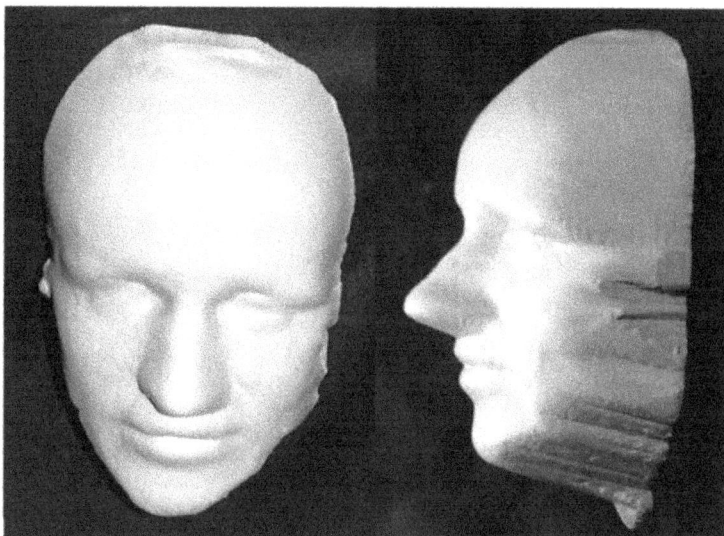

FIGURE 8.1 Early 'immobilizer' design based on DSP and 3D printed by Sanghera. Figure sourced with permission from [8].

required five days and considerable post-processing to remove supports and improve surface finish. Although at the time of the study it was clear that practical fabrication within clinical timeframes would await advancement in the printing technology, an accuracy to within 0.4 mm was demonstrated in comparing the design and the printed model, and the ABS material was shown to be similar to polystyrene at 6-MV photon beam quality.

Over a decade later, Fisher *et al.* [15] demonstrated the design of cranial immobilization based on CT data. As stated by the authors, the goal was to produce a technology so that there 'was no need to take plaster of Paris moulds'. Source CT data of a cranial phantom were acquired with 0.625-mm slice spacing, and a shell was designed following binarizing of the image, filling of holes, extending lateral edges to a surface, smoothing, and constructing a volume. The prototype immobilizer was printed using selective laser sintering (SLS) with PA2200 material. Other than proving feasibility of the printing itself, this work showed that 80% of points on the inner surface of the mask were within 4 mm of expected locations compared to the phantom geometry. Similar to that fabricated by Sanghera, the 'immobilizer' was a simple, solid shell, without perforations, attachment points, or other means for practical clinical use (Figure 8.2).

The same year, Laycock and team [16] presented a design based on 1.5T MRI data of a human volunteer with a fast spoiled gradient echo sequence. Image processing steps (Figure 8.3), performed in the Osirix package, were similar to those used by Fisher, including masking, segmentation, binarization, conversion to a hollow positive structure, creation of a negative shell, and conversion to tessellated STL file format. Both the positive cranial model and the negative shell were printed using jet fusion, with the former used to assess the fit of the latter. The same study assessed the change in dose due to the presence of the 3D printed shell, comparing various materials.

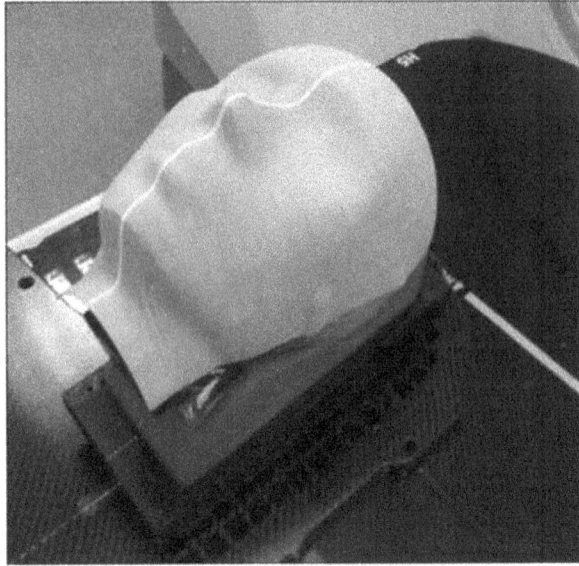

FIGURE 8.2   SLS-printed shell by Fisher et al. Figure sourced with permission from [15].

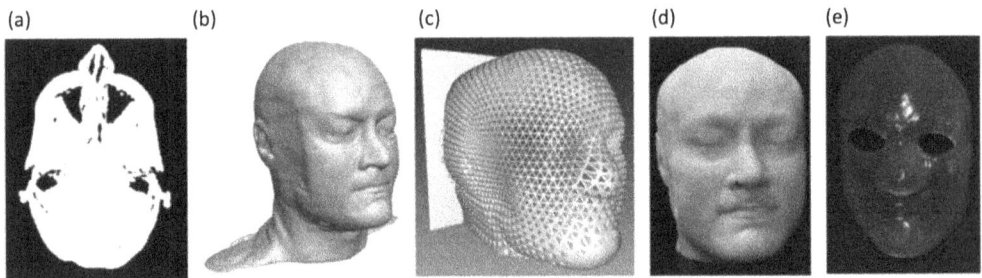

FIGURE 8.3   Immobilizer design and production from MRI data (a) showing creating of a volume (b), tessellation (c), printing of a positive (d), and a negative shell (e) from Laycock. Figure sourced with permission from [16].

While these early examples are basic in design, i.e., consisting of simple uniform shells of the anterior and lateral cranial surfaces, in 2018 Haefner *et al.* [17] presented 'a new approach' to immobilizer design, including highly engineered geometry and features that were more familiar to clinicians using TP systems, such as holes for eyes and mouth, a padded headrest, a baseplate/frame assembly with latches to enable actual fixation of a patient, and perforations to give the mask 'a friendlier appearance' (Figure 8.4). The design methodology was not provided in detail other than indicating that it was done using 'in-house software' based on T1 MRI data for eight human volunteers. The shell portion of the mask was 1.5 mm in thickness, i.e., somewhat thinner than typical stretched TP, and printed using FDM and ABS material. Notably, this was among the first demonstrations of 3D printing of shells that could actually immobilize the cranium, and pointed to the possibility of streamlining the design and fabrication processes using efficient digital tools.

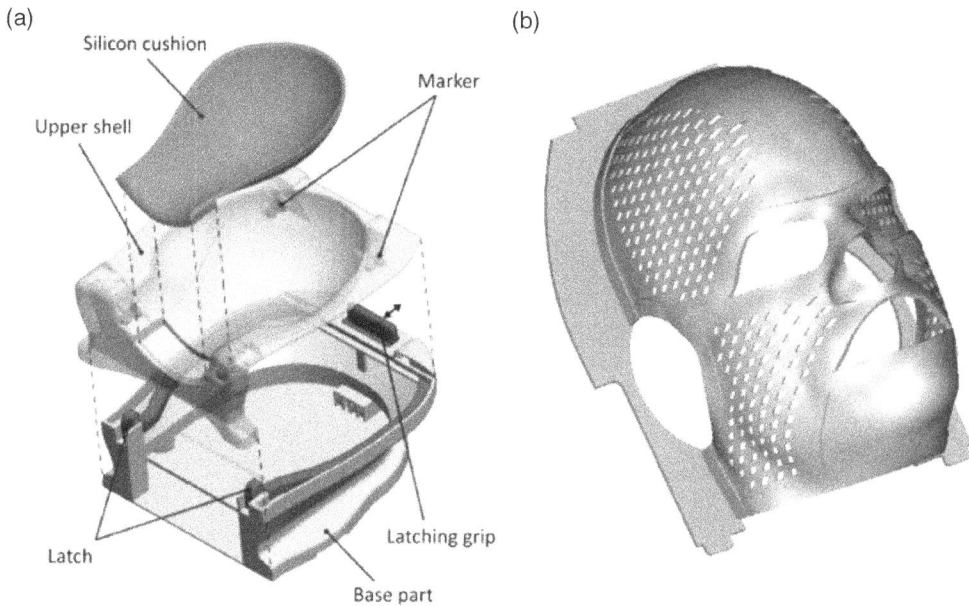

FIGURE 8.4 Immobilization base (a) and shell (b) produced by Haefner et al. (2018). Figure sourced with permission from [17].

Pham *et al.* [18] at the University of Montréal explored the disparate approach of 3D printing a positive of the patient's cranium as well as a customized headrest, and subsequently molding a conventional TP immobilizer over the positive cranial model. This was performed for 11 patients and additional CT scanning was performed to assess the similarity of patient position with the immobilizer applied to the positioning in the CT image from which the positive was formed. Findings showed discrepancies within 1 mm and 1 degree, validating an approach that involves a straightforward clinical process, e.g., involving just one planning CT session for the patient. While this method eliminates the direct printing of thin immobilizer shells (a challenging task for many 3D printing technologies) it does require fabrication of a full FDM-printed positive model for every patient and does not eliminate the labor and fabricator-dependent uncertainty involved in manual molding of TP mesh.

In 2022, Miron *et al.* [5] were motivated by a local survey reporting negative feedback from patients on the TP mask making process. This group developed a 3D printed immobilizer with the aim of increased patient comfort and reduced anxiety. The system was comprised of posterior and anterior components with large openings (Figure 8.5). The device was designed in the Mimics software (Materialise, Leuven, Belgium) based on patient MRI data and using templates in the software for adding facial cutouts. In addition, the design was integrated into the geometry of an MRI head coil. Four immobilizers were fabricated for volunteers using FDM and ABS. The focus of this study was to assess immobilization performance in comparison to a commercial cranial stereotactic immobilization system.

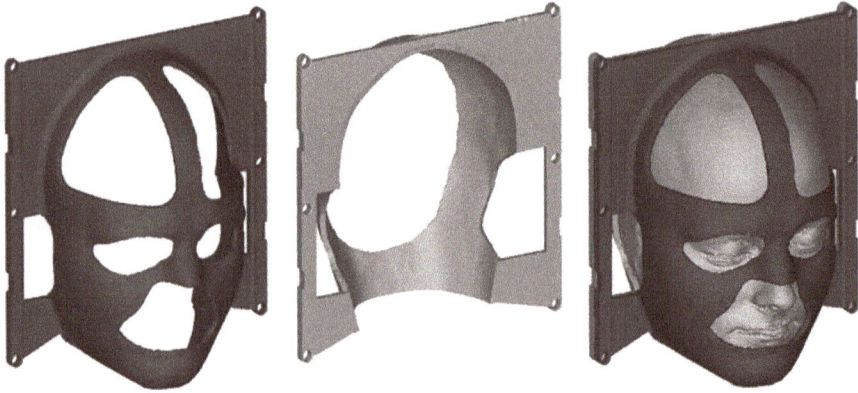

FIGURE 8.5 'Non-invasive' immobilizer design by Miron et al. Figure sourced with permission from [5].

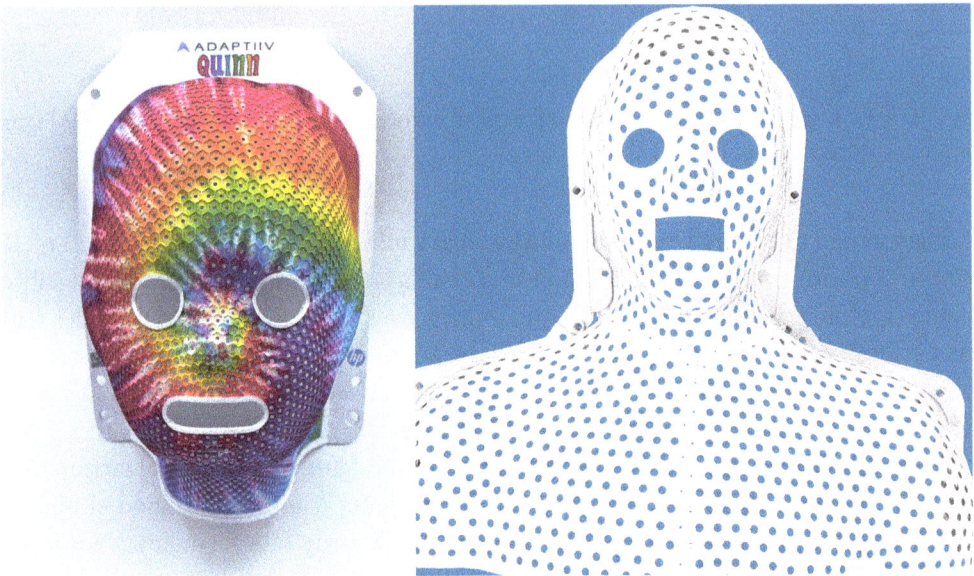

FIGURE 8.6 Multi Jet Fusion-printed cranial and head-and-neck immobilizers from Robar et al. (2022). Figure sourced with permission from [11].

In a collaboration with industry partners Adaptiiv Medical (Halifax, Canada) and HP (Corvallis, Oregon) in 2022, Robar *et al.* [11] demonstrated the first MJF-printed adult and pediatric cranial immobilizers (Figure 8.6). Three different MJF-printable media were compared, all based on polyamide 12 (PA12), a material that offers exceptional mechanical robustness, chemical resistance, biocompatibility, and high-quality surface finish. Immobilizer designs were based on CT phantom geometries. An advantageous material was identified for minimizing skin dose and used in the testing and fabrication of prototypes. Printed shells included wall thicknesses as low as 0.4 mm in order to minimize the skin dose received by the patient. A novel honeycomb metamaterial design was described in order to maximize stiffness of the shell while minimizing the amount

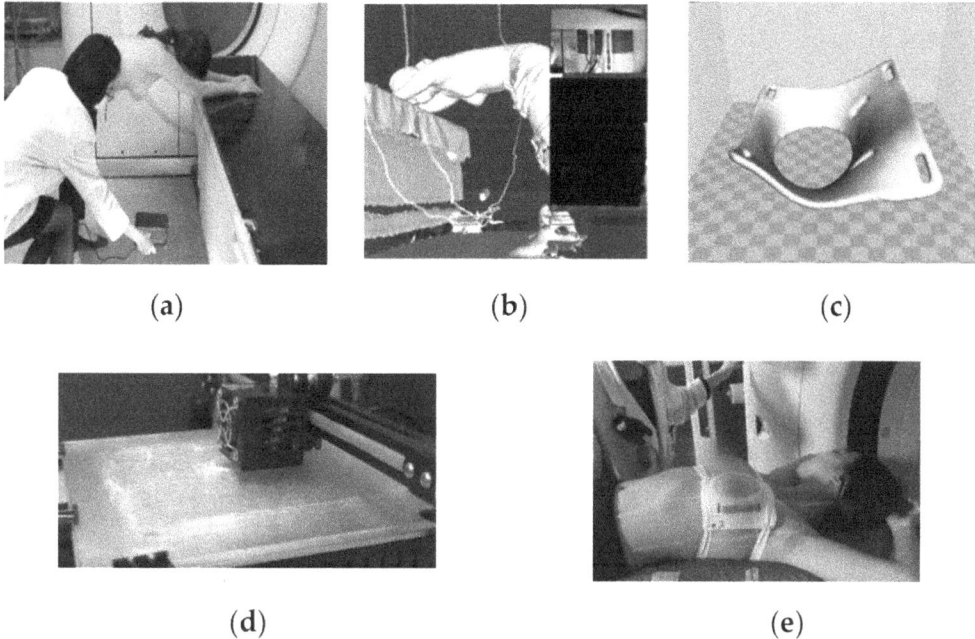

FIGURE 8.7   Process for the PERSBRA breast immobilizer showing optical imaging (a and b), the designed model (c), FDM printing (d), and application to the patient (e). Figure sourced with permission from [19].

of material required and radiological path length. The spatial accuracy of fabricated immobilizers was assessed, demonstrating agreement to within 3 mm. All immobilizers were compatible with S-frame baseplate systems.

3D printed immobilization may also be beneficial for extracranial sites as well, and Chen *et al.* [19] described a personalized breast holder (PERSBRA), with the goal of reducing radiation-induced heart disease (RIHD) by sparing the left anterior descending artery and heart during irradiation of the intact breast. As shown in Figure 8.7, in a 'standing forward' position, the skin surface is optically imaged in approximately 5 minutes. These data are used to form an immobilizing shell that is printed using FDM, which required 18 to 40 hours.

3D PRINTED MATERIALS AND SKIN DOSE

It is well known that traditional immobilizers, whether comprised of a TP mesh or a solid TP layer, e.g., a Perspex shell, will cause radiation dose buildup, that is, the dose received by the patient's skin will be higher than it would be without the immobilization. This buildup can be significant, for example, Laycock *et al.* reported a 54% to 80% increase of dose with various overlying immobilizer materials [16]. While superficial indications (e.g., skin cancer) may receive a high dose intentionally according to the treatment plan, for many clinical scenarios in treating the cranium, HN or breast, this dose is unwanted and may cause significant skin toxicity [20, 21]. The skin dose received by the patient will increase with both the electron density of the material used and the physical thickness,

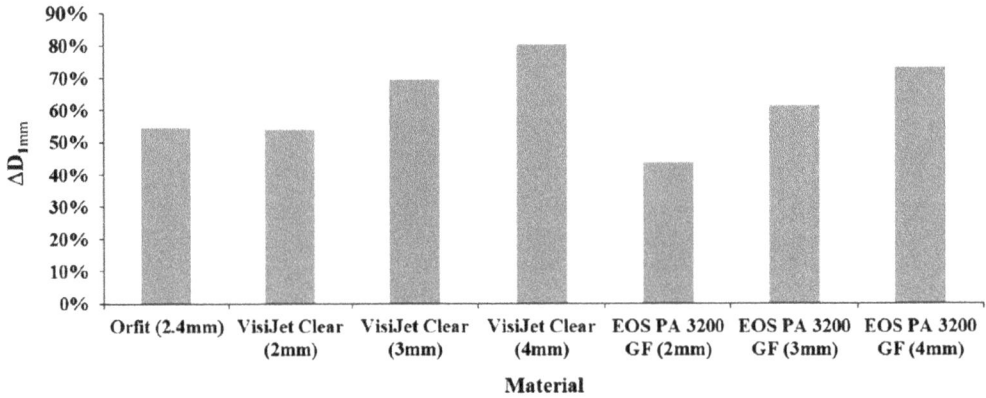

FIGURE 8.8   Increase of measured dose at 1 mm depth (relative to no buildup material), comparing traditional (Orfit) thermoplastic, to VisiJet Clear and EOS PA 3200 3D printing media. Figure sourced with permission from [16].

for both megavoltage photon and electron beams. The effective thickness will depend on the ray-line pathlength of the beam; thus beams oblique to the surface may be associated with increased buildup compared to normal incidence.

In considering materials for printed immobilizers, several authors investigated the dosimetric properties of various 3D printed media, and in some cases included comparison to status quo immobilization materials, e.g., TP mesh. An early examination was performed by Sanghera *et al.* [8] who noted comparable buildup between printed ABS and polystyrene over depths ranging from 1 to 6 mm.

Figure 8.8 shows findings by Laycock *et al.* [16] in which the percent dose increase was measured with a Roos chamber at a depth of 1.0 mm for various materials, relative to the dose measured with no buildup added. Comparison is made among a standard perforated TP shell (Orfit), and test materials comprised of VisiJet Clear as well as EOS polyamide (PA) 3200, two media available for the Z-Corp binder jet printer. Measured dose increased with thickness as expected, and the 2.0-mm samples caused either comparable or slightly less dose than the standard shell.

Robar *et al.* [11] investigated various MJF-printable materials based on PA12 nylon, measuring buildup curves for standard TP solid sheet, perforated TP shell, PA12 with glass beads, PA12 dark, PA12 light, polylactic acid (PLA), and PLA with hollow glass microspheres (HGM) combined in an extruded filament to lower its density. The results are shown in Figure 8.9. Measurement for the same physical thickness (3.2 mm) of samples yielded the comparison given in Figure 8.10, in which the measured dose has been normalized to that for standard perforated TP shell material. As shown in these figures, this study singled out a promising MJF material, PA12 light, which yields a lower dose than perforated TP, even though the PA12 light sample was non-perforated. The expectation is that perforating the PA12 light material may further lower the dose below that of standard TP mesh. In this same study, the authors developed a thin-walled honeycomb metamaterial design, demonstrating up to 40% surface dose reduction compared to standard TP mesh.

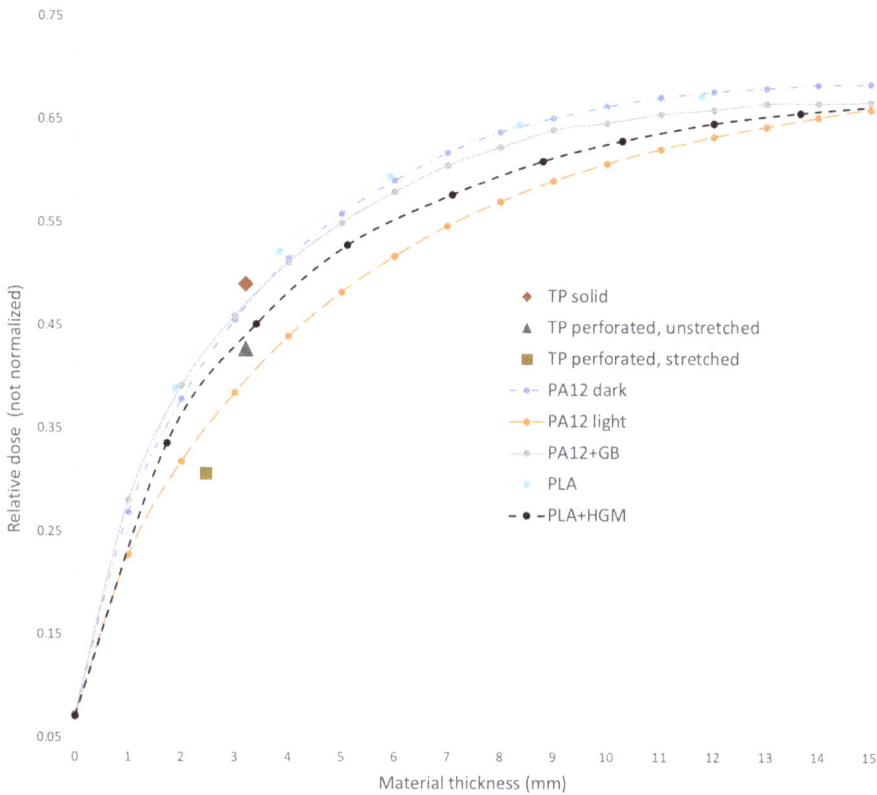

FIGURE 8.9   Parallel plate-measured relative dose below thicknesses of thermoplastic (TP) solid sheet, perforated thermoplastic, PA12 with glass beads, PA12 dark, PA12 light, polylactic acid (PLA), and PLA with hollow glass microspheres (HGM) added, showing more gradual buildup for the PA12 light material compared to other candidates. Figure sourced with permission from [11].

Asfia *et al.* also explored MJF printing [22], querying whether the printing color and orientation would affect the measured dose. Color did not have an effect at 6 MV but did produce a slight difference at 18 MV. Build orientation elicited a modest effect on dose, e.g., 3% change between 0- and 45-degree orientations, for a 6-MV beam at a measurement depth of 1 mm.

REPOSITIONING ACCURACY OF 3D PRINTED IMMOBILIZERS

Fortunately, multiple studies have provided a wealth of data describing inter- and intra-fractional repositioning accuracy of *status quo* TP immobilizers and these findings will serve as important benchmarks as innovators develop 3D printed solutions. In most series, mean and standard deviation statistics show positioning accuracy to within a few millimeters, but multiple studies demonstrate that larger outliers of positioning error will occur. Engelsman *et al.* [23] show intra-fractional patient motion up to 5 mm, although the mean among the patient cohort was 1.3 mm. Tryggestad *et al.* [24] observed mean inter-fractional translational shifts of 2 to 3 mm, with vector outliers up to 5 mm. In comparing two types of HN masks, Velec *et al.* [21] reported both inter- and intra-fractional

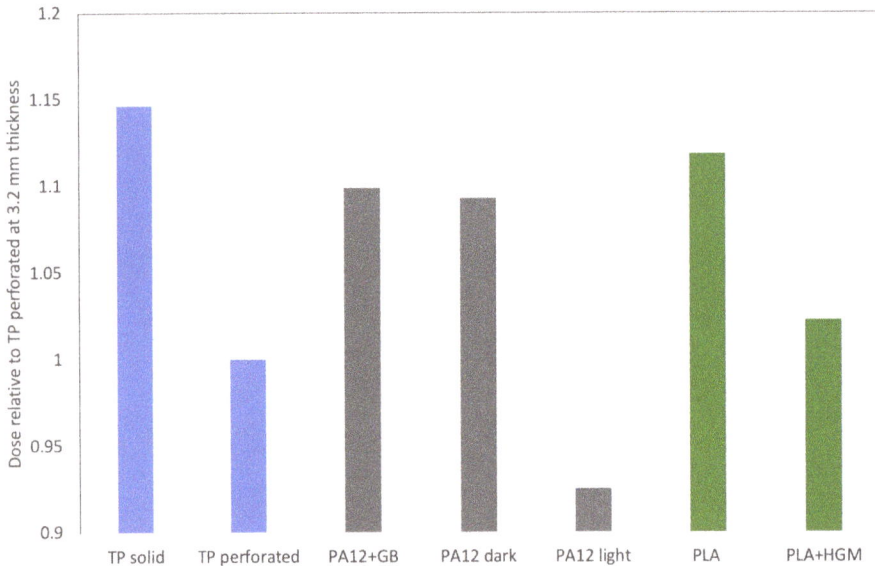

FIGURE 8.10   Comparison of measured dose for the same thickness (3.2 mm) of samples shown in Figure 8.9. Figure sourced with permission from [11].

error to be within 1 and 2 mm, with outliers up to approximately 9 mm. Gilbeau *et al.* [25] found a standard deviation of translation less than 2 mm and outliers of up to 4.5 mm in the cranium. For intracranial TP mesh masks, Boda-Heggemann *et al.* [26] reported a mean inter-fractional correction required of 4.7 mm. None of these studies demonstrated the extent to which poorly made masks will compromise positioning accuracy, but presumably inferior hand fabrication of immobilizers degrades performance. In turn, positioning error results in deterioration of the accuracy of dose received by the patient. For example, in radiosurgery, each 1 mm or error causes a loss of tumor coverage and dose conformity by 6% and 10%, respectively [27].

After developing the 3D printed immobilizer technology shown in Figure 8.4, in 2018 Haefner *et al.* [28] conducted a study in which eight healthy volunteers were imaged with repeat (n=10) MRI, removing and reapplying the immobilizer between scans, in order to simulate repositioning for fractionated treatment. Image data were reconstructed reconstructing with $1.25 \times 1.25 \times 1$ mm^3 voxel dimensions. Measured standard deviations of systematic and random errors were within 0.25 mm and 0.5 mm, respectively. The standard deviation of rotational error was below 0.3 degrees, with cranial pitch being the largest source. This work provided a first example showing that 3D printed immobilizers might rival or exceed the performance of TP mesh devices.

Several years later, Mattke *et al.* [9] used the same printed immobilization system to undertake a first clinical study of patients undergoing whole brain radiotherapy. Six patients were imaged over 10–12 fractions on Tomotherapy. Using megavoltage CT (MVCT) imaging, positioning offsets were recorded for each fraction. Results were compared to two control cohorts, one with TP mesh cranial immobilizers, and the second with standard HN masks. Results are shown in Figure 8.11, giving mean translational

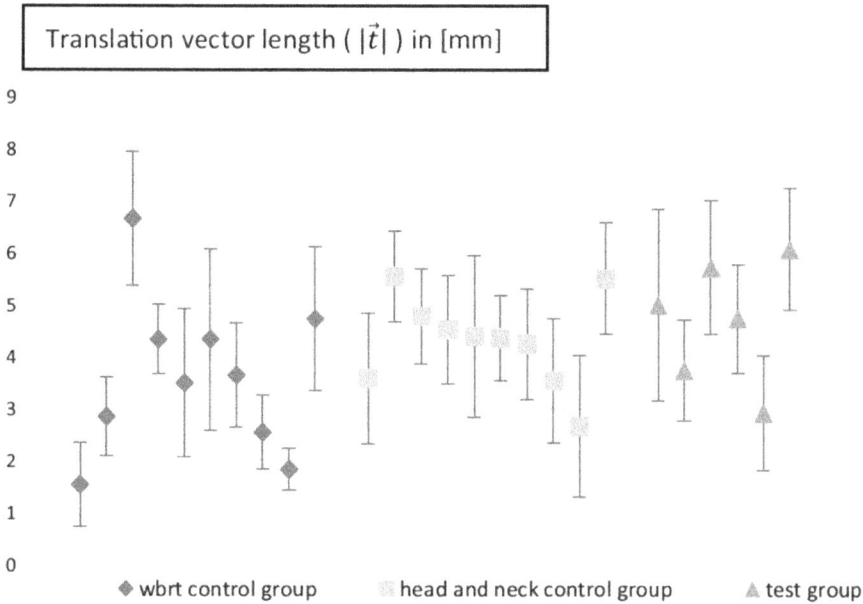

FIGURE 8.11 Comparison of mean translation vector length for whole brain and head-and-neck patients with thermoplastic immobilizers (diamonds and squares, respectively) and for patients with 3D printed immobilizers (triangles), from Mattke et al. Figure sourced with permission from [9].

vector length comparisons. For the test (3D printed immobilizer) group, the mean vector offset was 4.66 ± 1.65 mm. For the cranial and HN TP controls, the vector lengths were 3.61 ± 1.8 mm and 4.29 ± 1.43 mm, respectively. Mean rotational errors from this study are shown in Figure 8.12. Although the patient numbers were small in this study, the authors concluded that the repositioning errors were within the range of those that might be expected with traditional TP systems. Importantly, this investigation also proved the practicality of the workflow in the clinic. Imaging data were used without the need for the patient to be present during immobilizer fabrication, and an additional appointment was not required for pre-fitting of masks prior to the first fraction of treatment.

In another study, Miron *et al.* [5] 3D printed the anterior portion of a stereotactic radiotherapy (SRT) fixation immobilizer (Brainlab AG) as depicted in Figure 8.5. This 'non-invasive' shell was printed using FDM and 4.0-mm thick. Four volunteers received either this 3D printed mask (3DPM) or a standard TP SRT mask (SRTM). To compare the performance of these devices, subjects were imaged using motion-tracking MRI over 300 seconds. A first session was conducted with the volunteers quiescent, i.e., simulating compliant patients during treatment. In a second scan, subjects followed a motion protocol, during which they were instructed to attempt to translate or rotate their heads in a specific sequence. A subset of the results is shown in Figure 8.13. Average values of displacement were within ±1 mm for both the TP and 3D printed systems, however both the absolute deviations and standard deviations were improved using the 3D printed immobilizers.

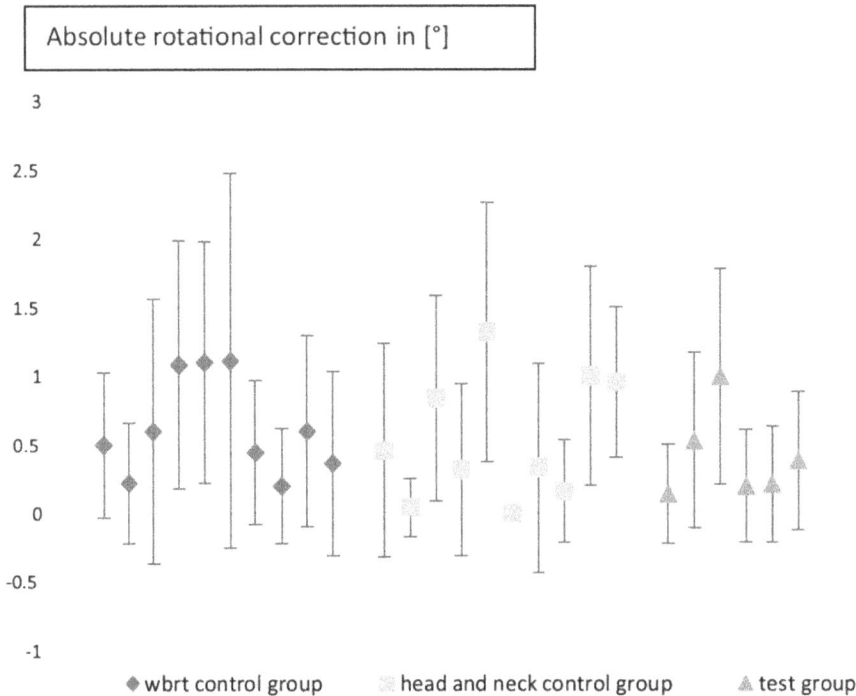

FIGURE 8.12 Comparison of absolute rotational corrections required for whole brain and head-and-neck patients with thermoplastic immobilizers (diamonds and squares, respectively) with 3D printed immobilizers (triangles), from Mattke et al. Figure sourced with permission from [9].

Limited examples exist of studies of repositioning accuracy for extracranial sites. For the PERSBRA system, ten patients were studied while undergoing whole breast irradiation [19]. Using the system depicted in Figure 8.7, patients were imaged without the immobilizer, with the immobilizer in place at the start of treatment, and then again with the immobilizer at the 6th day of the treatment course. By comparing the second and third datasets, this study showed intact breast repositioning accuracy of 6.7 ± 1.6 mm (anterior-posterior), 5.4 ± 1.5 mm (lateral), and 2.3 ± 1.4 mm (cranial-caudal). Comparison of contoured image datasets without and with the 3D printed immobilizer demonstrated improved sparing of the heart, left anterior descending (LAD) artery, and ipsilateral lung. Notably, the mean cardiac dose was reduced by approximately 27% through the positioning afforded by the personalized, printed immobilizer.

CLINICAL WORKFLOW INTEGRATING 3D PRINTED IMMOBILIZATION

Earlier in this chapter, the various potential advantages of 3D printed patient immobilization were outlined. However, following decades of using hand-fabricated TP to fashion these devices, a disruption of the *status quo* will require not only viable designs, materials, and 3D printing fabrication technology, but also a streamlined clinical workflow that does not introduce significant time or effort for the practitioners or patient. The following discusses various considerations in achieving this goal.

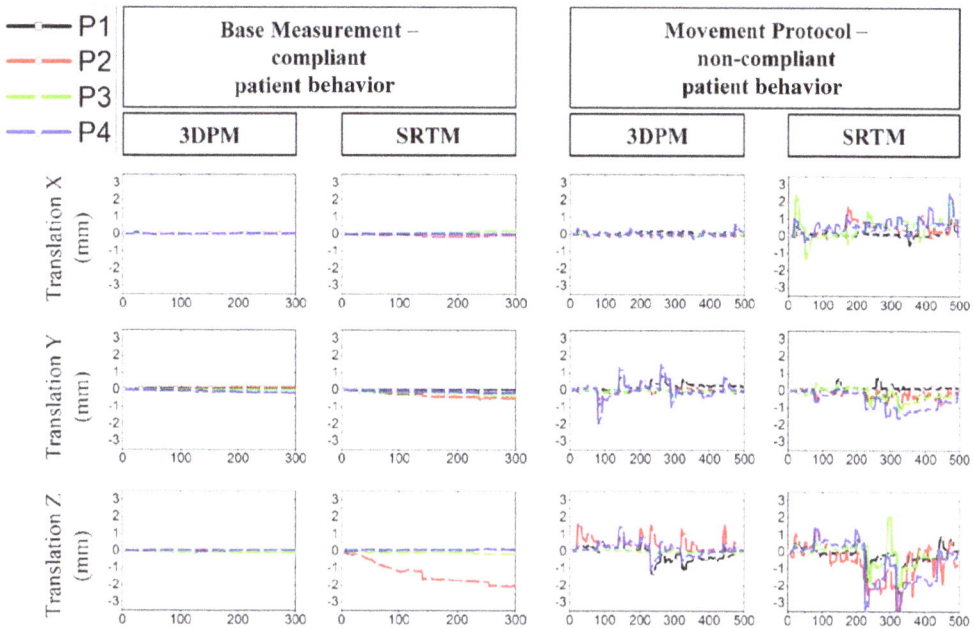

FIGURE 8.13   A subset of the results of the study by Miron et al. Patients were immobilized in either a standard stereotactic radiotherapy mask (SRTM) or a 3D printed mask (3DPM). Variability was measured with motion-tracking MRI. Scans were repeated with the subject quiescent (simulating compliant patients) or following instructions to translate or rotate the cranium in a movement protocol. Figure sourced with permission from [5].

Acquiring Source Imaging Data

Multiple examples of 3D printed immobilizer prototypes described in this chapter used 3D medical imaging data, e.g., either CT or MRI, as the basis for 3D printed immobilizer design. While it is true that most every patient undergoing RT receives CT imaging, and thus it may appear to be a natural candidate as source data, in fact using this dataset may not promote an efficient workflow. This is because while the CT data would be needed for the immobilizer design, optimally a second CT would be needed after fabricating the immobilizer, with the patient immobilized in the treatment position. This 'dual CT' conundrum is undesirable with regard to cost or efficiency, or the application of ionizing radiation. Thus a more likely approach involves the use of optical surface imaging. For example, optical surface imagers using photogrammetry or structured light [8, 10, 29–31] can capture the relevant cranial or HN anatomy in just a few minutes, without the need for ionizing radiation or an expensive medical scanner. Accessible optical imagers also provide accuracy and resolution that far exceed requirements for this application.

Some researchers [9] used MRI as the source data, but this would require its own imaging session for the patient with an expensive resource. Alternatively, if appropriate data are available in the image archive system, it could be used for rigid anatomies; however, these data must capture the external surface of the patient, which is not always the case, e.g., in diagnostic imaging studies. Moreover, the patient position must be representative (or made representative through data manipulation) of the patient in treatment position. While this may work in concept for the cranium, for HN cases, e.g., differences in neck extension between the source image data and the actual treatment position would prove problematic.

Immobilizer Software Design

A viable workflow integrating 3D printed immobilization will require efficient and robust software that designs the immobilizer based on 3D imaging data. While this remains in development at the time of writing, most of the examples in the literature have used non-approved and complex CAD software, much of which would be unworkable in the typical busy clinical environment. An example of progress toward producing of an automated application for this purpose is the work by Chen *et al.* [32] who described a fully automated framework for extraction of the surface and identification of facial features (eyes, nose, mouth) through atlas registration, to allow customization of the mask.

The requirements of an effective software application would include the capacity to:

- accommodate one or more formats of input data (e.g., tomographic or triangularized mesh formats)
- cope with the presence of noise in the data that would otherwise corrupt the surface delineation of the immobilizer;
- handle the scenario of missing data (e.g., in shadows cast during optical surface imaging);
- create topologies that will always fit the patient (e.g., avoiding concavities or other features that would make the immobilizer impossible to apply to cranial or HN anatomy);
- integrate with a generic headrest and baseplate, e.g., including fixation points;
- add features such as openings for eyes, nose, mouth, or for optical surface monitoring of skin surface;
- add labeling on the surface, e.g., patient identifiers, bar/QR codes or other; and
- produce an output format that is printable by an appropriate technology, e.g., MJF [11], or for ordering of the immobilizer with an on-demand (OD), approach, i.e., where the actual printing is outsourced to a provider who is equipped/certified to produce the device.

All of these requirements should be provided by a software application that is usable in a turnkey fashion by the typical practitioners, e.g., clinical medical physicists, dosimetrists, or radiation therapists.

Fabrication

Among all RT patient devices discussed in this book, including personalized photon or electron bolus, proton compensators, and surface or interstitial/intracavitary brachytherapy applicators, the 3D printed patient immobilizer is likely the most complex in its geometry. An immobilizer may feature a thin shell, perforations, materials with low dose buildup characteristics, an effective metamaterial design [11] providing rigidity and low buildup, attachment points to a base plate, and printed alignment markers or other labeling. It may also incorporate other devices, e.g., integrating a bolus in contact with the skin. The complexity of this printed device means that the highly accessible FDM or resin stereolithography printing technologies may not be likely candidates for this application. Even if immobilizers are reliably printable with these methods, the amount of post-processing (e.g., removal of supports, etc.) necessary may prove unfeasible. On the other hand, technologies such as SLS or MJF will be more suited to printing immobilizers [11].

Quality Assurance

Through digital design and fabrication, it can be expected that the accuracy of the immobilizer produced should exceed that possible through fabrication by hand, e.g., using molded TP. A robust, digital process should eliminate human error and be limited only by the accuracy of the source data in representing the true geometry of the patient. At the same time, quality assurance will be important in a clinical process. Figure 8.14 shows the result of a QC test where a MJF-printed immobilizer has been imaged after fabrication

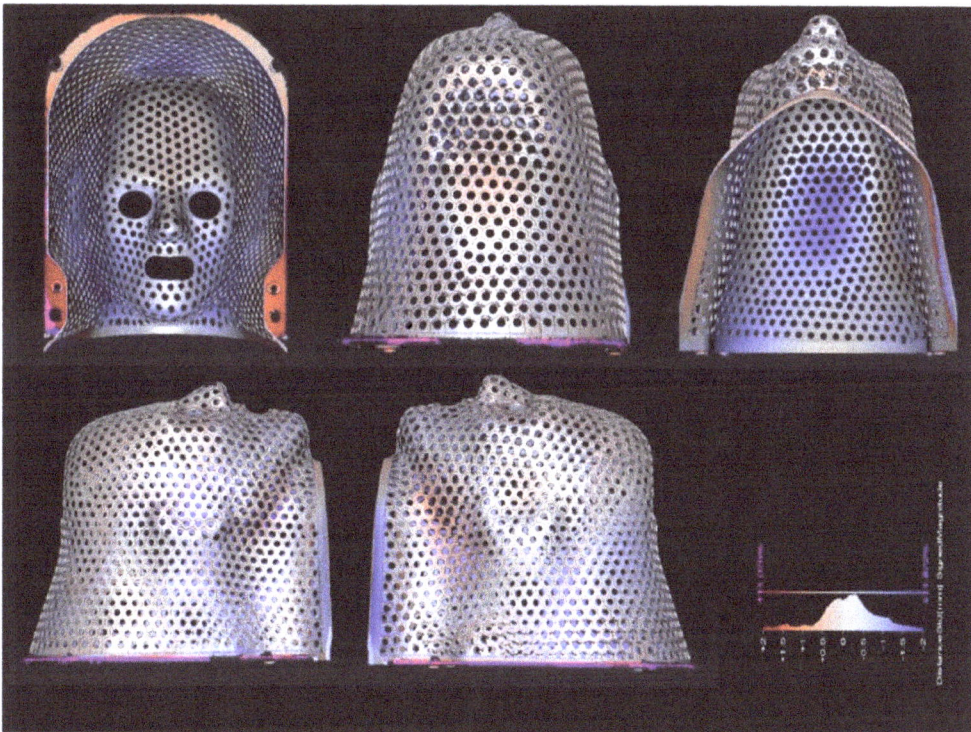

FIGURE 8.14   Shading showing difference between optical surface scan of an MJF-printed immobilizer and the source design. Figure sourced with permission from [11].

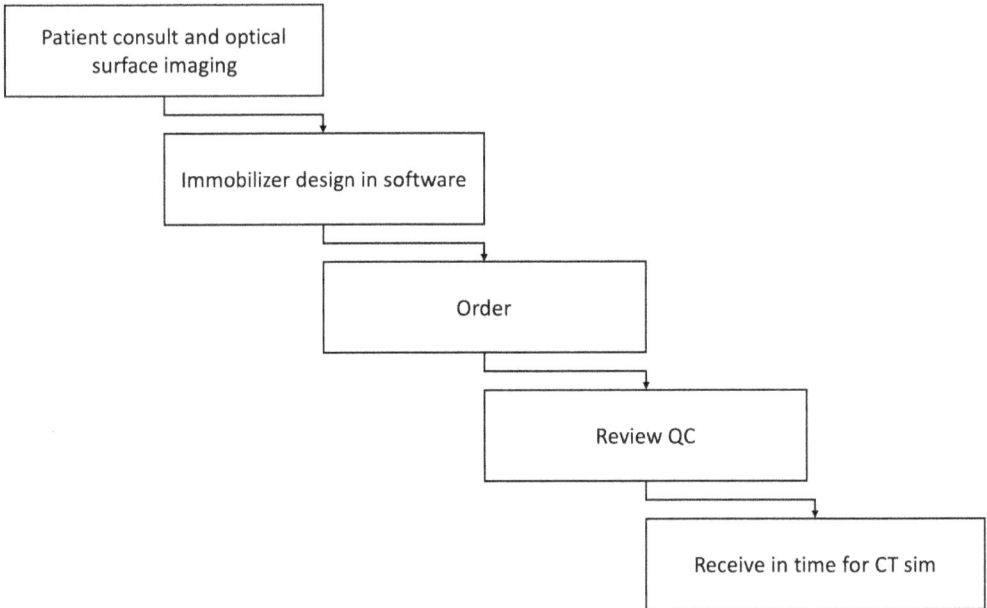

FIGURE 8.15   Example workflow for 3D printed immobilization in the clinic.

with high-resolution optical surface scanning, and the resultant scanned surface data are compared with the original design. The shading in this example shows dimensional accuracy of 97% of scanned points agree to within 2 mm.

A Complete Clinical Workflow for 3D Printed Immobilization

While 3D printed immobilization remains in the research and development stage at the time of writing, one can envisage an efficient workflow in the clinic that does not add significant time or effort, and in fact affords certain efficiencies and steps that promote a patient-centered process. To ensure adoption, this flow must align with the existing approach. Figure 8.15 depicts an example in which image data for immobilizer design are acquired early in the process, e.g., at the time of initial radiation oncology consult. This step would likely involve the patient being positioned simply on a generic head rest/immobilization baseplate and scanned with optical surface imaging in a few minutes. Once these data become available, they would be loaded by a dedicated application that would facilitate efficient immobilizer design by the clinical team, adding any desired features, e.g., perforations, openings, labeling, and attachment to the generic system. It is likely, given the required printing technology, that an OD order would then be placed. After printing, the OD provider would supply QC data, providing the medical physicists with an opportunity to view the result prior to receiving the device. Finally, the printed immobilizer is received by the clinical team. Importantly, providing a viable timeframe for manufacturing and shipping, the immobilizer would be available in time for the patient's CT simulation appointment (instead of having to fabricate a device at this time, tying up the CT resource and associated staff).

SUMMARY

This chapter has described various potential advantages introduced by 3D printing of patient immobilizers given the shortcomings of current methods to immobilize patients, and considering the technical advantages afforded by digital design and 3D printing processes. From the point of view of the clinical practitioner, the opportunity is twofold. First, 3D printing technology should introduce advantages in standardizing immobilizer quality, and particularly in the spatial accuracy in fitting to the patient. In turn this should enable more uniform performance in minimizing inter- and intra-fractional positioning error. Other features will introduce clinical advantages, e.g., the use of novel materials and metamaterials allowing minimization of skin dose and skin toxicity compared to today's TP devices. The second aspect is efficiency in the clinic, whereby laborious, manual methods may be retired. By leveraging 3D surface imaging and eliminating fabrication by hand, radiation therapy staff and CT simulation resources are alleviated. Finally, and critical to improving the patient experience, the immobilization fabrication method will become more aligned with other steps in the RT paradigm, that is, leveraging state-of-the-art digital technologies to enable minimally invasive and of high precision treatment.

REFERENCES

[1] Choong ES, Turner RN, Flatley MJ. Radiotherapy: Basic principles and technical advances. *Orthop Trauma*. 2014;28:167–171.

[2] Zhang L, Garden AS, Lo J, et al. Multiple regions-of-interest analysis of setup uncertainties for head-and-neck cancer radiotherapy. *Int J Radiat Oncol Biol Phys*. 2006;64:1559–1569.

[3] Klug N, Butow PN, Burns M, et al. Unmasking anxiety: A qualitative investigation of health professionals; perspectives of mask anxiety in head and neck cancer. *J Med Imaging Radiat Sci*. 2020;51:12–21.

[4] Clover K, Oultram S, Adams C, et al. Disruption to radiation therapy sessions due to anxiety among patients receiving radiation therapy to the head and neck area can be predicted using patient self-report measures. *Psycho Oncol*. 2011;20:1334–1341.

[5] Miron VM, Etzelstorfer T, Kleiser R, et al. Evaluation of novel 3D-printed and conventional thermoplastic stereotactic high-precision patient fixation masks for radiotherapy. *Strahlentherapie Und Onkologie*. 2022;198:1032–1041.

[6] Sharp L, Lewin F, Johansson H, et al. Randomized trial on two types of thermoplastic masks for patient immobilization during radiation therapy for head-and-neck cancer. *Int J Radiat Oncol Biol Phys*. 2005;61:250–256.

[7] Nixon JL, Brown B, Pigott AE, et al. A prospective examination of mask anxiety during radiotherapy for head and neck cancer and patient perceptions of management strategies. *J Med Radiat Sci*. 2019;66:184–190.

[8] Sanghera B, Amis A, McGurk M. Preliminary study of potential for rapid prototype and surface scanned radiotherapy facemask production technique. *J Med Eng Technol*. 2009;26:16–21.

[9] Mattke M, Rath D, Häfner MF, et al. Individual 3D-printed fixation masks for radiotherapy: First clinical experiences. *Int J Comput Ass Rad*. 2021;16:1043–1049.

[10] Douglass MJJ. Can optical scanning technologies replace CT for 3D printed medical devices in radiation oncology? *J Med Radiat Sci*. 2022;69:139–142.

[11] Robar JL, Kammerzell B, Hulick K, et al. Novel multi jet fusion 3D-printed patient immobilization for radiation therapy. *J Appl Clin Med Phys.* 2022;23:e13773.

[12] Lee N, Chuang C, Quivey JM, et al. Skin toxicity due to intensity-modulated radiotherapy for head-and-neck carcinoma. *Int J Radiat Oncol Biol Phys.* 2002;53:630–637.

[13] Ali I, Matthiesen C, Algan O, et al. Quantitative evaluation of increase in surface dose by immobilization thermoplastic masks and superficial dosimetry using Gafchromic EBT film and Monte Carlo calculations. *J X-ray Sci Technol.* 2010;18:319–326.

[14] Avanzo M, Drigo A, Kaiser SR, et al. Dose to the skin in helical tomotherapy: Results of in vivo measurements with radio chromic films. *Phys Medica.* 2013;29:304–311.

[15] Fisher M, Christopher A, Mohammad R, et al. Evaluation of 3-D printed immobilisation shells for head and neck IMRT. *Open J Radiol.* 2014;4:322–328.

[16] Laycock SD, Hulse M, Scrase CD, et al. Towards the production of radiotherapy treatment shells on 3D printers using data derived from DICOM CT and MRI: Preclinical feasibility studies. *J Radiotherapy Pract.* 2015;14:92–98.

[17] Haefner MF, Giesel FL, Mattke M, et al. 3D-Printed masks as a new approach for immobilization in radiotherapy – a study of positioning accuracy. *Oncotarget.* 2018;9:6490–6498.

[18] Pham Q-VV, Lavallée A-P, Foias A, et al. Radiotherapy immobilization mask molding through the use of 3D-printed head models. *Technol Cancer Res Treat.* 2018;17:1533033818809051.

[19] Chen C-P, Lin C-Y, Kuo C-C, et al. Skin surface dose for whole breast radiotherapy using personalized breast holder: Comparison with various radiotherapy techniques and clinical experiences. *Cancers.* 2022;14:3205.

[20] Siebers JV, Keall PJ, Wu Q, et al. Effect of patient setup errors on simultaneously integrated boost head and neck IMRT treatment plans. *Int J Radiat Oncol Biol Phys.* 2005;63:422–433.

[21] Velec M, Waldron JN, O'Sullivan B, et al. Cone-Beam CT assessment of interfraction and intrafraction setup error of two head-and-neck cancer thermoplastic masks. *Int J Radiat Oncol Biol Phys.* 2010;76:949–955.

[22] Asfia A, Novak JI, Mohammed MI, et al. A review of 3D printed patient specific immobilisation devices in radiotherapy. *Phys Imaging Radiat Oncol.* 2020;13:30–35.

[23] Engelsman M, Rosenthal SJ, Michaud SL, et al. Intra- and interfractional patient motion for a variety of immobilization devices. *Méd Phys.* 2005;32:3468–3474.

[24] Tryggestad E, Christian M, Ford E, et al. Inter- and intrafraction patient positioning uncertainties for intracranial radiotherapy: A study of four frameless, thermoplastic mask-based immobilization strategies using daily cone-beam CT. *Int J Radiat Oncol Biol Phys.* 2011;80:281–290.

[25] Gilbeau L, Octave-Prignot M, Loncol T, et al. Comparison of setup accuracy of three different thermoplastic masks for the treatment of brain and head and neck tumors. *Radiother Oncol.* 2001;58:155–162.

[26] Boda-Heggemann J, Walter C, Rahn A, et al. Repositioning accuracy of two different mask systems—3D revisited: Comparison using true 3D/3D matching with cone-beam CT. *Int J Radiat Oncol Biology Phys.* 2006;66:1568–1575.

[27] Guckenberger M, Roesch J, Baier K, et al. Dosimetric consequences of translational and rotational errors in frame-less image-guided radiosurgery. *Radiat Oncol Lond Engl.* 2012;7:63–63.

[28] Haefner MF, Giesel FL, Mattke M, et al. 3D-Printed masks as a new approach for immobilization in radiotherapy – a study of positioning accuracy. *Oncotarget.* 2018;9:6490–6498.

[29] Kang D, Wang B, Peng Y, et al. Low-Cost iPhone-assisted processing to obtain radiotherapy bolus using optical surface reconstruction and 3D-printing. *Sci Reports.* 2020;10:8016.

[30] Maxwell SK, Charles PH, Cassim N, et al. Assessing the fit of 3D printed bolus from CT, optical scanner and photogrammetry methods. *Phys Eng Sci Med.* 2019;43:601–607.

[31] Douglass MJJ, Santos AMC. Application of optical photogrammetry in radiation oncology: HDR surface mold brachytherapy. *Brachytherapy.* 2019;18:689–700.

[32] Chen S, Lu Y, Hopfgartner C, et al. 3-D printing based production of head and neck masks for radiation therapy using CT volume data: A fully automatic framework. *2016 IEEE 13th Int Symp Biomed Imaging ISBI.* 2016;403–406. https://ieeexplore.ieee.org/document/7493293

CHAPTER 9

3D Printed Radiation Detectors

Thalat Monajemi

INTRODUCTION

Radiation detectors are used widely in radiation oncology for quality control and assurance of the dosimetric and geometric integrity of radiation beams, for verifying and monitoring that radiation is delivered safely to patients, and in imaging. It is common practice that radiation oncology departments purchase commercially available detectors, then verify their function against other trusted detectors before deployment in the clinic. A significant body of research and development in radiation oncology is dedicated to elucidating the limitations of existing detectors by testing them in challenging measurement settings, e.g., in small radiation fields, on patient surfaces, and in high-energy particle beams. Required changes in the design of detectors are usually only achievable via collaboration with manufacturers. To date, the application of 3D printing in building novel radiation detectors in radiation oncology has not been as prevalent as clinical applications such as 3D printing of bolus, phantoms, or brachytherapy applicators. Like other applications, however, the relatively low cost, accessibility and capacity for rapid prototyping offered by 3D printing technology introduces the potential to provide radiation oncology departments with the freedom to build custom-designed and even patient-specific detectors.

The aim of this chapter is to report on the key innovations to date that focus on using additive manufacturing of detectors for use in radiation oncology.

GASEOUS DETECTORS

Air-filled ionization chambers are the most widely used and arguably the most versatile detectors in radiation oncology. The operational principle of an ionization chamber is that radiation enters the chamber, interacts with the gas in the central volume, and produces secondary charges [1]. An electric field is applied to the sensitive volume, which

 DOI: 10.1201/9781003288404-9

directs the secondary charges to a collecting electrode. The signal produced in the electrode is collected by an electrometer producing a readable integrated charge or current.

The first report on 3D printing to produce an ion chamber described a fused deposition modeling (FDM)-printed, small, single-wire drift tube used to measure cosmic ray muons [2]. The drift tube was printed using polylactic acid (PLA) to produce a gas volume in the shape of an inverted triangular prism with a base length of 28 mm, height of 24 mm, and tube length of 145 mm. A stainless steel anode wire was placed in the center of the tube, mid-print. At the time of writing, only two publications are available on the use of additive manufacturing in fabricating ionization chambers for use in radiation oncology. These efforts are summarized in this section.

Early 3D Printed Gaseous Detectors

One of the first reported [3] parallel plate ion chamber arrays produced via additive manufacturing is illustrated in Figure 9.1, which also depicts a cross section of a single detector element. The array consists of air-vented rectangular ionization chambers with dimensions 5×7 mm^2, each with a central conductive pin. Non-conducting parts of the detector were printed using acrylonitrile butadiene styrene (ABS), and conducting parts were printed using a conductive PLA filament (cPLA) [4]. cPLA and ABS could not be printed simultaneously as cPLA does not adhere well to ABS. Therefore, the conductive and non-conductive components were printed separately and then assembled in an interlocking fashion. FDM printing was chosen due to its accessibility and the freedom to print with conducting and non-conducting filaments.

A challenge in using new materials and designs for fabricating ion chambers, 3D printed or otherwise, is that electrical properties such as leakage, collection efficiency, change in resistivity, dielectric polarization, stability, or electric field uniformity are not

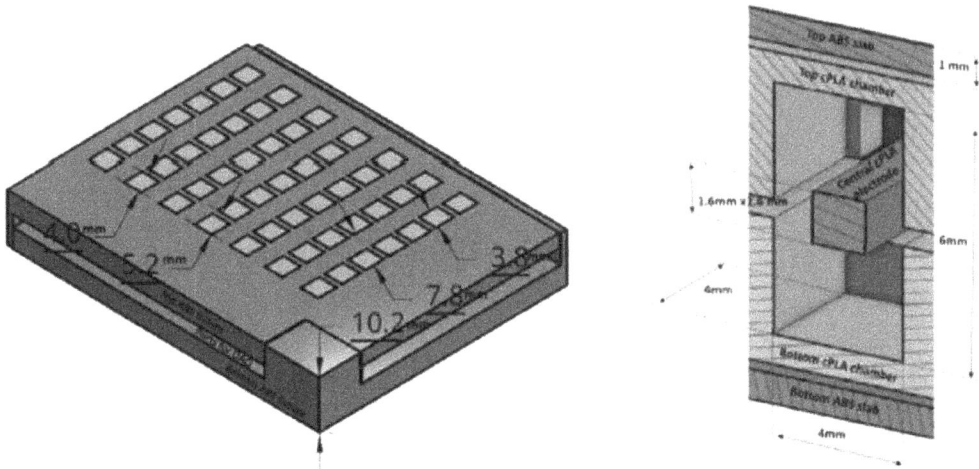

FIGURE 9.1   Designs of a 3D printed ionization chamber array (left) and cross-section through one of the chambers in the array (right). The array consists of insulating acrylonitrile butadiene styrene (ABS) and conductive polylactic acid (cPLA). Figure sourced with permission from [3].

yet well known. Fabrication via 3D printing could exacerbate these challenges by, e.g., adding directional dependence or nonuniform material changes.

The current–voltage curve of the array revealed a significant polarity effect (8%). Polarity effect [1] quantifies the amount by which the charge collected at the same voltage and one polarity differs from that of the opposite polarity. The early design shown in Figure 9.1 was fabricated using ABS insulating walls and highlighted the fact that the plastics used in 3D printing may distort electric fields applied to ion chambers due to charge accumulation or dielectric polarization. A subsequent design of this detector [5] consisted of 30 ×30 ionization chambers using a PLA frame for the electrodes with a 4×4 mm^2 spatial resolution. External electrodes consisted of cPLA, and internal electrodes of microwire.

RADIO-PHOTOLUMINESCENT GLASS DETECTORS

Radio-photoluminescent (RPL) glass detectors emit visible photons when excited by ultraviolet (UV) light after exposure to ionizing radiation. The most common RPL detector material is silver-activated phosphate glass. Ag$^+$ ions exist uniformly through the glass; holes and electrons released by ionizing radiation convert these ions to stable luminescent centers of Ag^{++} or Ag^0, respectively, at room temperature. The luminescence centers increase in proportion to the radiation dose. Following irradiation, this type of glass emits light with a prominent peak near the orange region of the spectrum, which is attributed to Ag^{++} and caused by electron transitions between energy levels of orbital electrons. The luminescence centers are not depleted even with repeated readout using UV light.

Early 3D Printed Radio-Photoluminescent Glass Detectors
Hashimoto *et al.* [6] have described 3D printing in the fabrication of RPL glass detectors that employed FDM to produce 3D dosimeters in two arbitrary shapes: a ring and an ear. Figure 9.2 shows the ear-shaped dosimeter, the image of the signal from this device, and the resultant measured dose distribution. Since no commercial RPL filaments were

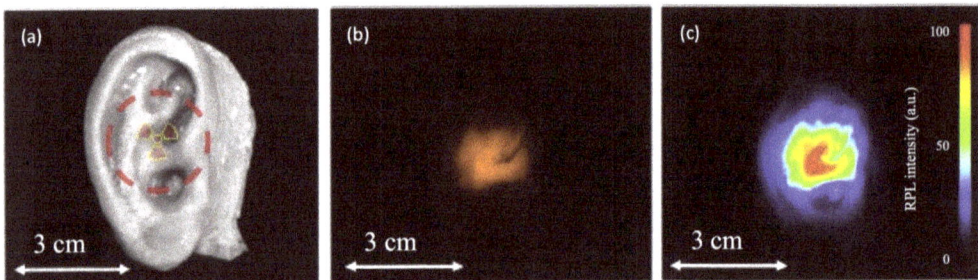

FIGURE 9.2 (a) Photograph of an ear-shaped dosimeter under LED lighting, (b) image from the RPL dosimeter signal indicating the irradiated region, and (c) dose profile from this image. Figure sourced with permission from [6].

available, this group fabricated their own printer filaments in-house. These filaments were composed of pulverized thermoplastic resin powder and powder RPL glass produced using a filament extruder. The glass powder was manufactured using commercially available raw materials including sodium metaphosphate, aluminum metaphosphate, and silver chloride, through mixing, heating, and cooling over 25 hours. The cooled RPL glass was turned into powder with an average size of 5 μm with a dry jet mill.

Three commercial thermoplastic resins have been tested for this application, PLA, ABS, and polycaprolactone (PCL) resin. PCL resin [7] is a biodegradable polyester with a melting point of 57°C and, unlike PLA or ABS, is not a typical material used for FDM printing. In the case where the thermoplastic resin was PCL, the filament was extruded at 70°C as opposed to 170°C in the case of ABS and PLA due to its lower melting point. The weight ratio of the RPL glass powder was 7.5%, producing a medium with an effective atomic number close to that of human tissue. Initial testing of the filaments by exposure to 30 Gy in a 90-kVp X-ray beam showed that PCL glass filament had the largest light intensity at 16.3 arbitrary units compared to 5.8 for ABS and 3.1 for PLA. In addition, this filament showed the greatest mechanical flexibility. Therefore, the ring and ear objects were printed with PCL.

PLASTIC SCINTILLATORS

The function of plastic scintillators is to convert the energy of incident radiation to optical photons that may be collected via a photodetector. When high-energy radiation interacts with a plastic scintillator, it ionizes the material. Plastic scintillators consist of a polymer containing aromatic functional groups and, most typically, two types of dissolved fluorescence dyes [8]. Since the amount of the dyes in the polymer is very small, e.g., a few percent by weight (wt%), essentially all excitations and subsequent relaxations occur in the polymer matrix. When the energy levels of the primary dye are matched to the matrix, rapid non-radiative energy transfer can occur from the matrix to the dye via a dipole–dipole interaction, called the Förster mechanism [9]. To avoid self-absorption of the emitted light and to ensure maximum transparency, a second wavelength shifting dye is added in a much lower concentration that absorbs the photons emitted by the primary dye and reemits them at a higher wavelength than the primary dye can absorb. Figure 9.3 illustrates the scintillation process.

High quality plastic scintillators can be produced by cast polymerization [10]. In this technique, a liquid monomer and the scintillating dyes are poured into a mold, heated, then cooled in a controlled and time-consuming process. Another method of production is injection molding [11] in which granulated plastic is mixed with the scintillating dyes. The mixture is loaded into a molding machine hopper and is directed continuously into a heated screw cylinder while being mixed. At the exit from the cylinder, the temperature reaches about 200°C immediately before being injected into the mold and cooled. Finally, scintillator extrusion is possible [12], where dry plastic pellets and dopants are fed into an extruder hopper under a nitrogen purge. The extruder melts, mixes, and delivers the scintillator at roughly 200°C into the profile die.

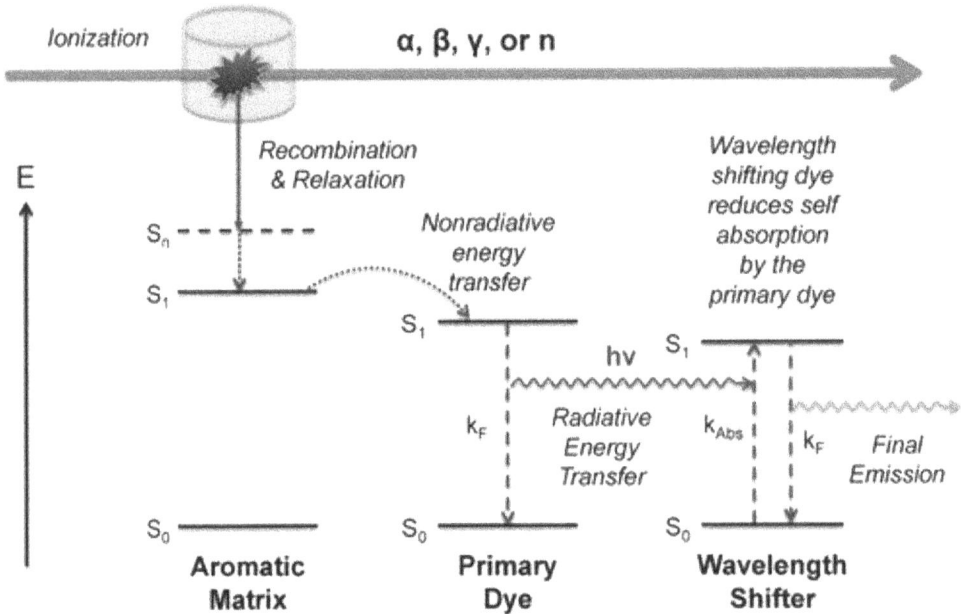

FIGURE 9.3 The process of energy transfer within a scintillator leading to emission of light. Figure sourced with permission from [28].

The First 3D Printed Plastic Scintillator

The first report on 3D printed plastic scintillators was published by Mishnayot *et al.* [13], and described stereolithography (SLA) to produce a printed sample that yielded light output of 30% of that of EJ-204 (Eljen, Limited), a familiar polystyrene based scintillator with efficiency of 68% of anthracene. The basis of the printed scintillator was an acrylic UV curable composed of SR9035 as the monomer, Lucirin TPO as the photoinitiator. Additional components were added to the formulation, including 2,5- diphenyloxazole, 1,4-bis(5-phenyl-2- oxazolyl)benzene, and naphtalene. The cup-shaped scintillator is shown in Figure 9.4.

Acrylic-based scintillators, such as the one used in this first report, are inherently less efficient than polystyrene-based scintillators that contain aromatic polymers [14]. Non-aromatic plastic acrylic scintillators are made by adding an aromatic co-solvent, typically naphthalene (10%–25% by weight). Naphthalene is an intermediate solvent that helps increase the scintillation efficiency of the acrylic-based polymers. Thus, the reduced efficiency of the printed scintillator in this study can be expected, and the researchers noted a further degradation of the sample over time, which they attributed to the sublimation of the naphthalene activator at high concentrations. Despite the lower signal, acrylic-based scintillators such as those in this study are more readily produced compared to styrene-based scintillators because styrene contains strong triplet quenchers that disturb the photopolymerization process [15]. The 3D printed scintillator described by Mishnayot *et al.* was not applied in radiation oncology but provided foundational information for further development.

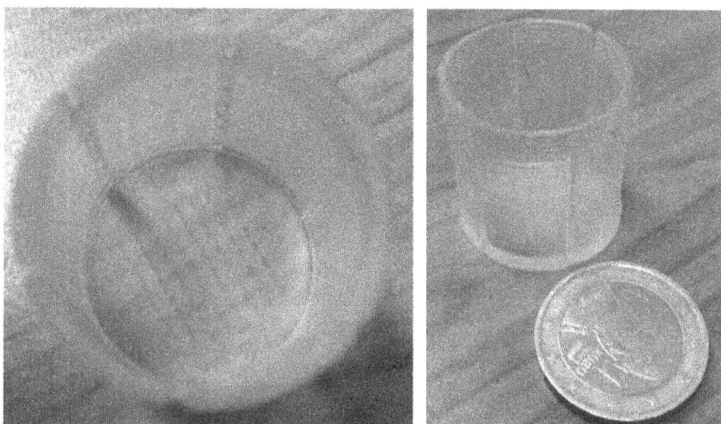

FIGURE 9.4   Cup-shaped acrylic scintillator printed by Mishnayot et al. Figure sourced with permission from [13].

Plastic Scintillators Cured by UV Light

Other applications of UV-cured 3D printed plastic scintillators in radiation oncology were based on modifications to the resin recipe by Mishnayot *et al.* [13]. Son *et al.* [16] described a modified resin that used an acrylic monomer and naphthalene instead of styrene. The scintillator was printed via digital light processing (DLP) with a UV LED light source of 385 nm. The resin was composed of BPA(EO)$_{15}$DMA (Bisphenol A (EO)15 dimethylacrylate) acrylic monomer, PPO (2,5-diphenyloxazole) as the primary dye, ADS086BE (2,7-Bis[2-(9-ethylcarbazol-4yl)yinyl]-9,9-dihexyl-9H-fluorine), as the secondary dye, TPO (Diphenyl(2,4,6-trimethylbenzoyl) phosphineoxide) as the photoinitiator, and 1-methyl-naphthalene [16]. Instead of 1,4-bis(5-phenyloxazol-2-yl) benzene (POPOP), a typical wavelength-shifting secondary dye, ADS086BE was used, which offers better solubility in the acrylic resin. TPO was added as the photoinitiator since its absorption length matched that of the UV LED light of the DLP printer at 385 nm.

Characteristics of a $1 \times 1 \times 1$ cm^3 printed sample were compared with the commercial plastic scintillator BC-408 (Saint Gobain). Figure 9.5 shows the effect of using ADS086BE as the secondary dye instead of POPOP. The peak emission wavelength is at 470 nm compared with BC-408 at 425 nm. The wavelength shifter, ADS086BE, is a yellow powder and the final scintillator product has a yellowish color instead of being clear. The transmittances of the BC-408 and fabricated scintillator were approximately 76% and 56% at maximum emission wavelengths of 425 and 470 nm, respectively. This difference in transmittance was attributed to the process of 3D printing, whereby a layer-by-layer polymerization of the scintillator affects the opacity of the sample. In contrast, in BC-408 the entire sample is polymerized at once.

This difference in transmission, along with the inherent inferior scintillation efficiency of acrylic monomers and the possible presence of oxygen introduced in the layer-by-layer polymerization process of DLP, resulted in a scintillation efficiency of approximately 68% compared with BC-408 (which has a light output of 64% of anthracene) for the 1 cm^3 sample. Oxygen can act as a strong quencher and cause degradation of the scintillator

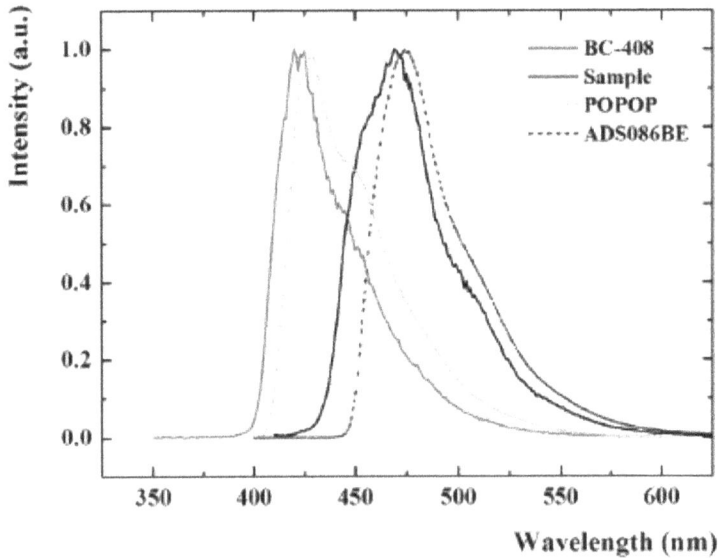

FIGURE 9.5 Comparison of wavelength spectra of a commercial plastic scintillator (BC-408), the fabricated sample, dissolved in cyclohexane POPOP or ADS086BE secondary dyes. Figure sourced with permission from [16].

efficiency [17]. Further studies of the scintillator [18] showed a similar decay time constant compared to BC-408. The 3D printed scintillator's performance was considered sufficient to be applied to applications with high dose rates such as radiation therapy.

Plastic Scintillators in the Shape of an Ionization Chamber

3D printing has been used to produce scintillator detectors replicating the geometry of familiar ionization chambers [19]. A plastic scintillation dosimeter with a shape identical to that of the ionization chamber PTW31010 (PTW-Freiburg, Germany) was printed. The 0.125 cc PTW31010 chamber has an active volume radius of 2.75 mm and length of 6.5 mm. The plastic scintillator was fabricated using a DLP 3D printer, curing 0.15-mm thick layers for 20 seconds each. As shown in Figure 9.6, the scintillator was wrapped in Teflon tape to reflect the scintillation light and covered with a 3D printed probe head. Scintillation light was directed to a photomultiplier tube using a silica optical fiber.

The scintillator was calibrated in a secondary standards lab under reference conditions in a Co-60 beam. The scintillator was used for measurement in the 16-mm beam of a Gamma Knife® Perfexion™ (Elekta AB, Stockholm, Sweden). The agreement of the dose rates from the Gamma Knife treatment plan and that measured with the scintillator was within 4.1%. The authors attributed this difference to the source intensity and geometry differences between the calibration and measurement conditions, and not to 3D printing-related factors.

Tumor-Shaped Plastic Scintillators

Other work used the versatility of 3D printing to replicate tumor geometry. In a study by Kim et al. [20] magnetic resonance imaging (MRI) data were used to design and print a scintillator in the shape of a vestibular schwannoma with a volume of 0.39 cm^3 (Figure 9.7).

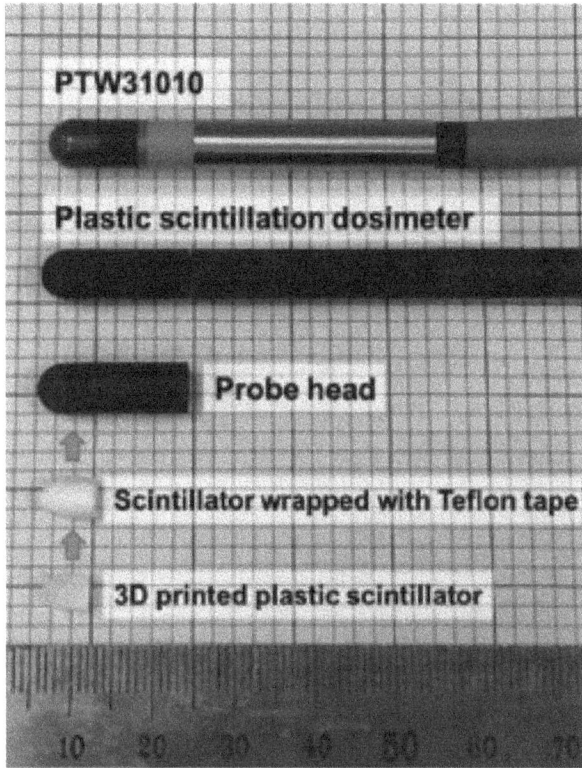

FIGURE 9.6 Plastic scintillation detector fabricated using 3D printing, compared to the PTW31010 ionization chamber. Figure sourced with permission from [19].

The tumor-shaped scintillator used the formulation of Son *et al.* [16]. The printing speed was approximately 20 seconds per layer, and a tumor-shaped scintillator with a height of 11.5 mm was printed in less than an hour. The outer surface of the tumor-shaped scintillator was coated with reflective paint consisting of titanium dioxide (TiO_2) pigment and black paint. The light output was read via an optical fiber and photomultiplier tube. Direct calibration at a secondary calibration lab and Monte Carlo simulation were used to calibrate this tumor-shaped detector.

Complex treatment plans are commonly verified through measurement of point dose values, or dose in a plane by using single detectors or detector arrays. The ability to print specific tumor shapes in a timely manner would provide radiation therapy departments with a third and importantly, a volumetric way of verifying planned dose distributions. The investigators suggest using the tumor-shaped dosimeter to verify the total energy deposited in the tumor allowing comparison to the value provided by the treatment planning system. In this study, while the measured energy determined with the calibration from the secondary calibration lab was 5.84 ± 3.56% lower than the calculated value, the energy measured using the Monte Carlo simulation calibration was 2.00 ± 0.76% higher than the calculated value in the Gamma Knife treatment planning system.

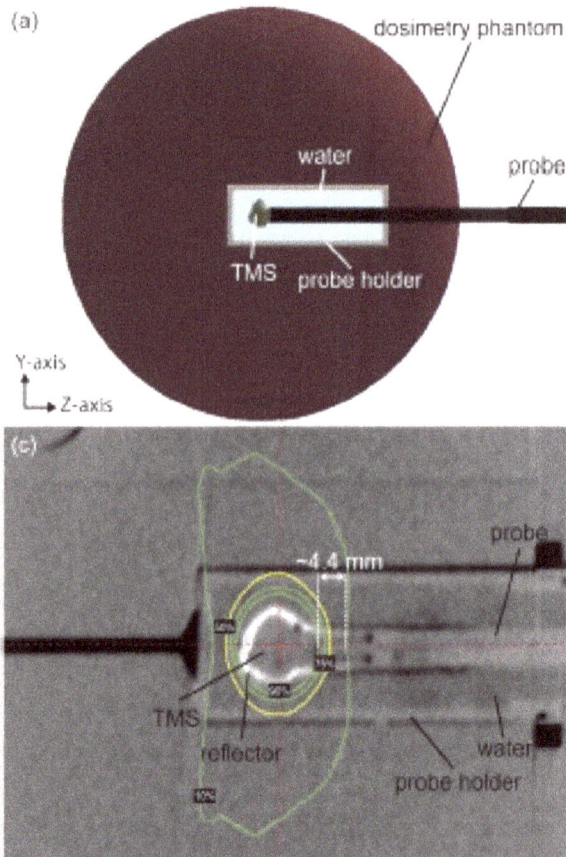

FIGURE 9.7   3D printed scintillator shaped to resemble a vestibular schwannoma within a dosimetry phantom (above) and with overlaid planned dose distribution (below). Figure sourced with permission from [20].

Isodose-Shaped Plastic Scintillators

Other investigators have considered producing scintillators to replicate calculated isodose volumes. Kim *et al.* [21] applied 3D printed scintillators to the challenging situation of measuring dose from small radiation fields. Plastic scintillating fibers are one of the few options for measuring doses in small fields, chosen for their small dimensions and water equivalence in their response to radiation [22]. The approach in this work was to use isodose-shaped plastic scintillators instead of scintillating fibers. Absorbed dose distributions were calculated by the treatment planning system (Leksell GammaPlan, Elekta AB, Stockholm, Sweden) for the 4- and 8-mm collimators in a Gamma Knife, in an 8 cm-radius phantom. Replicating to the calculated dose distributions, two sets of scintillators were printed. One modeled the 97.2% isodose surface and another the 95.6% isodose surface (Figure 9.8). The resin for this acrylic-based scintillator was that presented by Son *et al.* [16]. One scintillator had a maximum dimension of 1.5 mm and a volume of 0.003 cm^3. The other had a volume of 0.005 cm^3. The scintillator was 3D printed via

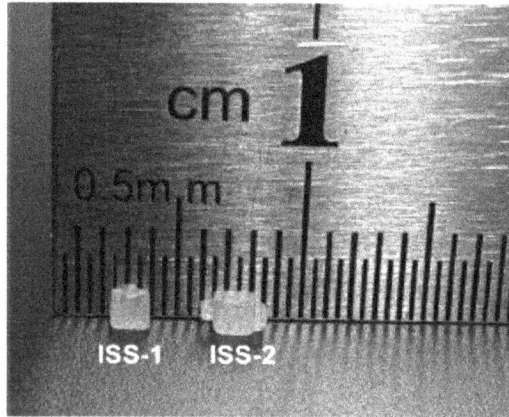

FIGURE 9.8   Two scintillators 3D printed to match the 97.2% (left) and 95.6% (right) isodose surfaces for the 4-mm collimated field from the Gamma Knife. Figure sourced with permission from [21].

DLP that hardens resin with a spatial resolution of 0.05 mm/pixel. The scintillators were covered in reflective paint and connected to a temperature-controlled photomultiplier tube via an optical fiber.

The treatment planning system determined the ratio of the energy absorbed in each total scintillator volume to that calculated for the central voxel. Thus, rather than using, e.g., a small point detector with low light output, this approach allowed the investigators to use scintillators with larger volumes yielding greater signal-to-noise ratio, and to infer the dose at the center point of the scintillator. It is notable that these isodose-shaped scintillators were capable of measuring output factors with uncertainties comparable to a PTW T60019 (PTW, Freiburg, Germany) micro-diamond detector.

Plastic Scintillators Printed Using Fused Deposition Modeling

The fabrication of the scintillators discussed above required developing in-house resins and curing those resins layer by layer with UV light. One limitation of this approach is that it is challenging to polymerize styrene-based monomers that offer high efficiency of light output. In contrast, FDM, i.e., extrusion of a polymer through a heated nozzle, makes printing the more efficient and styrene-based scintillators accessible. The other advantage of FDM is the possibility of printing multiple materials simultaneously. Currently FDM printing is also the most accessible mode of 3D printing and offers great potential for the widespread use in a radiation oncology setting.

Plastic Scintillator Filaments

At the time of writing, no commercial FDM scintillator printing filaments are available. The feasibility of using PLA, a widely used material in FDM printing, as the base matrix for plastic scintillators was explored in 2020 by Hamel *et al.* [23]. This feasibility study focused not on 3D printing but on plastic scintillators based on renewable polymers. Polystyrene is considered nonbiodegradable and obtained from petroleum products with an estimated lifetime of more than a thousand years. PLA, on the other hand, is derived from starches. The scintillator consisted of 2,5-diphenyloxazole (PPO) as the primary fluor and 1, 4-bis(2-methylstyryl) benzene molecules (bis-MSB) as the secondary fluor in a PLA matrix. The addition of PPO was motivated by the fact that PLA has an aliphatic structure as opposed to polystyrene, which has an aromatic structure. Therefore, naturally, PLA does not display a strong fluorescent yield and will not transfer much energy to the primary dye in its excited state. PPO was therefore added in high concentration to overcome this shortcoming of the PLA polymer base. The scintillation output was only 500 photons/MeV when irradiated in a Co^{60} beam. The scintillator exhibited only 13% transmittance at the peak emission wavelength of 424 nm. At the same wavelength, EJ-200 (Eljen Technology), a PVT-based commercial plastic scintillator, showed a 76% transmission and an efficiency of 10,000 photons/MeV. Since PLA is commonly used in FDM printing, this proof-of-concept work may represent a starting point for more studies toward developing suitable scintillator filaments with favorable scintillation properties.

Also in 2020, custom-made polystyrene-based BCF-10 (Saint Gobain, Ohio, USA) scintillating fibers were used as filaments to print $1 \times 1 \times 1$ cm^3 scintillator samples for application in radiation oncology [24]. Although cladded BCF-10 is a commercially available product, the filament used in this work was non-cladded, with a diameter of 3.0 mm. In scintillating fibers, cladding is a coating material with a lower refractive index than the scintillator and is used to reflect the light into the fiber via total internal reflection. However, when used in 3D printing, the cladding would interfere with the homogeneity of the printed scintillators.

Berns and colleagues [25] reported on the development of plastic scintillator filaments consisting of polystyrene doped with p-terphenyl and POPOP. To overcome the difficulty in handling a polystyrene filament due to its hardness, byphenyl, a plasticizer component, was added to the mixture. The percent by weight of byphenyl was decided in a trial-and-error process to maximize the light yield and transparency of the flexible filament.

In 2022, the first report [26] on fabricating an optically reflective filament was published. Although not a plastic scintillator, the filament may be essential in enhancing scintillation collection efficiency and is a relevant development. The reflective filament was produced by dispersing several commonly used reflective pigments into polymer pellets and then extruding the mixture. Based on the measurements of reflectivity, the best results were obtained for samples with 10 to 30% titanium dioxide, TiO_2 reflective pigment with polystyrene or PMMA with approximately 90% reflectivity.

3D Printed In Vivo Dosimeters

Most detectors found in radiation oncology departments are best suited to measuring radiation in quality control and assurance applications, i.e., in the absence of a patient. As a result, the design of most detectors is such that they are either too rigid, fragile, bulky, or cumbersome to use directly on patients, limiting the routine clinical use of *in vivo* dosimetry. In 2022, the first report on using 3D printed plastic scintillators as *in vivo* dosimeter arrays was published by Lynch *et al.* [27]. Bolus and immobilization devices are routinely used in radiation therapy, and 3D printing is increasingly employed in their fabrication, as described in Chapters 1, 4, and 5 of this book. In concept these common patient devices could be comprised of or could contain plastic scintillating materials. The concept is illustrated in Figure 9.9. Using dual-material FDM printing,

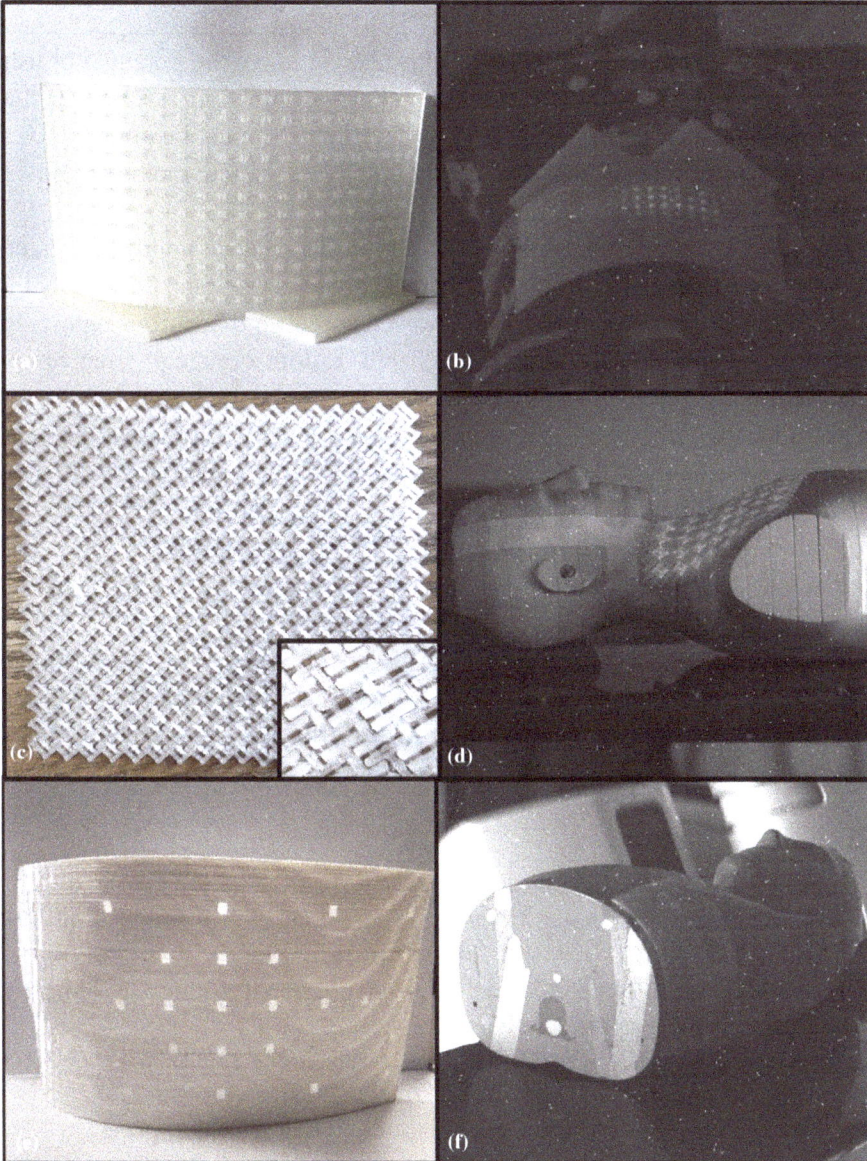

FIGURE 9.9   3D printed patient-customized bolus containing polystyrene scintillating elements, showing (a) a regular array of 3-mm scintillating elements in a bolus, (c) an interlocking flexible mesh with segments printed using scintillating materials, (e) a customized bolus with scintillating elements at chosen locations relative to the dose distribution, and (b, d, and f) illustrating the optical signal captured by the sCMOS camera during treatment delivery. Figure sourced with permission from [27].

Lynch *et al.* included plastic scintillators printed within the surface of a patient bolus [27]. The readout of the scintillation light was achieved by low-noise sCMOS cameras located in the treatment room. Preliminary work showed promising results compared to Monte Carlo calculations. However, dosimetry via optical camera readout is challenging and development is ongoing.

FUTURE WORK

Although the developments highlighted in this chapter show the potential of using 3D printing to fabricate radiation detectors for radiation oncology, research in this area remains in its early stages. Further study and development must be done to investigate detector designs, printing materials and techniques, signal readout methods, and detector performance.

As a fabrication method, 3D printing is exceptionally versatile in producing detectors with complex or customized geometries with a broad range of materials. Numerous examples of printed detectors now exist. However, based on the various reports to date, two challenges have emerged. The first is reliable readout of signals from 3D printed detectors. While 3D printing may enable a radiation oncology department to build an array of ionization chambers, for example, accurate readout of these chambers will require further development. The second challenge is the calibration of printed detectors. This is particularly difficult given the arbitrary and potentially complex geometries that may be produced. In such cases, the treatment planning system or Monte Carlo calculation might be leveraged to calibrate the detector's response with the known geometry of the detector, for example.

In summary, as described in this chapter, 3D printing provides a powerful catalyst for development of novel devices ranging from gaseous detector arrays to scintillation detectors, and further development is warranted to translate these technologies to the clinic.

REFERENCES

[1] Andreo P. *Fundamentals of ionizing radiation dosimetry*. John Wiley & Sons; 2017.

[2] Fargher S, Steer C, Thompson L. The use of 3D printing in the development of gaseous radiation detectors. *Epj Web Conf*. 2018;170:01016.

[3] Brivio D, Naumann L, Albert S, et al. 3D printing for rapid prototyping of low-Z/density ionization chamber arrays. *Med Phys*. 2019;46:5770–5779.

[4] Kwok SW, Goh KHH, Tan ZD, et al. Electrically conductive filament for 3D-printed circuits and sensors. *Appl Mater Today*. 2017;9:167–175.

[5] Albert S, Brivio D, Aldelaijan S, et al. Towards customizable thin-panel low-Z detector arrays: Electrode design for increased spatial resolution ion chamber arrays. *Phys Med Biol*. 2020;65:08NT02.

[6] Hashimoto T, Sato F, Tamaki S, et al. Fabrication of radiophotoluminescence dosimeter with 3D-printing technology. *Radiat Meas*. 2019;124:141–145.

[7] Zheng S, Lü H, Chen C, et al. Epoxy resin/poly(ethylene oxide) (PEO) and poly(ε-caprolactone) (PCL) blends cured with 1,3,5-trihydroxybenzene: miscibility and intermolecular interactions. *Colloid Polym Sci*. 2003;281:1015–1024.

[8] Birks JB. *The theory and practice of scintillation counting.* Elsevier, 1964;321–353. https://doi.org/10.1016/C2013-0-01791-4

[9] Förster T. Zwischenmolekulare Energiewanderung und Fluoreszenz. *Ann Phys.* 1948;437:55–75.

[10] Harper CA, Petrie EM. *Plastics materials and processes.* John Wiley and Sons, 2003;xi–xxxii.

[11] Karyukhin AN. *Injection molding scintillator for ATLAS Tile calorimeter.* 1996.

[12] Pla-Dalmau A. *Extruded plastic scintillator for the MINOS calorimeters.* Batavia, IL (United States); 2001.

[13] Mishnayot Y, Layani M, Cooperstein I, et al. Three-dimensional printing of scintillating materials. *Rev Sci Instrum.* 2014;85:085102.

[14] Moser SW, Harder WF, Hurlbut CR, et al. Principles and practice of plastic scintillator design. *Radiat Phys Chem.* 1993;41:31–36.

[15] Green W. Industrial photoinitiators a technical guide. 2010;115–138.

[16] Son J, Kim DG, Lee S, et al. Improved 3D printing plastic scintillator fabrication. *J Korean Phys Soc.* 2018;73:887–892.

[17] Knoll GF. *Radiation detection and measurement.* John Wiley & Sons; 2010.

[18] Kim D, Lee S, Park J, et al. Performance of 3D printed plastic scintillators for gamma-ray detection. *Nucl Eng Technol.* 2020;52:2910–2917.

[19] Lee S, Kim TH, Jeong JY, et al. Dose rate measurement of Leksell Gamma Knife Perfexion using a 3D printed plastic scintillation dosimeter. *Nucl Eng Technol.* 2020;52:2334–2338.

[20] Kim TH, Lee S, Kim DG, et al. A feasibility study of using a 3D-printed tumor model scintillator to verify the energy absorbed to a tumor. *Nucl Eng Technol.* 2021;53:3018–3025.

[21] Kim TH, Yang HJ, Jeong JY, et al. Feasibility of isodose-shaped scintillation detectors for the measurement of gamma knife output factors. *Med Phys.* 2022;49:1944–1954.

[22] Das IJ, Francescon P, Moran JM, et al. Report of AAPM Task Group 155: Megavoltage photon beam dosimetry in small fields and non-equilibrium conditions. *Med Phys.* 2021;48:e886–e921.

[23] Hamel M, Lebouteiller G. Attempting to prepare a plastic scintillator from a biobased polymer. *J Appl Polym Sci.* 2020;137:48724.

[24] Lynch N, Monajemi T, Robar JL. Characterization of novel 3D printed plastic scintillation dosimeters. *Biomed Phys Eng Express.* 2020;6:055014.

[25] Berns S, Boyarintsev A, Hugon S, et al. A novel polystyrene-based scintillator production process involving additive manufacturing. *J Instrum.* 2020;15:P10019–P10019.

[26] Berns S, Boillat E, Boyarintsev A, et al. Additive manufacturing of fine-granularity optically-isolated plastic scintillator elements. *J Instrum.* 2022;17:P10045.

[27] Lynch N, Robar JL, Monajemi T. Camera-based radiotherapy dosimetry using dual-material 3D printed scintillator arrays. *Med Phys.* 2023;50:1824–1842.

[28] Hajagos TJ, Liu C, Cherepy NJ, Pei Q, et al. High-Z sensitized plastic scintillators: A review. *Adv Mater (Weinheim).* 2018;30, no. 27:e1706956.

CHAPTER 10

3D Printed Phantoms in RT

Tsuicheng David Chiu, David Parsons,
Zhenyu Xiong, Robert Reynolds, and You Zhang

INTRODUCTION

Throughout the history of medicine, advancements have resulted from multi-disciplinary collaborations between scientists, engineers, physiologists, and physicians. Much of this technological progress has required a combination of ingenuity and technical craftsmanship in developing medical devices. The traditional development process of a new medical instrument has been limited by the complexity of design and fabrication, inventors' skills and experience, available materials, and the time and effort required to prototype. Under these constraints, developing a new apparatus has been difficult or possibly untenable for a single practitioner or institution. Historically, the cost to develop a customized device for a single patient treatment has been prohibitive. However, over the past decade, 3D printing has become accessible and has evolved considerably with respect to the versatility of the technology, leading to major shifts in prototyping and manufacturing [1–3]. 3D printing has introduced the possibility for an individual or small team to design and fabricate a novel and customized device with a reasonable learning curve and at an affordable cost. In addition, the technology has unlocked rapid prototyping, which allows iteration on designs.

In recent years, 3D printing technology has been embraced by innovators in medicine [2, 4–7]. The accessibility of the technology has narrowed the gap between medical and non-medical specialties, allowing collaboration by radiologists, radiological technologists, engineers, physicists, surgeons, and biologists. A small development team is now able to design a new instrument, and to realize a prototype within days. This expedient process results in rapid iteration of innovation and development that can lead to improvements in patient treatment. Common applications can be found in surgical planning, biocompatibility assessment, 3D printed prostheses, hospital quality management, treatment quality assurance (QA), treatment machine QA, procedure risk assessment, model verification and validation, among others. In this chapter, 3D printed phantoms used in radiotherapy will be discussed. These novel phantom technologies play various roles in patient

DOI: 10.1201/9781003288404-10

immobilization, treatment verification, equipment QA, motion studies, imaging studies, validation of procedures, and training.

3D PRINTED PHANTOMS IN RADIATION THERAPY

3D printing technology can help to fabricate medical phantoms that were previously difficult or impossible to produce through other means. Commonly, medical phantoms provide realistic models of human anatomy used for imaging studies and radiation therapy (RT) planning, for example. These phantoms can be customized to closely mimic the characteristics of a particular patient's anatomy, such as size, shape, and density. This allows for more accurate imaging and RT planning, which can lead to improved treatment outcomes for patients. Medical phantoms can be used for training and education purposes as well, allowing healthcare professionals to practice and perfect imaging methods, interventional procedures, or RT techniques. Phantoms can also be made to mimic abnormal anatomy, such as tumors, providing tools that can aid in the development and evaluation of new imaging and therapy techniques. 3D printing technology can contribute significantly to the planning and administration of imaging procedures and a broad range of therapeutic interventions.

3D PRINTING MEDICAL PHANTOMS: MATERIALS AND METHODS

While the previous chapters of this book have described materials that are mostly directly printed, e.g., through deposition, curing or fusing, this section expands the material selection to include those that are not directly printed but are integrated into phantoms at other steps of fabrication. Medical phantoms can be fabricated using a wide variety of materials, including polyvinyl chloride (PVC), polyvinyl alcohol (PVA), silicone, polylactic acid (PLA), polymer resin. Each material has its own unique properties and benefits, and the choice of material will depend on the specific application and desired characteristics of the phantom. For example, PVC is a popular choice for phantoms used in RT planning because it yields similar X-ray attenuation properties to human tissue. PVA is a water-soluble material often used as a support material in 3D printing and can be dissolved after the printing process. Silicone is a flexible and durable material available with selectable hardness that can be used to create phantoms that closely mimic the feel of human tissue. PLA is a biodegradable thermoplastic and a popular choice in 3D printing. Resin is a versatile material that can be used to create detailed and highly accurate phantoms. We will explore the properties and advantages of each of these various materials in more detail throughout this section, as well as the fabrication methods used to create medical phantoms with 3D printing technology.

3D Printing Technologies for Fabrication of Phantoms

Chapter 2 of this book describes various 3D printing technologies in detail, as well as the range of printable media for each. Here we briefly revisit several printer and material options that have been common candidates for printing of medical phantoms.

Fused Deposition Modeling (FDM)

FDM is a type of 3D printing that uses heated thermoplastic filament extruded through a nozzle to build an object layer by layer on a heated build plate. It is used widely for prototypes, models, and functional parts due to its accessibility and affordability. Common FDM media include PLA, acrylonitrile butadiene styrene (ABS), polyethylene terephthalate glycol (PETG), thermoplastic polyurethane (TPU), and thermoplastic elastomer (TPE). Each material involves various advantages and disadvantages, and these are listed in Table 10.1 in the context of fabrication of imaging phantoms. Mechanical properties can vary depending on the specific types or brands of the materials.

Stereolithography (SLA)

SLA is a 3D printing technology that uses a liquid resin material that is selectively cured by a UV laser or other light source to create an object layer by layer. For example, a laser is directed onto the surface of the liquid resin, curing and solidifying the resin in the desired shape. The build platform is then lowered by a small increment and the next layer of liquid resin is then added on top. This process continues until the entire object is formed. SLA printing is known for its high resolution and precision, producing smooth and detailed objects. However, the media used are often more expensive than FDM filaments and the post-processing for the finished product is also more complex. It is commonly used for jewelry, dental and medical models, and other high-precision applications. In phantom fabrication, SLA is a good tool to generate a part when fine detail is required.

Binder Jet, Inkjet and Multi Jet Fusion Printing

These technologies deposit liquid droplets of binder or fusing agent over a layer of material to cause selective fusion according to the design of the object. In Multi Jet Fusion (MJF; HP), a fusing agent is selectively applied to an 80-µm polymer powder layer, effectively printing in small and discrete voxels. Immediate application of thermal energy fuses the voxels receiving the fusing agent, and unlike other printing methods, successive layers are also fused together forming a cohesive 3D object as the printing proceeds. These technologies are capable of producing objects with very high resolution and highly complex geometries using a wide range of materials, including polymers, ceramics, and metals. They offer the capacity to print using multiple materials, and in the case of MJF, varying material mechanical, radiological [8], optical or electromagnetic properties voxel-by-voxel. MJF also enables color printing on the top surface, allowing custom labeling, images, or patterns.

FABRICATION TECHNIQUES FOR MEDICAL PHANTOMS

There are two main approaches used in the fabrication of medical phantoms: direct 3D printing and casting. Depending on the design and materials, direct 3D printing of a phantom may be preferred as it offers the advantage of designing and manufacturing the phantom with a streamlined and highly digital method, largely eliminating fabrication by hand. However, the selection of 3D printable materials is finite, and available options may not provide the required mechanical, aesthetic, or radiological properties. For example, highly flexible materials are difficult to achieve with most printing technologies. As described in Chapter 4 in the context of silicone patient bolus, the alternative of casting allows 3D printing of a mold into which a chosen material is poured. This approach leverages the resolution and versatility of 3D printing in producing detailed geometries and extends the range of usable materials. In many examples, the material to be used in casting can also be customized by changing its composition.

Direct 3D Printing

Direct 3D printing is a method that creates medical phantoms through the printing itself, allowing for intricate shapes and geometries, as well as the incorporation of diverse materials into the design. This technique is popular for fabrication of medical phantoms in imaging, RT, and surgical training, offering advantages of speed, flexibility, and the capacity to customize designs to meet specific needs. It is a streamlined prototyping approach, providing an expedient approach to design, printing, and revision.

Casting

Alternatively, a custom mold can be 3D printed and subsequently filled with a chosen material, like silicone, for example, to form the final medical phantom or component of a phantom. This technique offers greater control over the material properties and allows fabrication of medical phantoms with varied textures and densities. The process demands extra manual steps, however, and the casting process requires dedicated techniques and skills. Casting is a popular method for creating medical phantoms for RT and surgical training. In the following section we describe common methods used in this approach and provide detail on both hot and room-temperature casting.

Media for Casting Using 3D Printed Molds

Polyvinyl Chloride (PVC). PVC is a synthetic plastic polymer that is used widely in various applications, including construction, electrical, electronic, and medical industries. It offers several advantageous properties, including durability, chemical resistance, weather resistance and low cost. PVC is highly resistant to wear and tear, making it a good choice for high-stress applications. It is resistant to many chemicals, including acids, bases, and salts, making it suitable for use in harsh chemical environments. It is also resistant to moisture, heat, and UV radiation, making it suitable for outdoor use. Several of these characteristics make PVC a viable choice in the fabrication of medical phantoms, where it is desirable due to its low cost, ease of processing, and capacity to be molded into various shapes and sizes. High environmental resistance gives PVC-based phantoms a significant shelf life. To achieve desired properties, PVC can be blended with other materials, such as silicone or TPE. The requirements of a medical phantom must be considered to determine whether PVC is appropriate. For example, if the phantom will be used for medical imaging, the formulation must provide a realistic signal during image acquisition, e.g., X-ray attenuation for radiographic imaging, acoustic impedance for ultrasound (US), or spin relaxation time for magnetic resonance imaging (MRI). If it is used for dosimetric purposes in radiation oncology physics, it must demonstrate accurate radiological characteristics such as attenuation coefficient or stopping power.

Polyvinyl Alcohol (PVA). PVA is well-suited to fabrication of US and MR imaging phantoms due to its acoustic properties and the ability to create devices with specific properties that accurately simulate human tissue. It is capable of providing sufficient signal from hydrogen in MRI [9]. By providing an appropriate enclosure sealing the PVA material, it can be used to fabricate phantoms with acceptable longevity. Additionally, PVA can be used to create phantoms with specific elasticity or viscosity, closely simulating human tissue. PVA is often used in combination with other materials, such as gelatin, to create phantoms with desirable properties. One advantage of PVA is its water solubility, which makes it easy to dissolve and remove from the phantom after use. It is biodegradable, making it an environmentally friendly option. However, it exhibits a low heat and UV resistance, making it unsuitable for use in phantoms that will be exposed to high temperatures or UV radiation. PVA is also hygroscopic, meaning that it absorbs moisture from the air, a behavior that can negatively impact its mechanical properties. PVA is water-soluble and degrades over time, which can lead to changes in a phantom's properties and, for example, will affect the accuracy of results obtained from imaging or dosimetry phantoms. Proper storage and maintenance are required to ensure the longevity and stability.

Silicone. Silicone is a highly desirable material due to its unique properties, such as high temperature resistance, excellent electrical insulation properties, and biocompatibility. It is highly versatile and can be easily molded into various shapes and forms, making it a popular choice in a wide range of industries. However, it is comparatively costly and difficult to recycle. Additionally, its low resistance to UV radiation can cause it to degrade over time, which limits usefulness in applications that require long-term durability. Careful consideration of these factors is necessary when using silicone as a material for various applications. Soft silicone has been used in the fabrication of medical phantoms due to its elasticity and ability to accurately simulate mechanical properties of human tissue. It can be formulated to match specific densities and mechanical properties, making it an ideal material for creating phantoms used in imaging and RT, such as breast phantoms for mammography, or for bolus materials in RT treatment. Silicone does involve shortcomings such as low shear strength, allowing deformation or tear under stress. Achieving consistent properties in large-scale production can be challenging, necessitating robust quality control (QC).

Agar. Agar is a versatile material that can be molded into various shapes and sizes, making it a popular choice for the fabrication of medical phantoms due to its low cost, biocompatibility, and high water-holding capacity. One potential drawback is its relatively low strength and rigidity, which may make it less suitable for applications requiring high durability. Additionally, agar is sensitive to temperature and humidity, which cause changes in its mechanical properties over time. Agar can be prone to microbial growth if not stored properly, underscoring the importance of proper storage and handling. Despite these limitations, agar remains a popular and versatile material for a wide range of applications.

Hot Casting

When fabricating a medical phantom using PVC, the raw material, in either pellet or liquid form, must be heated to a high temperature of between 175°C and 200°C. This process is necessary to melt the PVC and make it pliable, allowing it to be molded into the desired shape. Once heated, the PVC is poured into a heat-resistant mold that has been designed to create the shape of the medical phantom. The mold is then left to cool and harden. It is important to note that working with heated PVC requires a high level of caution due to the extreme temperatures involved. Special equipment, such as heat-resistant molds and protective gear will be necessary to safely handle the material. The high temperatures also make it challenging to achieve consistent properties in large-scale production, which can affect the accuracy of the medical phantom. It is important to exercise caution when working with heated PVC, as the high temperatures can release fumes that are potentially harmful when inhaled. A fume hood is highly recommended when fabricating PVC medical phantoms. Proper ventilation and personal protective equipment, such as respirators, should be used to minimize exposure to potentially harmful gases.

When fabricating a medical phantom using PVA, the raw material, available either as a powder mix/water combination or liquid PVA solution, must be heated to a temperature between 50°C and 70°C to allow it to become pliable. The mechanical properties of a PVA cast are related to PVA concentration. Higher concentrations will provide more hardness but require higher heating temperatures to adequately dissolve PVA. Once heated, the PVA is poured into a heat-resistant and waterproof mold. After pouring, the PVA must undergo a series of freeze-thaw cycles to solidify and achieve the desired mechanical properties. The freeze cycle will be done typically at −15°C, and thawing will occur at room temperature. This cycle is repeated multiple times to create a stable and consistent PVA medical phantom. To facilitate the process, a stirring heating plate with a beaker is required to keep the PVA solution in a homogenous state. Proper care must be taken when working with heated PVA, as the material can cause burns and can be messy during the pouring process.

Fabricating agar for medical phantoms is similar to using PVA, although agar does not require the freeze-thaw cycle. The agar mixed with water is heated to a temperature of approximately 90°C to 100°C until it is fully dissolved. Once dissolved, the agar is poured into a heat-resistant and waterproof mold, then left to cool and solidify. After solidifying, the agar can be further refrigerated to achieve the desired texture and mechanical properties. Agar is most often used in combination with gelatin to create medical phantoms with a realistic tissue-like texture.

Room Temperature Casting

Casting silicone using a two-part mixing technique at room temperature involves combining two components, the base and the catalyst, in a specific ratio to trigger a chemical reaction that causes the silicone to cure and harden. First, the base and catalyst are combined until the mixture is completely uniform to avoid any defects or inconsistencies in the final product. Once mixed, the silicone is poured into the mold and left to cure at room temperature. The curing time will depend on factors such as the type of silicone being used, the size of the mold, and the desired hardness of the final product. Typically, room temperature silicone casting will require a few hours to several days for curing.

To achieve a high-quality product and to ensure safety during the fabrication process, it is crucial to mix the silicone components accurately and work in a well-ventilated area. Additionally, degassing the silicone mixture is an important step to eliminate any trapped air bubbles, which will cause defects or unevenness in the final product. The degassing process involves using a vacuum chamber to create a low-pressure environment, allowing air bubbles to expand and rise to the surface of the mixture. After the vacuum is released, the homogenous mixture can be poured into the mold. The degassing duration will depend on the type of silicone and the size of the mixture, typically requiring between 1 and 10 minutes. While not all types of silicone require degassing, the manufacturer's instructions should be followed for best results.

Cured silicone is typically not adhesive to most other materials. This can be a benefit in situations where there may be spillage or excess silicone, as it can be left to fully cure before being easily removed from surfaces. Unlike some adhesives or other materials that may be difficult to clean up once spilled, cured silicone can be simply peeled or scraped away from the surface. However, it is important to note that there are some materials that may be more prone to adhering to cured silicone, such as certain plastics or silicone surfaces. It is always recommended to consult the manufacturer's instructions or run a test on a small area for the specific type of silicone being used, to ensure proper handling and cleanup procedures.

3D PRINTED PHANTOMS FOR MEDICAL IMAGING

A wide array of imaging modalities is used in medicine. Radiation oncology employs planar radiographic imaging, fluoroscopy, computed tomography (CT), MRI, US, positron emission tomography (PET), single photon emission tomography (SPECT), angiography, and others. These distinct imaging technologies require specific QA and QC testing, and historically, generic phantoms have been available for this purpose. However, 3D printing introduces the potential to develop new phantom types, as well as phantoms that are customized to reflect specific patient anatomies, or to test certain characteristics of an imaging system that are not addressed by standard tools. The human body is complex, of course, and creating a physical phantom that accurately represents anatomy, in terms of the response of an imaging system, is a significant challenge. For example, using just one or two materials in a direct 3D printing or casting process to simulate all tissues in the human body will be limiting. Nevertheless, phantoms created with 3D printing have proven to be valuable tools for testing and optimizing medical imaging procedures [6, 9–11].

Imaging Phantoms: Design Goals

Designing a 3D printed phantom to test an imaging system requires careful consideration of several factors, including the intended purpose and the modality for which it will be used. The purpose of the phantom may vary, from testing the accuracy of medical imaging equipment to simulating different pathologies or conditions for research or training purposes. The imaging modality will dictate the required properties and characteristics in the phantom material. For example, a phantom for CT imaging will require materials with representative photon interaction cross sections over the X-ray energies of interest. An MRI phantom will require materials with realistic proton density and materials giving realistic spin-lattice and spin-spin relaxation responses. A PET or SPECT phantom may require realistic radiologic properties as well as the ability to hold injectable radionuclides. A US phantom will include structure with realistic acoustic impedance. The phantom may also need to be durable, reusable, or modular to accommodate different imaging scenarios.

There exist various options available to manipulate the physical and radiological characteristics of medical phantoms, particularly for imaging phantoms. These options include, for example, changing the FDM 3D printing infill to alter the phantom's density, adding different polymers into SLA resin to change its solidification properties, adjusting the concentration of materials such as PVC, PVA, and agar/gelatin to mimic corresponding densities, and adding different components during silicone casting to simulate different textures. By manipulating these factors, researchers and medical professionals can create phantoms with different characteristics that can be used to test and optimize medical imaging equipment and techniques.

Material Selection According to Imaging Modality

The selection of appropriate materials plays a crucial role in achieving acceptable results in phantom fabrication. Before embarking on the design process, it is essential to understand how different materials respond to various imaging modalities. This knowledge forms the foundation for making informed decisions during the phantom design phase. Table 10.1 provides a comparison between commonly used phantom materials for US, CT, and MRI. By understanding the strengths and limitations of different materials in relation to specific imaging modalities, one can make informed decisions that will ultimately lead to more functional and realistic phantom designs. In addition, it is important to consider other factors such as cost, availability, and the feasibility of fabrication when selecting phantom materials. The desired properties of the phantom, such as durability, flexibility, and tissue-mimicking characteristics, where relevant, should also be considered.

EXAMPLES OF 3D PRINTED PHANTOMS

In this section, we highlight a diverse array of phantoms fabricated using 3D printing, focusing on aspects such as their intended purpose, design, material selection, and the fabrication methods employed. A review of applications of 3D printing in radiation oncology reported that 3D printing of phantoms has been among the most frequent [12] and thus there are many descriptions of inventive new devices. The examples chosen for this section provide an appreciation of the range of applications possible, the variety of printing/casting techniques and materials, challenges related to phantom design and

TABLE 10.1   Useful Properties of FDM Filaments, SLA Resins, Molded Silicone, and Molded PVC, PVA, and Agar in Phantoms for Imaging with Ultrasound, Computed Tomography, and Magnetic Resonance Imaging

3D Printing Technology	Ultrasound (US)	Computed Tomography (CT)	Magnetic Resonance Imaging (MRI)
FDM filaments and SLA resins	High impedance mismatch between most of 3D printing materials and water. Useful only for making enclosures/cases.	3D printed plastic materials mimic rigid bony structures in the human body, offering a realistic representation for medical simulations and research. By adjusting the infill percentage and pattern, these materials can be customized to adjust signal (Hounsfield Units, HU) in CT imaging, ensuring accurate and diverse testing scenarios.	Given that regular plastic is not detectable in MRI images, employing FDM filaments or standard SLA resins serves as an excellent method for creating void features, such as grid patterns, inside phantoms, which aid in conducting magnetic field distortion tests.
Silicone	Limited US penetration due to high acoustic attenuation compared to water-based materials.	Versatile material for simulating various soft tissues, with its adjustable density allowing for customization to meet diverse requirements.	Many silicone products are oil-based and contain hydrogen particles, enabling them to provide signal in MRI images. Different silicone formulations can yield varying signal responses; however, these signals may diminish over time as the oil gradually vaporizes.
PVC/PVA/Agar	Effective materials for fabricating US phantoms. Acoustic properties are close to those of soft tissue and water.	Effective materials for making CT phantoms. The density and signal response are close to soft tissue and water.	Effective materials for making MRI phantoms. They contain hydrogen leading to strong signal response.

fabrication, and the value of innovative phantoms in advancing various aspects of technology and medical practice.

A Phantom for MRI Calibration (MR-CBCT Phantom)

The magnetic resonance-cone beam computed tomography (MR-CBCT) phantom [9] was created as a calibration tool with the purpose of evaluating and remedying magnetic field distortion in MRI. This multi-platform phantom utilizes CBCT images as reference images for correcting geometric distortion present in MR images. The primary objective of the design was to ensure that the geometric features in both CBCT and MR images are spatially consistent. By analyzing these features, it is possible to assess the distortion and to create deformation metrics that can be applied, in this case, to MR images of animals being imaged in preclinical studies.

The fabrication of this small-scale phantom required several materials to establish signal contrast in both CBCT and MRI (Figure 10.1). A significant challenge was to

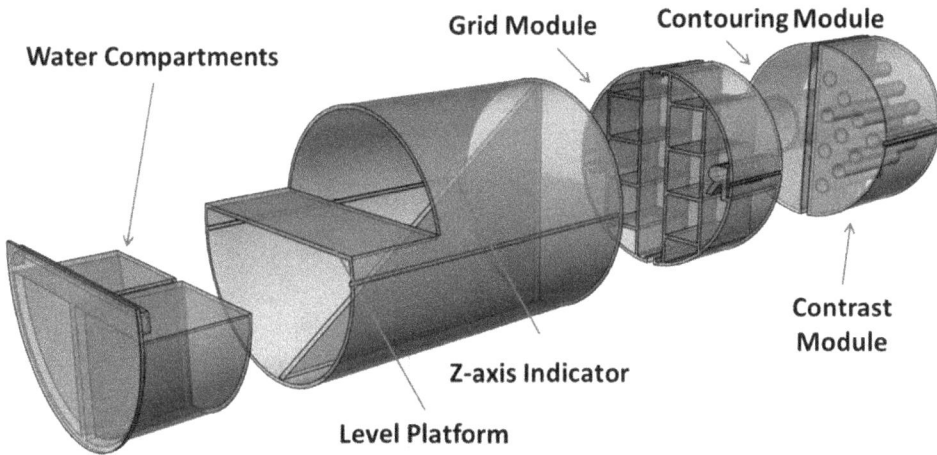

FIGURE 10.1   Schematic design of the MR-CBCT phantom. Figure sourced with permission from [9].

generate sufficient hydrogen signal during MR scanning. The materials employed in the design included PLA for the structures, silicones, glass rods, marble, air, and water (to provide contrast and to boost the hydrogen signal). The CBCT images yielded distinct Hounsfield Unit (HU) differences between the glass marble and rods, silicones, and air. However, on MR images, the various silicones used retained distinct intensities, while the glass marble and rods, along with PLA and air, appeared as voids (Figure 10.2).

The phantom was designed with dimensional accuracy as a priority for geometric calibration. The 3D printer selected for this work ensured precision. The grid module was used to evaluate transverse distortion, while the outer shell and z-axis indicator ensured out-of-plane accuracy. Additionally, a leveling platform was integrated into the design to allow accurate and relocatable setup, given that a curved scanning cradle was utilized in the study. The phantom was developed with a modular design, allowing for the incorporation of additional features by replacing different module components.

Given the multiple materials involved, the fabrication process was complex and required specific skills to assemble the phantom, rather than a direct and automated 3D printing approach. Additionally, achieving water-tightness in an FDM PLA print presented a challenge that needed to be overcome. Overall, the phantom proved to be a valuable tool in preclinical studies and demonstrated the importance of careful material selection and design considerations in achieving accurate calibration in MRI.

Head-and-Neck Phantom with Novel FDM Materials

Attenuation of X-ray photons is the relevant material property in CT scanning, where the density of a material affects its signal in an image. An innovative approach to fabricating a head-and-neck phantom (Figure 10.3) used different percentages of bismuth infusion in native ABS filaments to create variable radiodensities [10]. The results showed that ABS filaments infused with higher concentrations of bismuth provided greater radiopacity on CT images, emulating bone density. This study highlighted viable methods

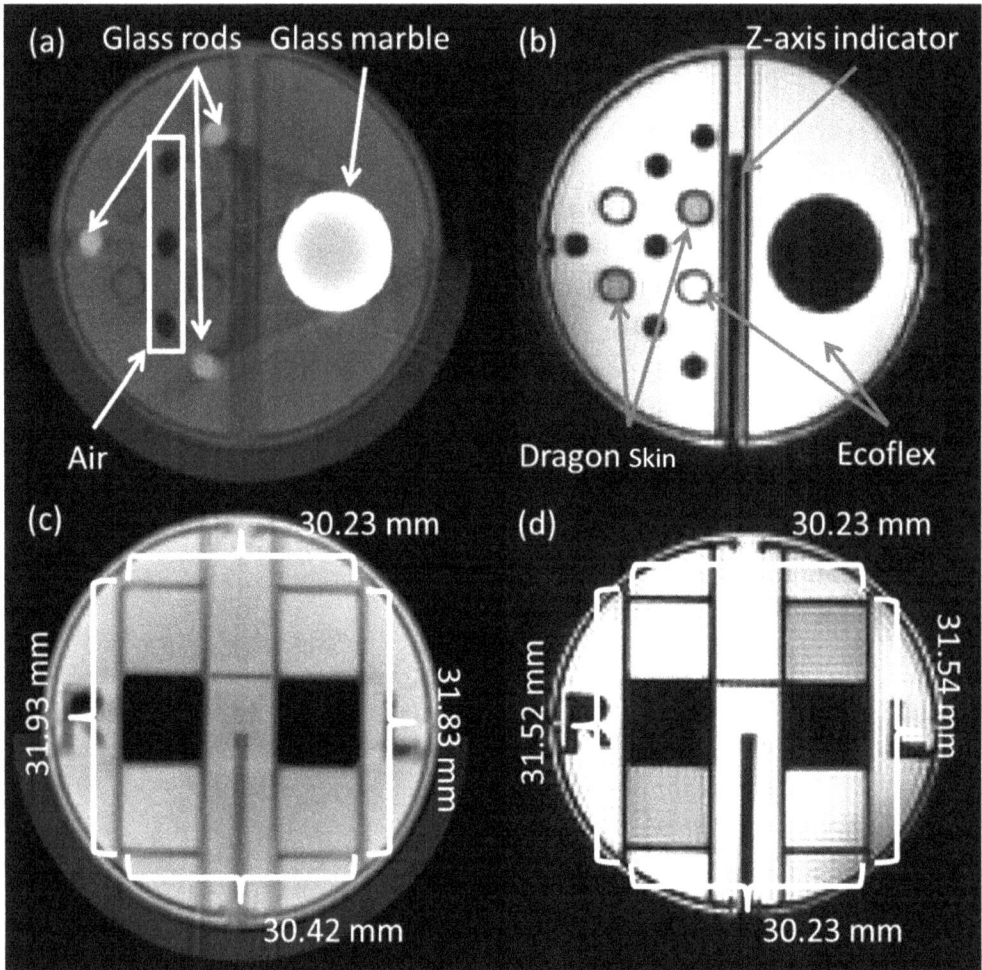

FIGURE 10.2 CBCT and MR images from the MR-CBCT phantom showing (a) CBCT and (b) MRI of contouring and contrast modules, and (c) CBCT and (d) MRI of the grid module. Figure sourced with permission from [9].

for the creation of custom anatomical phantoms as it provided a means of manipulating radiodensity for specific imaging purposes. These findings could also lead to the development of new materials with enhanced radiopacity.

The study utilized both native ABS and modified ABS materials. Native ABS closely matches the density of water (1.01–1.03 g/cm³) and is suitable for 3D printing soft tissue in anatomical phantoms. The modified ABS was produced by altering a commercial bismuth-infused ABS filament (2.7 g/cm³), allowing for the creation of ABS filaments with adjustable density (ranging from 1.2 to 2.5 g/cm³) by mixing bismuth ABS with ABS resin in varying percentages, depending on the design goals.

To create a head-and-neck phantom, CT image data of a patient were used, and both soft tissue and bone were segmented. This delineation was necessary to facilitate use of dual extruders for printing the phantom, printing with either native ABS or bismuth-infused

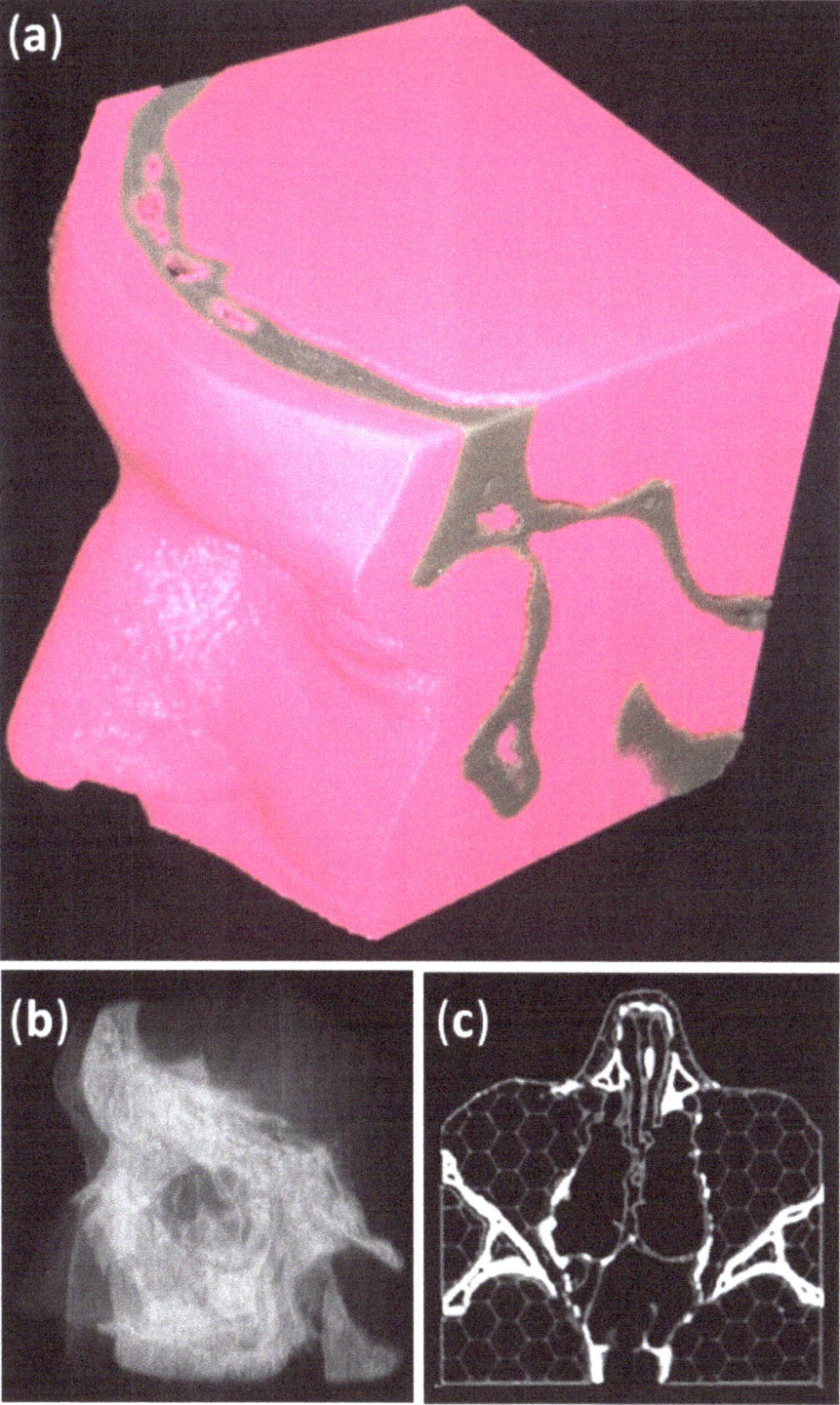

FIGURE 10.3   3D printed naso-cranial phantom printed with custom ABS materials providing simulation of tissue and bone in CT imaging. Figure sourced with permission from [10].

ABS. While the density of native ABS is similar to that of soft tissue, it was found that the energy attenuation response differs, thus, various infill percentages were tested to achieve an appropriate mean HU in imaging. This study serves as an excellent example of innovation of both printable materials and fabrication methods to address a specific need in medical imaging.

Multi-Modality Breast Phantom

This study [11] described the development of a multi-modality (CT, MRI, and US) breast phantom using tissue-equivalent materials and 3D printing techniques. The objective was to produce a versatile phantom for QC testing. By reproducing the radiodensity and anatomical characteristics of real breast tissue (Figure 10.4), the aim was to provide a

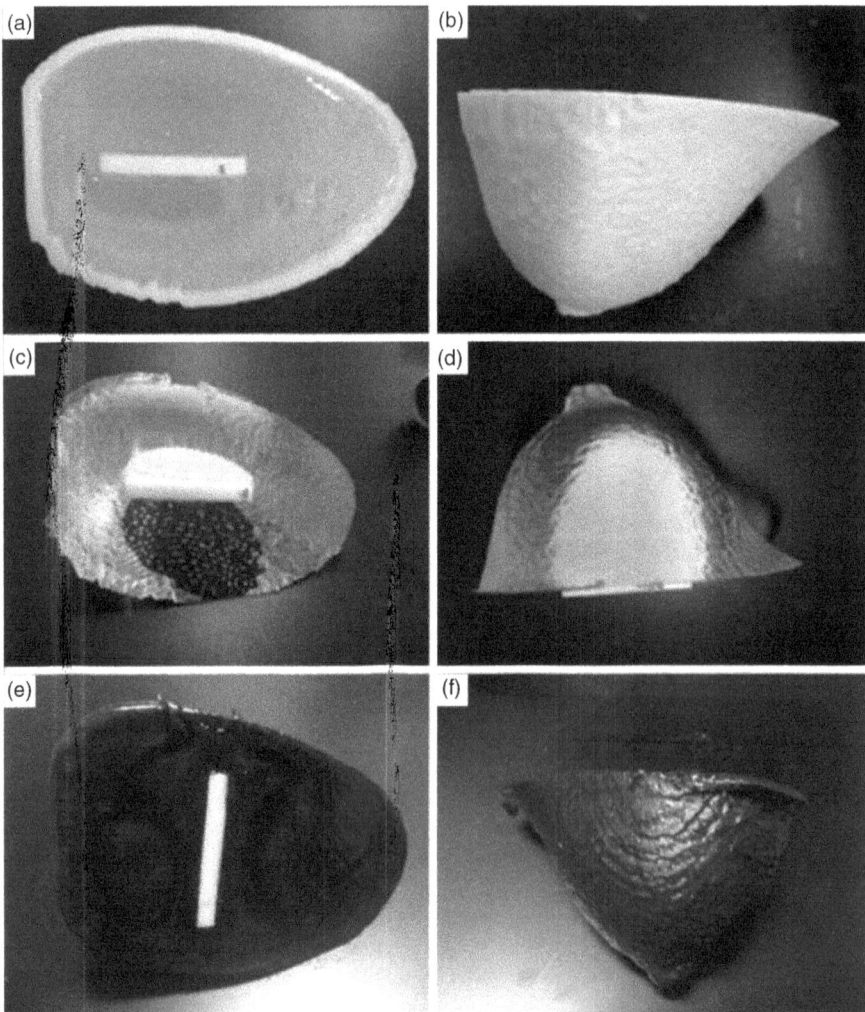

FIGURE 10.4 The breast phantom showing the mold (a and b), a PVC phantom for mammography and MRI (c and d), and US phantom fabricated using PVC, softener, and graphite powder (e and f). Figure sourced with permission from [11].

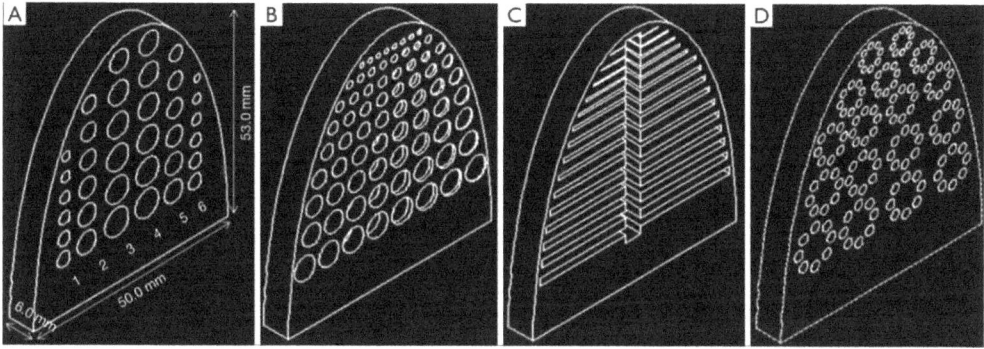

FIGURE 10.5   Design of the breast phantom inserts including simulated tumors (a), cylinders to test depth resolution (b), fibers (c), and microcalcifications (d). Figure sourced with permission from [11].

dependable and standardized platform for evaluating the performance and accuracy of breast imaging systems. The phantom was designed to incorporate various structures commonly observed in the female breast, including microcalcifications, fiber lesions, and tumors of different sizes. These features were incorporated in a modular design (Figure 10.5).

To accurately represent breast tissue, PVC material was chosen for its acoustic properties that closely resemble soft tissue, making it ideal for US imaging. Additionally, PVC contains hydrogen, allowing it to be visible on MR images. To mimic typical breast texture observed in US images, graphite powders were added into the phantom, resulting in images that simulate the speckle pattern seen in real US scans. This addition enhances the realism and fidelity of the phantom when used for assessing US imaging performance. To introduce realistic tumor structures, custom lesions of various dimensions were created using 3D printed ABS material. These lesions enable the evaluation of the imaging modalities' abilities to detect and characterize tumors of varying sizes and characteristics.

The multi-purpose breast phantom was designed to address the needs of mammogram screening, with compatibility between mammography, MRI, and US imaging modalities. The inclusion of a simple rigid tumor module enabled effective evaluation from a single direction, enhancing the versatility and utility of the phantom. In concept, this phantom is configurable to emulate various clinical scenarios, for example, the density of PVC or silicone materials can also be adjusted to simulate variable density of breast tissue.

Prostate Phantom for Brachytherapy Training

While the examples above highlight several versatile imaging phantoms, in this work a realistic prostate phantom was developed to allow hands-on simulation practice and education in interstitial brachytherapy [13]. The primary objective was to equip trainees with the necessary manual skills for ultrasound-guided prostate high dose rate (HDR) or low dose rate (LDR) treatment, as well as practice in interpreting real-time imaging. The phantom aimed to eliminate the need for trainees to practice on patients and allowed them to become familiar with the procedure without time pressures. The prostate phantom not only offered an effective training solution but also served as a cost-effective alternative to purchasing expensive and disposable phantoms.

The prostate phantom included several simulated anatomical features, including the urethra, seminal vesicles, prostate, rectum, and background tissue. To ensure these organs-at-risk (OARs) were visible on US images, a combination of materials was employed during the fabrication process to achieve intensity differences in imaging. The bulk of the phantom was constructed using PVC, chosen for its minimal acoustic attenuation, simulating the background tissue and the prostate itself. To differentiate the prostate from the background, fine mason powders were added during the casting process. These powders created speckles within the prostate in US imaging, enhancing its visibility relative to background. To provide a robust structure for US probe insertion and to maintain the integrity of the surrounding tissue, a higher density of PVC was used to create the tissue around the simulated rectum. This denser PVC material offered increased strength and stability during training sessions. The urethra and seminal vesicles were fabricated using silicone, despite it not being the primary choice for US phantom construction. However, considering the small size of the urethra and seminal vesicles, the impact on US imaging was minimal.

This work demonstrates an innovative approach employing 3D printing indirectly in the fabrication process. All components of the phantom were cast using 3D printed molds, ensuring precise replication of each OAR. Depending on the OAR, a set of molds was employed, including those 3D printed directly or created through double casting using heat-resistant rubber. The resulting phantom closely mimics the anatomy of the human prostate, making it an excellent tool for training in HDR or LDR prostate brachytherapy. The phantom successfully replicates the conditions encountered in the operating room, requiring operators to identify and track the inserted needles and to avoid damaging the urethra during guidance by US (Figure 10.6), in the presence of typical image artifacts. The fabrication process of the phantom (Figure 10.7) involved casting in layers, where the

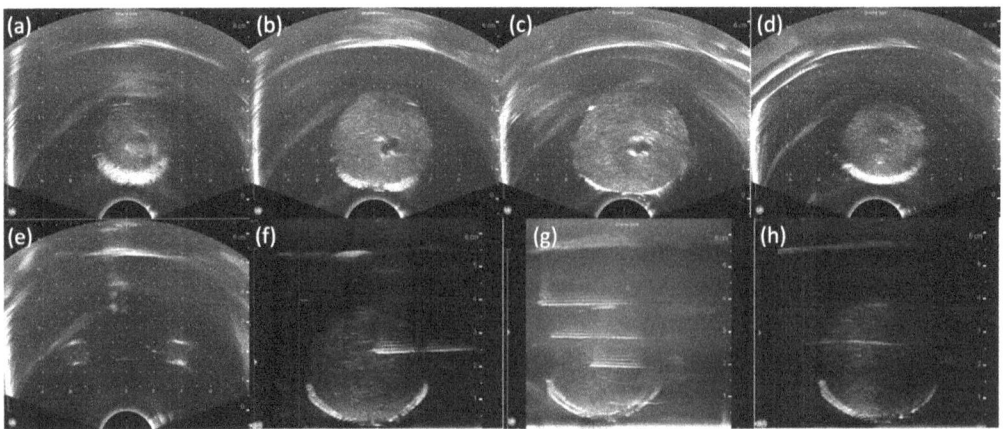

FIGURE 10.6 (a to d) US images of the prostate from the apex to base in axial views, (e) urethra and seminal vesicles superior to the prostate base, (f and g) view of needle insertion, and (h) needle track artifacts after needle removal. Figure sourced with permission from [13].

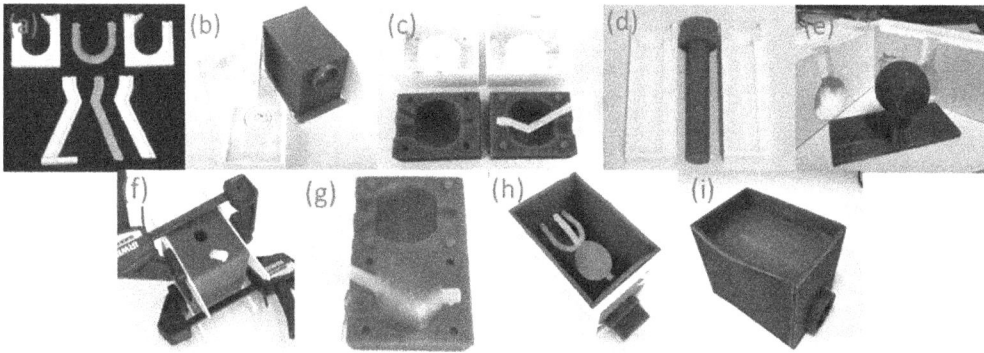

FIGURE 10.7   Construction of the prostate phantom showing (a) simulated urethra (bottom) and seminal vesicles (top), (b) the phantom case, (c) prostate casting molds with urethra, (d) the probe insert, (e) a prostate positioning tool, (f) the setup for prostate casting, (g) the final prostate with urethra (h) the setup prior to final casting, and (i) the final phantom. Figure sourced with permission from [13].

first layer extended to the top of the rectum, the next to the half height of the prostate, and the final layer extending to the top of the phantom. This technique facilitated precise placement of the prostate and seminal vesicles at desired locations within the phantom, allowing realistic training geometries to be created.

With regard to design and fabrication, this phantom offers a cost-effective alternative compared to some commercial solutions, however its fabrication required specific manufacturing skills as well as significant labor. The fabricating process involved hot casting, which imposes limitations on material selection for the phantom case, which may be improved by using heat-resistant materials.

Pneumatic-Driven Anthropomorphic Breathing Phantom for CT and MRI

In order to replicate realistic breathing motion in an anthropomorphic phantom, a model based on a real patient's thoracic anatomy was created (Figure 10.8) [14]. To overcome the challenges of simulating deformable breathing motion in a cost-effective and MR-safe device, a pneumatic-driven system was devised. This system utilized a Raspberry Pi-controlled air pump to regulate the airflow into and out of 3D printed lungs, thereby mimicking the process of breathing. To ensure accuracy and realism, ribs, sternum, and spine were incorporated into the phantom. As a result, the expansion of the lungs was directed toward the inferior and partially anterior directions, replicating the natural breathing motion observed in real patients. This coordinated lung expansion, in conjunction with the movement of the diaphragm, created a faithful simulation of respiratory motion. By integrating the pneumatic-driven system and considering the anatomical structures involved, the anthropomorphic phantom was capable of replicating various breathing patterns and motion. This innovation provided a practical and cost-effective solution for achieving simulating respiratory motion in a safe and controlled manner, making it a valuable tool for a wide range of medical applications, such as imaging, RT, and treatment planning.

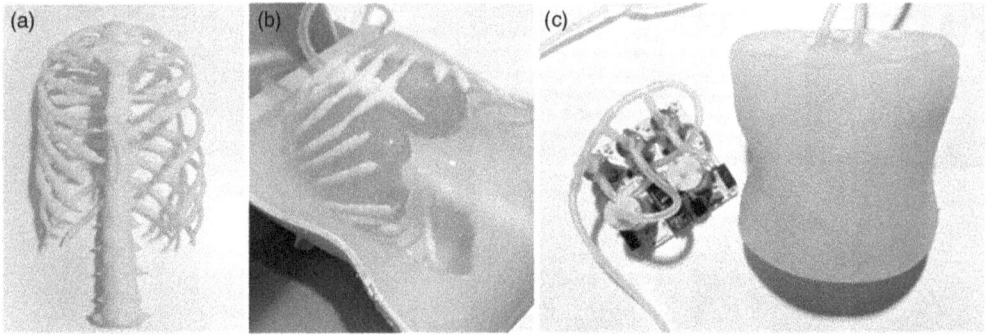

FIGURE 10.8 The pneumatic thorax phantom showing the SLA-printed bone structure (a), the complete phantom (b), and the phantom with its pneumatic connection (c). Figure sourced with permission from [14].

The anthropomorphic phantom developed for this study included various anatomical structures, such as spine, ribs, spinal cord, liver, lungs, and tumor. The incorporation of multiple OARs increased the complexity of the design and posed challenges during fabrication. The fabrication process involved the use of different materials, including two types of silicone, 3D printed bony structures, elastic lungs, and cast soft liver and tumor structures using PVC and PVA. The bony structures were 3D printed using Formlabs Rigid 10k resin, which has a density of 1.63 g/cm³. In CT imaging the HU observed for the bony structures was lower than expected due to an unrealistic effective atomic number of the materials (the atomic number of bone falls within the range of 12 to 14 [15], while acrylic-based resin typically has an atomic number of approximately 6). The liver was cast using PVC, and a silicone volume was inserted to simulate the tumor. The lungs were 3D printed using Formlabs Elastic resin and sealed with silicone around the air tubing to ensure airtightness. The lung volume could be increased by 40% to 60% by adjusting the thickness of the lung wall. For the muscle and spinal cord, Eco-flex 00-10 silicone material was used, while the skin was cast with Dragon Skin 20 (Smooth On, Inc.). Each OAR exhibited different intensities on CT and MR images, facilitating easy delineation for imaging purposes.

This breathing phantom was developed to provide a research platform for image reconstruction algorithms, motion management techniques, and treatment gating methods in RT. By using an air pump to control lung volume expansion, the phantom realistically represented the translation and deformation of lung and abdomen tissues, mimicking the complex mechanics of human respiration. The breathing pattern could be customized for individual patients, facilitating personalized motion studies. To ensure compatibility with CT and MRI, the materials used in the phantom were carefully selected. The air pump and controller, kept outside the imaging suite, allowed for precise control of the air flow, enabling MRI scans (Figure 10.9) to be performed without interference. While the construction process was laborious, the cost to manufacture the phantom was reported to be reasonably low.

This anthropomorphic breathing phantom holds significant research value, especially considering the lack of commercially available MRI-compatible anthropomorphic

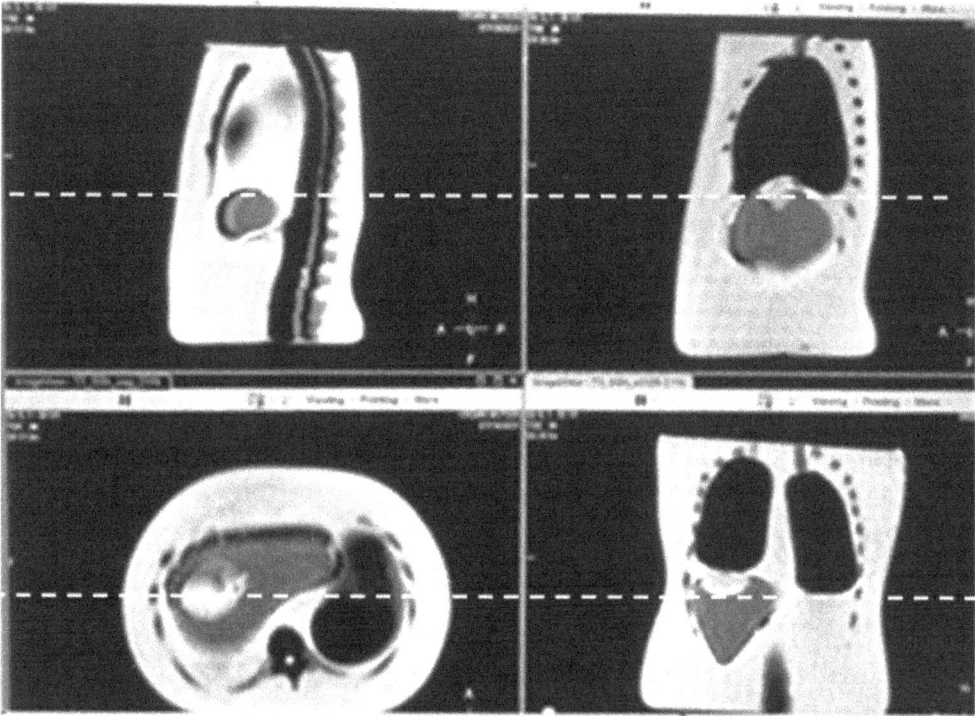

FIGURE 10.9   MRI images of the breathing phantom. Figure sourced with permission from [14].

motion phantoms. One potential limitation of this phantom is the incapacity to support dosimetric measurement, as it is not readily compatible with the insertion of dosimeters.

Kidney Phantom for Education and Training

In the field of surgical planning, simulation, instrument development, and training, realistic organ models have proven highly valuable. Urological surgery, for example, requires *in vitro* organ phantoms that accurately replicate the complexities of the human kidney. However, existing animal models and simulator systems fall short in representing the intricate morphology and physical properties of human organs. These limitations have prompted the need for innovative approaches to fabricate organ phantoms that offer a more realistic representation. In one innovative study [16], a novel fabrication process was described that enables the creation of a human kidney phantom with realistic anatomical structures and physical characteristics. The fabrication process combines 3D wax printing and polymer molding, allowing for the precise replication of the kidney's anatomical features. The resulting soft phantoms are designed in detail to mimic the properties of human kidney tissues.

High resolution cadaveric CT data were used for the design of the kidney phantom. Instead of creating a single phantom that aims to accommodate multiple imaging modalities such as CT, US, and endoscopy, the researchers opted to fabricate separate phantoms with distinct materials within the same design. Three materials were employed: silicone (Ecoflex 00-20), agar (4% agarose), and Polydimethylsiloxane (PDMS). These materials yielded appropriate HU values on CT. The silicone and agar kidneys exhibited an elastic modulus properties close to that of human kidney tissue, resulting in acceptable US images. However, agar demonstrated superior US image quality due to its lower acoustic attenuation. On the other hand, PDMS demonstrated the closest tensile strength to kidney tissue, making it more durable during endoscopy procedures without easily damaging the phantom.

The fabrication methods for the kidney phantom were innovative in that they employed dissolvable materials to simplify the double casting process (Figure 10.10). An inner mold, which represented the kidney's internal structure, was 3D printed using wax. This inner mold was then placed within outer molds, which were also created using 3D printed wax and designed to replicate the kidney's external shape. To fabricate the phantoms, three different materials, silicone, agar, and PDMS, were cast into the molds. By using an ethanol solution heated to 70°C, the inner molds made of wax could be easily dissolved, allowing for the removal of the inner structure, leaving behind the desired phantom.

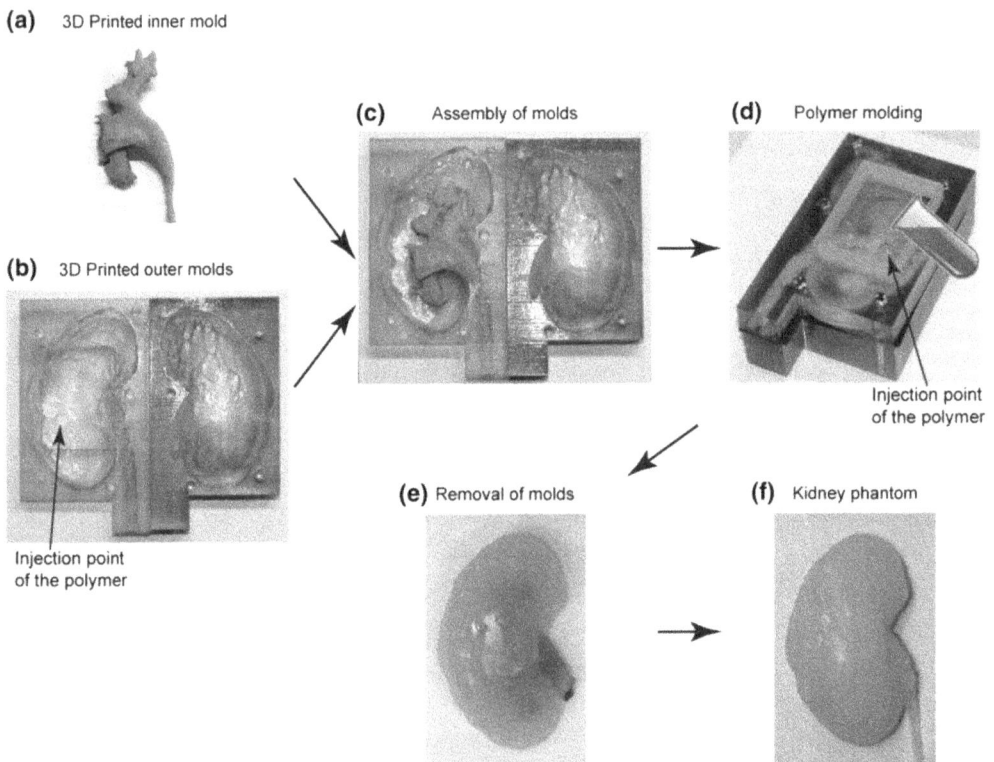

FIGURE 10.10   Workflow for kidney phantom fabrication showing (a) printing a wax inner mold, (b) printing an outer mold in photopolymer, (c) inserting the wax mold and assembling the upper and lower outer molds, (d) pouring and degassing liquid polymer, (e) removal from mold and dissolving of inner mold in ethanol, and (f) the final phantom. Figure sourced with permission from [16].

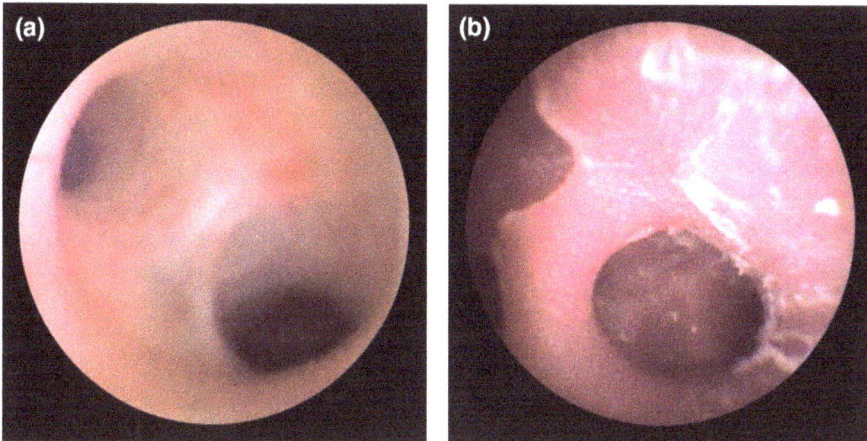

FIGURE 10.11   Validation for endoscopic imaging, comparing a view of the upper calyces in (a) a human kidney and (b) the kidney phantom. Figure sourced with permission from [16].

The study reports that the kidney phantoms were effective for the imaging modalities considered. Figure 10.11 shows a comparison of endoscopic images between a human and phantom kidney, for example. While the findings indicate that that the agar kidney is realistic in terms of mechanical properties, it posed challenges during endoscopy procedures due to its susceptibility to damage from the endoscopy probe and accessories. As for other phantom examples described above, fabrication was laborious, especially given the need for separate phantoms per imaging modality, and the requirement of direct printing of the inner mold for each. One option may be to create a mold for this inner structure, allowing the production of multiple copies in an efficient manner.

DISCUSSION AND CONCLUSION

Over the past decade, the field of 3D printing has witnessed significant advancements, transforming the landscape of prototyping and fabrication. These advancements include the development of new materials with specialized properties, the refinement of printing methodologies for enhanced precision and speed, and the simplification of user interfaces to make the technology more accessible to a new and diverse population of users. As a result, the barriers to bringing novel ideas to life have been greatly lowered, enabling individuals from various backgrounds to harness the power of 3D printing for their creative endeavors.

In the realm of medical applications, one area where 3D printing has made a profound impact is the development of medical phantoms. These phantoms serve as valuable tools in addressing specific challenges encountered in imaging, and in various treatment interventions including RT. By utilizing 3D printing technology, researchers and designers can fabricate phantoms with intricate and customized structures that closely resemble human anatomy. The achievable level of precision and customization allows for more accurate simulations, aiding in the planning and optimization of treatment.

However, it is important to note that the success of a medical phantom design is not solely dependent on the choice of 3D printer utilized. While the printing technology itself provides a powerful means of fabrication, essential to the production of a useful device is the careful selection of materials and fabrication methods. Each material used in the fabrication process introduces distinct properties that can significantly impact the performance and functionality of a phantom. Researchers must gain a thorough understanding of these materials and their characteristics to make informed decisions during the design process. Important considerations include the desired structural complexity, mechanical properties, and the signal obtained from various imaging modalities. Appropriate fabrication methods must be selected, including direct printing, casting, and post-processing procedures.

REFERENCES

[1] Berman B. 3-D printing: The new industrial revolution. *Bus Horizons*. 2012;55:155–162.

[2] Filippou V, Tsoumpas C. Recent advances on the development of phantoms using 3D printing for imaging with CT, MRI, PET, SPECT, and ultrasound. *Méd Phys*. 2018;45:e740–e760.

[3] Thakar CM, Parkhe SS, Jain A, et al. 3d Printing: Basic principles and applications. *Mater Today Proc*. 2022;51:842–849.

[4] Amor-Coarasa A, Goddard L, DuPré P, et al. *3D printing for the radiologist*. Elsevier, 2022;143–156. https://doi.org/10.1016/C2019-0-04024-1

[5] Andreadis II, Gioumouxouzis CI, Eleftheriadis GK, et al. The advent of a new era in digital healthcare: A role for 3D printing technologies in drug manufacturing? *Pharmaceutics*. 2022;14:609.

[6] Bieniosek MF, Lee BJ, Levin CS. Technical note: Characterization of custom 3D printed multimodality imaging phantoms: 3D printed imaging phantoms. *Méd Phys*. 2015;42:5913–5918.

[7] Russ M, O'Hara R, Nagesh SVS, et al. Treatment planning for image-guided neurovascular interventions using patient-specific 3D printed phantoms. *Proc SPIE—the Int Soc Opt* Eng. 2015;9417:941726–941726–11.

[8] Robar JL, Kammerzell B, Hulick K, et al. Novel multi jet fusion 3D-printed patient immobilization for radiation therapy. *J Appl Clin Med Phys*. 2022;23:e13773.

[9] Chiu TD, Arai TJ, III JC, et al. MR-CBCT image-guided system for radiotherapy of orthotopic rat prostate tumors. *PLoS One*. 2018;13:e0198065.

[10] Ceh J, Youd T, Mastrovich Z, et al. Bismuth infusion of ABS enables additive manufacturing of complex radiological phantoms and shielding equipment. *Sensors Basel Switz*. 2017;17:459.

[11] He Y, Liu Y, Dyer BA, et al. 3D-printed breast phantom for multi-purpose and multi-modality imaging. *Quant Imaging Med Surg*. 2019;9:63–74.

[12] Rooney MK, Rosenberg DM, Braunstein S, et al. Three-dimensional printing in radiation oncology: A systematic review of the literature. *J Appl Clin Med Phys*. 2020;21:15–26.

[13] Chiu T, Xiong Z, Parsons D, et al. Low-cost 3D print–based phantom fabrication to facilitate interstitial prostate brachytherapy training program. *Brachytherapy*. 2020;19:800–811.

[14] Chiu T, Ho S, Visak J, et al. Developing a pneumatic-driven, dual-modal (MR/CT) and anthropomorphic breathing phantom for image-guided radiotherapy. Poster presentation at the AAPM 2022 Annual Meeting, with proceedings online, 2022. https://w4.aapm.org/meetings/2022AM/programInfo/programAbs.php?sid=10772&aid=65594

[15] Griffiths HJ. Tissue substitutes in radiation dosimetry and measurement. No. 4. *Radiology.* 1989;173:202–202.

[16] Adams F, Qiu T, Mark A, et al. Soft 3D-printed phantom of the human kidney with collecting system. *Ann Biomed Eng.* 2017;45:963–972.

CHAPTER 11

Operationalizing 3D Printing in the Radiation Oncology Department

Brian Overshiner and James L. Robar

PLANNING FOR 3D PRINTING IN THE CLINIC

Given the range of 3D printable devices in the radiation therapy setting, there may exist multiple motivations for establishing a 3D printing resource. A comprehensive review of 3D printing in radiation oncology by Rooney *et al.* [1] reported a broad array of applications including (in order of decreasing frequency in the literature) printing quality assurance (QA) phantoms, brachytherapy applicators, patient bolus in photon, electron and photon radiotherapy, preclinical animal irradiation, compensator blocks, and patient immobilization. In most articles cited in this review, authors described various advantages that will be realized, including patient comfort, improved accuracy, streamlined work-flow, and cost-effectiveness.

The prospect of 3D printing to create custom devices in the clinic will be seen as an exciting venture to personnel, but multiple issues warrant consideration during the formation of the program. Key questions that need to be addressed in the planning stages include the following.

- What devices will be printed? Patient bolus? Brachytherapy applicators? Patient immobilization? Dosimetry or QA phantoms?

- Are these devices for use by staff only, e.g., phantoms and tools, or will they be applied in treating patients?

- What are the specific goals in 3D printing the proposed devices? Improved accuracy? Improved versatility in treatment delivery? Increased efficiency? How are these goals measurable?

DOI: 10.1201/9781003288404-11

- Accordingly, what printing media are needed? Will these materials necessitate specific provisions, e.g., sterilization and biocompatibility?

- Should 3D printing be performed in-house, or outsourced to an on-demand (OD) service?

- If printing is to be done at the point-of-care (POC), what 3D printing equipment is within budget and can it be operated by staff in the department?

- For POC printing, what are the facility requirements to accommodate this equipment including space, ventilation, and facilities for post-processing? Who will operate and maintain the printing equipment?

- If printing is to be outsourced through an OD service, who is the service provider, and can this provider satisfy the technical requirements as well as timelines associated with clinical processes?

- What human and technical resources will be needed to provide QA of the devices produced?

- What are the costs involved, and is reimbursement applicable?

Thus, while there are multiple considerations in developing a program, most decisions will be driven by the primary question, i.e., the range-specific devices that will be produced. An accurate and complete answer to this question will inform decisions downstream, guiding the selection of printing equipment, software, space resources, sterile processing, staffing, and other operational costs. Oversights in the planning process can lead to, for example, a department purchasing an expensive 3D printer only to discover that it is incapable of meeting the required reliability, accuracy, or material compatibility requirements. Similarly, a clinic may assume an overly narrow view at the inception of the program, e.g., foreseeing printing patient bolus only, and over time may wish to extend the range of devices printed. Where possible, a long-term view of the role of 3D printing in the clinic should be taken.

REGULATORY REQUIREMENTS AND RISK MANAGEMENT

For practitioners using POC printing in-house, the institution is ultimately responsible for the quality of the devices produced. However, equipping a facility to include 3D printing hardware and software must involve determining whether regulatory-approved (or medical device registered) equipment/applications will be required. For example, regulatory-approved software applications to produce 3D printed patient accessories in radiotherapy are now available (e.g., 3DBolus, Adaptiiv Medical, or 3D Systems). While the literature references numerous non-regulatory-approved computer-aided design (CAD) packages, in many cases these have been used only in research settings and may not be permitted for regular clinical use [2]. In the United States, with the emergence of in-house medical 3D printing, the Food and Drug Administration (FDA) released 3D printing guidelines for producing medical devices [3]. Prior to that, the FDA also issued technical considerations for the end-to-end process including design, manufacture, and testing, as it relates to 3D

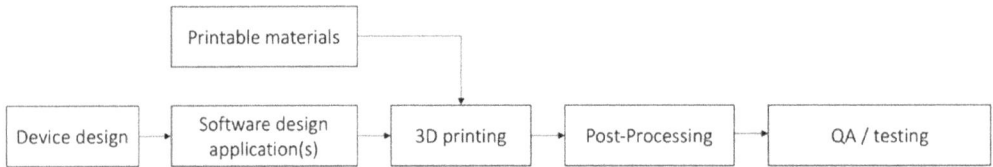

FIGURE 11.1   A typical 3D printing process.

printing [4]. A typical process includes design considerations, control over materials, fabrication using 3D printing, post-processing, and QA, as depicted in Figure 11.1.

As more data are collected and regulations are released for POC additive manufacturing, it is recommended to use validated and approved equipment, including software applications, 3D printers, and printing media. An institution's risk management department or legal counsel may be involved in the planning phase to assist in decision-making and to provide guidance protecting the practitioner, the patient, and the organization. Discussions with risk management may also consider the key decision between POC and OD printing.

POINT-OF-CARE VERSUS ON-DEMAND 3D PRINTING

In POC printing, a department will commission one or more 3D printers, calibrate and maintain this equipment, and undertake the actual printing in-house. An OD approach typically involves device design in the department, e.g., interfacing with the treatment planning system (TPS), and sending the design output to an offsite printing service. Some printing providers are well equipped to handle the requirements of radiation oncology applications (e.g., specific to material uniformity and spatial tolerances of devices) and may even be certified to produce medical devices. Choosing between POC and OD involves multiple considerations.

Opting for POC printing may limit the range of printing technologies to those that are lower in cost and simpler to operate. Fused deposition modeling (FDM) and stereolithography (SLA) printers will be likely options. While the POC approach offers the advantage of control over the timing of printing, which typically requires hours to overnight [5], FDM and SLA printers will limit the selection of materials as well as the achievable complexity of printable devices. With FDM and SLA, a range of solid or flexible polymers will be available, e.g., polylactic acid (PLA), thermoplastic polyester (TPE), thermoplastic polyurethane (TPU), and others. For FDM, there will be few options that will be sterilizable with autoclave [6], as discussed in Chapter 3 of this book. Material uniformity is important for patient devices such as bolus, and FDM-printing typically yields values within ± 100 Hounsfield units (HU) when devices are CT imaged. Outliers in uniformity will occur if the printer is not operating to specification, for example, and FDM extrusion issues can cause low-density regions or voids within bolus. While printing of bolus and many brachytherapy applicators will be possible at the POC, highly complex geometries, for example, shell immobilizers [7], as described in Chapter 8, may prove challenging or impossible with high reliability. In contrast, an OD service may provide industrial-grade printing technologies that would be otherwise inaccessible at the POC, as well as different materials and higher performance specifications. For example, Multijet Fusion (MJF, HP) fuses small particles of polymers in voxels on the order of 80–100 μm and therefore shows no striation in printed devices. It offers exceptional material uniformity, typically ± 10 HU when CT imaged. Both biocompatible and sterilizable materials are available.

An important consideration in the POC-versus-OD decision is cost. For 3D printing in general, it has been reported that the digitization and automation of manual processes in the clinic results in cost efficiency [1, 8]. While an immediate concern may be the consumable expense of ordering printed parts in the OD approach, this equation is more nuanced. For example, an exemplary cost comparison is shown in Figure 11.2. The POC option involves capital costs for hardware and software, HR costs to operate the service, consumable costs for materials and parts, as well as overhead in establishing the resource within the department. Given the time-critical nature of producing patient devices and possible failure modes (e.g., for FDM), facilities often operate more than one printer, which multiplies some of the costs. The OD scenario eliminates many of these line items, but of course will involve the recurring cost of the printed devices themselves. In this option, it is common that the HR cost of device design step remains since this step is completed in-house. After receiving the part, the quality control (QC) requirements may be reduced for the OD option if this is provided by the printing service. For example,

	Point-of-care (POC)	On-demand (OD)
Capital costs	3D printers	
	Design software	Design software
	Slicer software	
	Outfitting space (power, ventilation)	
HR costs	Device design	Device design
	Device printing	
	Device printing, failed prints	
	Device QC	+/- (QC may be provided)
	Printer calibration, repair, maintenance	
	Mould filling and handling	
Consumable costs	Printing media	OD printing and shipping
	Elastomer pouring media (e.g., moulds)	
	Printer parts and replacement	
Overhead	Space, electricity, ventilation, etc.	
	Staff training on 3D printers and maintenance	

FIGURE 11.2 Capital, human resource, consumable, and overhead cost comparison between POC and OD printing options. This example comparison considers an operation that includes direct printing of devices, e.g., patient bolus, as well as printing molds to be filled with skin-safe silicone. Note that quality control (QC) costs may be reduced if the OD service validates part dimensions, uniformity, and density, for example.

some providers may optically scan the produced part to assess spatial fidelity, and may compare measured to expected mass and volume issuing a QC certificate of analysis (CoA) (e.g., Adaptiiv Medical/HP).

Depending on the jurisdiction of the department, reimbursement may be applicable to support a portion of the 3D printing operation. In the United States, the situation is variable with respect to reimbursement codes, government mandates, and insurance regulations. Should reimbursement be an option, meeting with finance experts on billing processes during the planning stages may be advantageous in supporting sustainability of a 3D printing operation.

CLINICAL WORKFLOW

Integrating 3D printing into a clinical workflow to produce patient-personalized devices will involve some new steps for the department, but the process will be reminiscent of that used for manually produced devices over many years in the clinic. That is, the device is requisitioned, manufactured, subject to QA, and finally applied to the patient. Figure 11.3 illustrates a team approach to 3D printing that is already common among many radiation oncology departments. Upon reviewing the anatomy of the patient, the radiation oncologist may have enough foresight to request the device (e.g., bolus, applicator, or other) and may complete this early in the process, e.g., at the time of patient consult. Well-organized departments will include this requisition within the oncology information system, e.g., Aria (Varian Medical Systems), Mosaiq (Elekta), or other. It may occur, however, that the radiation therapist (RT) identifies the need for a customized patient device at the time of CT simulation. An example of this is observation of a complex patient surface for fitting of bolus. Similar may occur at the time of treatment planning, where a dosimetrist or medical physicist will recognize the benefit of 3D printing. For example, a dosimetrist may recognize that a 'synthetic' bolus added in planning software is unlikely to actually fit the patient in reality, or may raise the need to create a modulated electron bolus (MEB) to improve dose conformity. Typically, the design of the device occurs during treatment planning or shortly thereafter. Some device design applications will interface directly with the TPS through a DICOM or other interface. The 3D printing itself may be done at the POC, e.g., overseen by an RT, dosimetrist, medical physicist, medical physics assistant, or a technician. Alternatively, the designed device will be transmitted immediately to the OD provider. Once fabricated, QA is performed, e.g., to verify the dimensional accuracy and material uniformity of the device. If an OD printing service is used, QC testing on the device may be performed with issuance of a CoA. Part of the required QA will occur at the treatment unit, e.g., by

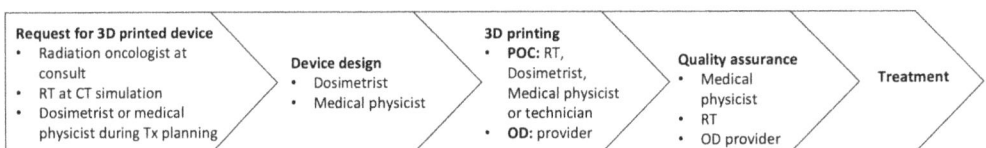

FIGURE 11.3   A team approach to incorporating 3D printing into the radiation therapy process.

verifying positioning and fit of the device on the patient visually and through onboard imaging, e.g., cone beam CT. Finally, the 3D printed device will be used throughout the treatment course.

Communication is key throughout this workflow to ensure that it proceeds smoothly and meets required timelines. Optimally, digital care paths will be employed, i.e., with the steps depicted in Figure 11.3 included as activities or appointments. This is a linear process with events occurring sequentially, thus completion of each step must trigger the next. Some applications for 3D printed device design include a portal for OD ordering, allowing for checking on the timing of fabrication, QC, and shipping of devices.

SELECTING 3D PRINTING TECHNOLOGIES

3D Printers

Additive manufacturing has existed since the 1980s, and various technologies have been developed as described in Chapter 2 of this book, each with its own printable materials, performance specifications, efficiencies, and costs. Lu *et al.* [9] provided a comparison of powder bed fusion, material extrusion, material jetting, and photopolymerization methods with a view to printing polymer-based bolus. Orton *et al.* compared FDM, SLA, Polyjet, MJF, and SLS in terms of stopping power, HU uniformity/repeatability, and other metrics in the context of proton therapy [10], an application for which the spatial accuracy and uniformity of the printed device (e.g., compensator) are crucial.

A useful comparison of technologies must have the intended application in mind. For example, if the aim is direct printing of patient bolus only, a wide variety of printing technologies can be considered. If the objective is not to print bolus directly, but rather to print molds into which flexible bolus elastomer is to be poured, options may broaden further, given that material uniformity will not be of particular interest, and flexible printing media will not be required. If the intention is also to print surface brachytherapy applicators with in-printed catheter tunnels, then the printing technology selected might require achieving spatial resolution/fidelity on the order of 0.1 mm instead of 0.5 mm, for example. If, on the other hand, the goal is to print gynecological applicators, the focus

	Fused Deposition Modeling (FDM)	Stereolithography (SLA)	Multi Jet Fusion (MJF)
Printer cost	Low	Low	High
Likely mode of access	POC or OD	POC or OD	OD
Spatial resolution (example)	0.5 mm	0.1 mm	0.1 mm
Format of materials	filament	resin	polymer powder, fusing agents
Average material uniformity	Acceptable with outliers	Acceptable	Excellent
Build success rate	Moderate	Moderate to high	High
Autoclave sterilizable materials	Very few	Yes	Yes
Biocompatable materials	Yes	Yes	Yes
Flexible materials	Yes	Yes	Yes
Typical applications in RO	Photon bolus, electron bolus, elastomer bolus moulds, surface brachytherapy applicators	Photon bolus, electron bolus, elastomer bolus moulds, surface and gynecological brachytherapy applicators, proton compensators	Photon bolus, electron bolus, elastomer bolus moulds, surface and gynecological brachytherapy applicators, patient mesh immobilization

FIGURE 11.4 Comparison between FDM, SLA, and MJF printing technologies, listing attributes of interest to radiation oncology applications.

will be narrowed to those that offer high spatial resolution, as well as both biocompatible and sterilizable materials.

Figure 11.4 shows a comparison of three example technologies: FDM and SLA, which are probable POC printers, and MJF, which is more likely accessed through OD service. This is provided as an example only; the actual specifications and performance of various printers will depend on the models selected.

Several 3D printer manufacturers such as Formlabs and Ultimaker are now advertising their machines as FDA compliant when using specified software and procedures [11] and it is reasonable to expect this trend to continue as regulatory requirements evolve.

Software Applications

A high-level depiction of typical data flow for 3D printing in the radiation therapy department is shown in Figure 11.5. Commonly, the process begins at the TPS, where the user (e.g., dosimetrist or medical physicist) has a full view of the relevant patient anatomy including the target volume and organs-at-risk. This TPS may be for external beam planning, e.g., where a 3D printed photon bolus or MEB is required, or for brachytherapy, where the aim may be to fabricate a customized high dose rate (HDR) applicator with in-printed source trajectory tunnels. In either case, the output from the TPS will be a set of delineated structures, which may include a first representation of the device of interest.

At this stage, the description of the desired structure is incomplete with regard to fabricating a physical object and additional operations will be required to convert that structure into a printable device. These are handled by the *design application*, which may perform a range of functions including data import, smoothing (e.g., to avoid slice artifacts from the source DICOM data), cropping (e.g., to provide a flat build surface for FDM printing), cleaving (for devices that must be fitted on a patient in two or more parts), the addition of catheter tunnels (for HDR brachytherapy applicators), and inclusion of other features such as cavities for shielding or *in vivo* dosimeters, spatial marking such as cross-hairs or fiducials to aid in alignment, as well as orientation or patient labeling. As shown in Figure 11.5, the data flow between the TPS and design software may be bi-directional, i.e., the design object may be pushed back to the TPS so that the final geometry and material description is captured in the final treatment plan and is accounted for in the dose calculation. The principal output of the design software is a file suitable for 3D printing (e.g., STL or 3MF formats) or issuance of a print order to an OD service. Multiple options are available for design software applications. The design application may be highly versatile and complex (e.g., CAD applications) requiring specific skill sets in the clinic, or may be more dedicated and designed for turnkey clinical use (e.g., Adaptiiv Medical 3DBolus and 3DBrachy).

Variants to the data flow in Figure 11.5 are possible. For example, if a patient's image (e.g., CT or MRI) data are available and the design application is capable, the process may actually begin at the design stage rather than in the TPS. In this scenario, the imaging data for the patient would be imported immediately into the design application. Assuming there is sufficient *a priori* knowledge of the required geometry of the device (e.g., the

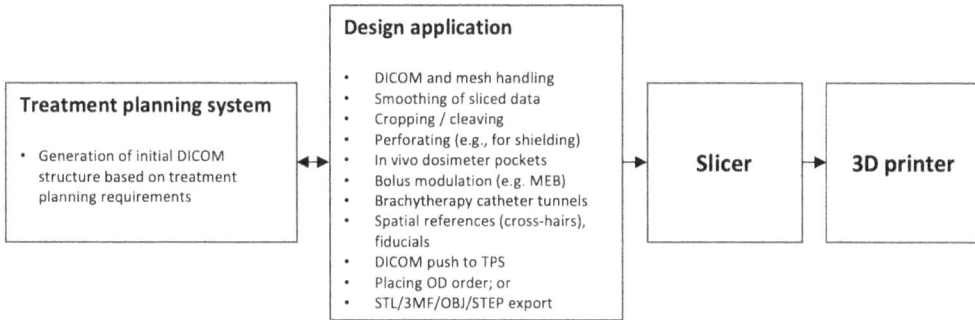

FIGURE 11.5   Software applications and data flow for 3D printing in a radiation therapy department.

location, thickness, and extent of a bolus), the design can be performed upfront. This allows the process of device design and fabrication to begin immediately and the TPS steps can follow, potentially importing the designed device into the treatment plan.

A *slicer* software application receives the output from the design application and converts this (typically triangularized mesh) format into one that can be printed. In the case of FDM printing, for example, this results in a series of G-codes that control the trajectory of the extruder as it deposits material layer by layer. This software will also specify other parameters such as the hot-end extrusion temperature, the temperature of the build plate, the speed of the extruder during printing and non-printing translation, among others. Relevant to devices such as bolus, it will also specify printing instructions for the interior of printed volumes, i.e., whether these volumes are largely hollow, filled with a pattern at a certain *infill factor*, or solid. Boluses generally need 100% infill (or as close to this value as possible). Slicers also generate *support structures* that are printed to support parts of the model that would otherwise collapse during fabrication, e.g., overhangs, designed to be removed during post-processing. Settings for controlling the presence (or absence) of support structures are important for multiple applications in radiation oncology. While support structures might be needed for many bolus topologies, for applications requiring hollow regions, it must also be possible to print regions devoid of support structures. For example, hollow tunnels are needed for brachytherapy applicators and hollow voids are needed in molds. While open-source slicer applications are available, some 3D printers must be paired with dedicated slicer applications. In reviewing 3D printing technologies, it is important to evaluate the features of the slicer software application to ensure that it will satisfy requirements according to the device(s) to be fabricated.

QUALITY ASSURANCE AND END-TO-END TESTING

The process depicted in Figure 11.5 involves the TPS, design software, and slicer software, as well as hardware components, i.e., the 3D printer itself. Fortunately, radiation oncology departments are already well versed with QA of complex systems, i.e., testing of the data flow in radiation therapy including imaging, treatment planning, and delivery. *Unit testing* is possible for each individual component of the process in Figure 11.5, as is end-to-end testing (e2e) of the full workflow. Both unit testing and e2e testing should be defined and carried out at frequencies defined by the department, as well as after change of settings (e.g., in slicer or printer configuration) or software/hardware upgrades.

Unit Testing

Unit testing isolates the smallest testable parts of an application or process, examining the output of these parts for known inputs. For example, for the process of Figure 11.5, the following unit tests could be performed.

1. **Import from treatment planning to design software.** If image and structure data are transferred from the TPS to device design software, simple geometric structures (e.g., cubic, rectangular, or simple curved structures) can be defined in the TPS, transferred, and inspected for accuracy upon import by the design software. This can include validation of dimensions, inclusion of fine detail, possible sampling errors. If the material property (e.g., relative electron density) is set in the TPS, this may be verified after import.

2. **Design software to triangular mesh or DICOM output.** Similarly, a regular object in the design software can be exported, and this output (e.g., STL, 3MF, or other) can be read by a standard mesh handling software, inspected for accuracy and measured with digital tools. If the design software allows push of the final object back to the planning system, this structure should be reviewed in the TPS. If this structure should have an assigned material property (HU or relative electron density), this should be checked.

3. **Slicer.** After importing the model into the slicer software, the ready-to-print model can be reviewed, again for dimensional accuracy and completeness. This tests possible artifacts or errors introduced in the slicing process.

4. **3D printing.** A *benchmark phantom* can be loaded directly by the slicer application and printed with the standard set of printing parameters used in clinical operation. The concept of a benchmark phantom is that it emulates actual patient devices in approximate shape and complexity, but is easily measurable after printing (e.g., with calipers or micrometer). For example, the benchmark phantom in Figure 11.6 (Adaptiiv Medical Technologies) includes features of a bolus, in-printed *in vivo* dosimeter pockets, and brachytherapy catheter tunnels, as well as measurable guides in the x-, y-, and z-dimensions. Measured dimensions (i.e., lengths, widths, thicknesses, diameters) should be compared to expected design values, and a tolerance should be applied, along with pass/fail criteria. This printed model can also be imaged with CT to check for HU uniformity.

End-to-End Testing

End-to-end testing evaluates the entire system including all software and hardware components and interfaces between them. Medical physicists in radiation oncology departments will be familiar with e2e testing given requirements in stereotactic

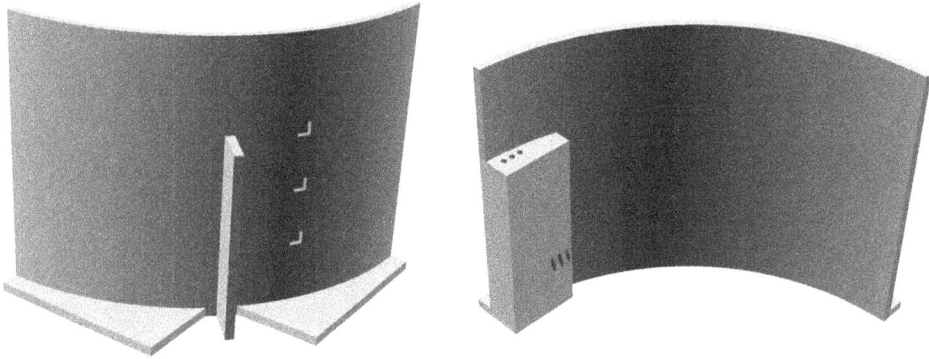

FIGURE 11.6 Example benchmark phantom. The curved section emulates a bolus in terms of shape and thickness but is physically measurable after printing. Rectangular sections are included in x-, y-, and z-dimensions for dimensional validation. The print also includes details used in patient devices, e.g., pockets for embedded dosimeters, and curved catheter tunnels for brachytherapy applicators (with permission from Adaptiiv Medical Technologies, Halifax, Canada).

radiosurgery, for example, whereby a phantom geometry will be subject to imaging, treatment planning and localization, image guidance, and treatment delivery, following the full patient process closely. In this case, the results of the e2e test (e.g., targeting accuracy, delivered dose) are measurable and subject to action and tolerance levels. Similar can be performed on the workflow of Figure 11.5. A reference structure can be defined in the planning system. As for the benchmark phantom, this should be reminiscent of actual devices to be produced, yet easily measurable, at least for dimensional accuracy. The e2e process is then followed using the same configurations and settings as would be used for design and fabrication of a patient device. After printing, the resultant device is inspected, measured (for dimensional accuracy and HU uniformity for example), and compared to the initial input design.

The QA process described above assumes POC printing. If an OD service is used, appropriate QA procedures are still required; however, the slicer and 3D printing steps will be outsourced. The OD provider should be able to receive a benchmark phantom input and send the fabricated model to the department for inspection and measurement. In addition, the OD provider may perform their own QC testing for every patient device produced and may issue the results in the form of a CoA to the clinical department. An example of a CoA for a chestwall bolus is shown in Figure 11.7, giving spatial fidelity results based on high-resolution optical scanning, as well as comparison of mass and design density to expected values.

PRINTING FACILITIES IN-HOUSE: SPACE AND SAFETY

If a department elects to print at the POC, requirements for the space housing the printers, ventilation, and power will be applicable and should be considered in the planning stages.

Azimi and colleagues [12] showed that FDM printing produces both ultrafine particles (UFPs of less than 100 nm in dimension) and volatile organic compounds (VOCs). This

	NUMBER: Form-Q-71		Version V00	
▲ADAPTIIV	TITLE: Certificate of Analysis – 3D Printed Accessory			Page 1 of 2
	EFFECTIVE DATE : DRAFT			

Catalogue Number ADPT-ONDEM-3DPRT
Accessory Serial Number 2022 - 01 - 20 - SAMPLE
                        YY   MM   DD   Order ID
Patient ID MN0006012439
Date of Manufacture 2022-01-20
Accessory Description Simple Bolus Chest Wall – NSH; Order Tracing ID: **NSH - 03022022 - MN0006012439**

Part 1. Spatial Fidelity

Optical Scanning Results

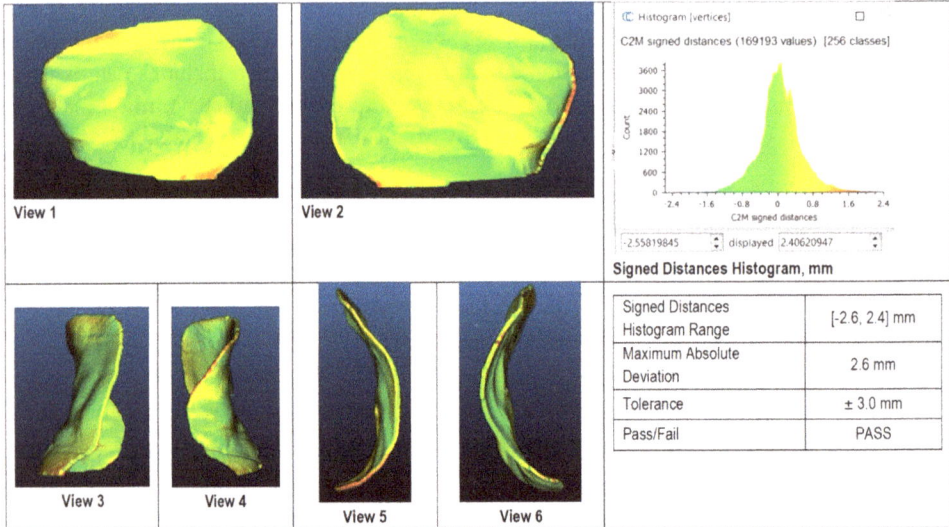

	STL/Designed	Measured	Difference
Volume	255.88 cc		
Mass	286.6 g	293.3 +/- 0.1 g	6.7 g (2.3 %)
Density	1.12 g/cc	1.15 +/- 0.001 g/cc	0.026 g/cc (2.3 %)

FIGURE 11.7   Certificate analysis for a chestwall bolus, showing results of high-resolution surface optical scanning, and a frequency histogram of signed distances from the design to the fabricated part, with applied tolerances. In addition, the mass and design density are compared to expected values (with permission from Adaptiiv Medical Technologies, Halifax, Canada).

report illustrated that emission rates will depend on the filament type, the printer, and other variables such as the nozzle and bed temperatures. For example, Figure 11.8 demonstrates that acrylonitrile butadiene styrene (ABS) FDM printing results in the highest emission rate of UFPs and PLA produces the lowest, with various other filaments between these extremes. The same study demonstrated example temporal profiles of UFP concentrations. An example for ABS is shown in Figure 11.9, which illustrates a variable concentration during printing an exponential decay of concentration over 1–2 hours after print completion.

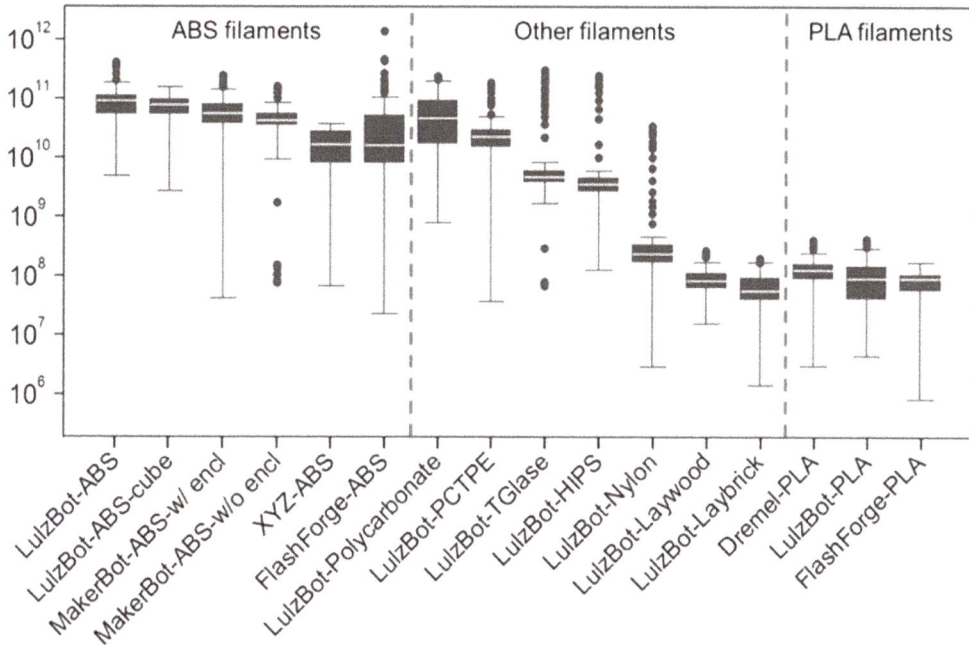

FIGURE 11.8   Ultrafine particle (UFP) emission rates (in UFP per minute) for various 3D printer and filament combinations, where boxes show 25th and 75th percentile values, with the median in between. Whiskers indicate upper and lower adjacent values and circles show outliers. Figure sourced with permission from [12].

Note: Here ABS is acrylonitrile butadiene styrene, PCTPE is plasticized copolyamide thermoplastic elastomer, TGlase is a transparent resin, HIPS is high-impact polystyrene, Laywood is a simulated wood material, Laybrick is a simulated brick material, PLA is polylactic acid.

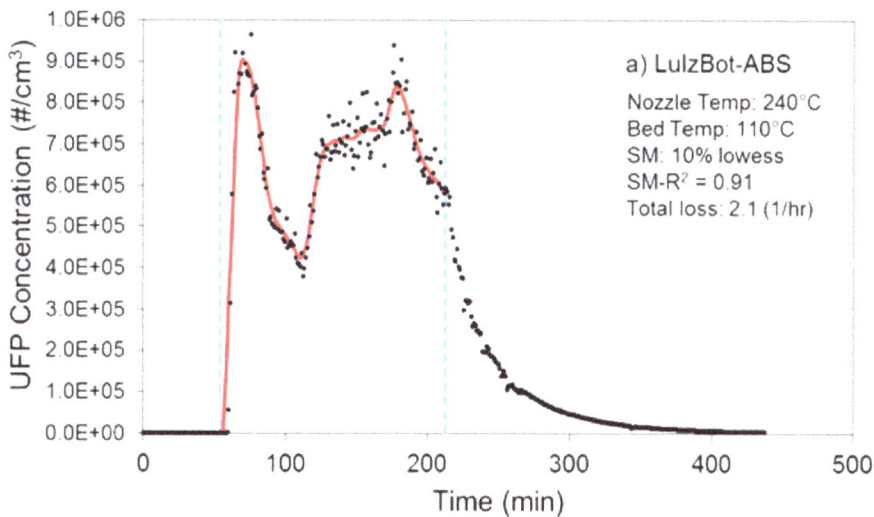

FIGURE 11.9   Time course of UFP concentration where printing with ABS occurred between the vertical dashed lines. The profile of this concentration depended on both material and printer. Notable is the decay of concentration for over 100 minutes following completion of the print. Figure sourced with permission from [12].

This report also quantified VOC emission rates for 16 different printer/media combinations, measuring emissions of 19 different compounds. The VOC emitted in highest quantity was Caprolactam, released when printing with Laywood, Laybrick, plasticized copolyamide thermoplastic elastomer (PCTPE), and nylon. The second highest VOC emission was styrene, released when printing ABS. Lowest values were obtained during PLA printing, which emits Lactide. ABS emissions are concerning given that this material is a fairly common choice in FDM printing, and Styrene VOC can be harmful. However, unless there are compelling reasons to include it, ABS printing should be avoidable in a radiation oncology department. In any case, ventilation is important in equipping a printing lab [14]. Commercial enclosures are available for 3D printers, and some of these include both filters and extraction fans.

As for any laboratory in the hospital environment, workplace safety should be consulted in establishing a 3D printing facility. Aside from ventilation, this discussion will help to define any required safety protocols, availability safety data sheets (SDS), personal protective equipment (PPE) requirements, fire-suppression measures, and required signage, e.g., alerting staff to moving parts and hot surfaces. This consultation should consider not just the printing process, but safety issues during post-processing steps. For example, unused resins must be disposed of correctly and not poured down drains. Chemicals used in post-processing may have their own storage, use, and disposal requirements. A valuable resource on this topic is the National Institute for Occupational Safety and Health (NIOSH) guidelines for 3D printing safety in the workplace [13].

Additional Space Requirements

Aside from ample space for housing the 3D printers, additional room should be allocated in the same area to store printing materials (e.g., filaments or resins), for printed models, and for benchtop space used in post-processing of printed parts. If SLA printing is used, this post-processing may require ample room for UV curing and part cleaning. There may be a need for hand tools or simple power tools, e.g., Dremels or other, for removal of support structures. If the program also includes pouring of silicone elastomer into 3D printed molds, e.g., for flexible bolus, space should be allocated for this on easily-cleaned surfaces. This may also require space for mixing of elastomer, and potentially for a desication chamber for removing air bubbles. Printing technologies beyond FDM and SLA, such as PolyJet, may introduce other facility needs, e.g., a water jet to clean off support material.

As discussed above, if the department opts for OD printing, it will be relieved of all facility requirements, an advantage that should be factored into capital equipment and operational cost analyses.

SUMMARY

Integrating 3D printing into a busy radiation oncology department may be challenging at first, but ultimately transformative in streamlining workflows, eliminating manual fabrication and associated human error, and enabling creation of patient devices that were previously impossible. Detailed planning is key, and this process should include all stakeholders including healthcare practitioners, technical staff, and leadership. The specific goals for the 3D printing operation will drive program design, and if planned well, the program established should keep pace with the rapid evolution of this promising approach in radiation oncology.

REFERENCES

[1] Rooney MK, Rosenberg DM, Braunstein S, et al. Three-dimensional printing in radiation oncology: A systematic review of the literature. *J Appl Clin Med Phys*. 2020;21:15–26.

[2] Song WY, Robar JL, Morén B, et al. Emerging technologies in brachytherapy. *Phys Med Biol*. 2021;66:23TR01.

[3] FDA. 3D printing of medical devices [Internet]. [cited 2020 Mar 26]. Available from: www.fda.gov/medical-devices/products-and-medical-procedures/3d-printing-medical-devices

[4] FDA. Technical considerations for additive manufactured medical devices [Internet]. [cited 2016 May 10]. Available from: www.fda.gov/media/97633/download

[5] Ehler E, Sterling D, Dusenbery K, et al. Workload implications for clinic workflow with implementation of three-dimensional printed customized bolus for radiation therapy: A pilot study. *PLoS One*. 2018;13:e0204944.

[6] Cunha JAM, Mellis K, Sethi R, et al. Evaluation of PC-ISO for customized, 3D printed, gynecologic 192-Ir HDR brachytherapy applicators. *J Appl Clin Med Phys*. 2014;16:5168.

[7] Robar JL, Kammerzell B, Hulick K, et al. Novel multi jet fusion 3D-printed patient immobilization for radiation therapy. *J Appl Clin Med Phys*. 2022;23:e13773.

[8] McCallum S, Maresse S, Fearns P. Evaluating 3D-printed bolus compared to conventional bolus types used in external beam radiation therapy. *Curr Med Imaging*. 2020;17:820–831.

[9] Lu Y, Song J, Yao X, et al. 3D printing polymer-based bolus used for radiotherapy. *Int J Bioprinting*. 2021;7:414.

[10] Orton E, Engelberts C, Orbovic R, et al. Characterization of CT Hounsfield units uniformity of 3D-printed materials for proton therapy [Internet]. 2020. Available from: https://virtual.aapm.org/aapm/2020/eposters/302708/elizabeth.orton.characterization.of.ct.hounsfield.units.uniformity.of.html?f=menu%3D17%2Abrowseby%3D8%2Asortby%3D2%2Amedia%3D2%2Atopic%3D23602

[11] Goehrke S. Materialise mimics in print certification program clears ultimaker and form labs for medical 3d printing [Internet]. 2018. Available from: www.fabbaloo.com/2018/11/materialise-mimics-inprint-certification-program-clears-ultimaker-and-formlabs-for-medical-3d-printing

[12] Azimi P, Zhao D, Pouzet C, et al. Emissions of ultrafine particles and volatile organic compounds from commercially available desktop three-dimensional printers with multiple filaments. *Environ Sci Technol*. 2016;50:1260–1268.

[13] NIOSH. 3D printing safety at work [Internet]. [cited 2023 Jun 7]. Available from: www.cdc.gov/niosh/newsroom/feature/3Dprinting.html

[14] The importance of ventilation and your 3D printing workspace [Internet]. 3D Printing Canada. [cited 2023 Jun 7]. Available from: https://3dprintingcanada.com/blogs/news/the-importance-of-ventilation-and-your-3d-printing-workspace

Index

Note: Page locators in **bold** and *italics* represents tables and figures, respectively. Footnotes consist of the page number followed by "n" and the footnote number e.g., 54n32 refers to endnote 32 on page 54.

For Product Safety Concerns and Information please contact our EU
representative GPSR@taylorandfrancis.com
Taylor & Francis Verlag GmbH, Kaufingerstraße 24, 80331 München, Germany

9 781032 264578